AF849750

ENTEROVIRUS INFECTIONS AND TYPE 1 DIABETES MELLITUS

Enterovirus Infections and Type 1 Diabetes Mellitus

Luis Sarmiento-Pérez
and
Eduardo Cabrera-Rode

Nova Science Publishers, Inc.
New York

Copyright © 2007 by Nova Science Publishers, Inc.

All rights reserved. No part of this book may be reproduced, stored in a retrieval system or transmitted in any form or by any means: electronic, electrostatic, magnetic, tape, mechanical photocopying, recording or otherwise without the written permission of the Publisher.

For permission to use material from this book please contact us:
Telephone 631-231-7269; Fax 631-231-8175
Web Site: http://www.novapublishers.com

NOTICE TO THE READER

The Publisher has taken reasonable care in the preparation of this book, but makes no expressed or implied warranty of any kind and assumes no responsibility for any errors or omissions. No liability is assumed for incidental or consequential damages in connection with or arising out of information contained in this book. The Publisher shall not be liable for any special, consequential, or exemplary damages resulting, in whole or in part, from the readers' use of, or reliance upon, this material.

Independent verification should be sought for any data, advice or recommendations contained in this book. In addition, no responsibility is assumed by the publisher for any injury and/or damage to persons or property arising from any methods, products, instructions, ideas or otherwise contained in this publication.

This publication is designed to provide accurate and authoritative information with regard to the subject matter covered herein. It is sold with the clear understanding that the Publisher is not engaged in rendering legal or any other professional services. If legal or any other expert assistance is required, the services of a competent person should be sought. FROM A DECLARATION OF PARTICIPANTS JOINTLY ADOPTED BY A COMMITTEE OF THE AMERICAN BAR ASSOCIATION AND A COMMITTEE OF PUBLISHERS.

LIBRARY OF CONGRESS CATALOGING-IN-PUBLICATION DATA

Sarmiento-Pérez, Luis.
Enterovirus infections and type 1 diabetes mellitus / Luis Sarmiento-Pérez, Eduardo Cabrera-Rode.
p. ; cm.
Includes bibliographical references and index.
ISBN 13: 978-1-60021-339-7
ISBN 10: 1-60021-339-1
1. Diabetes -- Etiology. 2. Enterovirus diseases. I. Cabrera-Rode, Eduardo. II. Title.
[DNLM: 1. Diabetes Mellitus, Type 1 -- etiology. 2. Enterovirus Infections -- complications. WK 810 S246e 2006]
RC660.S27 2006
616.4'62 -- dc22 2006021281

Published by Nova Science Publishers, Inc. ✣ New York

To those persons with diabetes and their relatives

Contents

PREFACE

Luis Sarmiento-Pérez and Eduardo Cabrera-Rode

We used to think that chronic and infectious diseases were separate. Several chronic diseases once attributed to lifestyle and genetics are now known to be caused or exacerbated by infectious agents. These include stomach ulcers and certain types of cancer and arthritis. At least 15 % of all cancers worldwide are a consequence of chronic infectious disease, the most important of which are hepatitis B and C viruses (liver cancer); the human papillomavirus (cervical cancer) and the *Helicobacter pylori* bacterium (stomach cancer). Evidence is mounting for other, still unproven associations between infectious agents and chronic diseases. These findings are prompting health professionals to rethink ways of preventing or minimizing long-term illness and disability. Understanding the links between virus and the emergence of chronic diseases such as type 1 diabetes will provide new opportunities to address and counter a significant public health challenge.

Type 1 diabetes mellitus results from autoimmune destruction of pancreatic islet β cells. The incidence of the disease is increasing at a rate of 2-3 % per year in the developed world, in which type 1 diabetes carries an increased risk of morbidity and premature death from a range of diabetic complications, including cardiovascular disease, renal failure and blindness. Diabetes as a single disease (of which type 1 represents 10-15%) is estimated to consume 8-10% of the National Health Service acute services budget. Of major concern are the increasing incidence of the disease in young children, and the emergence of latent autoimmune diabetes in adults.

Although the discovery of islet cell autoantibodies in 1974 shaped thinking on the pathogenesis of type 1 diabetes, leading to its classification as autoimmune in nature, the etiology of the disease remains unknown. Disease-associated genes are clearly important, but numerous studies, especially those on monozygotic twins, show that heritable factors alone account for only 30-50 % of disease susceptibility. Attention has therefore focused on environmental factors that might trigger and/or accelerate disease. Among the possible external candidates, the enterovirus has attracted the greatest attention as a putative trigger or accelerant of disease.

Enteroviruses have been examined for their possible role in the etiology of type 1 diabetes for nearly 40 years. It is now evident from studies in several countries that enterovirus infection accompanies or precedes the onset of diabetes in many individuals. These evidences include the isolation of coxsackievirus B4 from the pancreas of a child at diagnosis of type 1 diabetes, several epidemiological and prospective studies showing that some cases of type 1 diabetes are strongly associated with enterovirus infections, seasonal incidence studies, case-control studies that show an increased prevalence and levels of IgM antibodies to enterovirus in newly diagnosed patients. Other evidences involves several case studies in which diabetes develops after an enterovirus infections, increased T cell response to enterovirus antigens in type 1 diabetic patients, suggestions that enterovirus infections during pregnancy might initiate the events leading to childhood diabetes, and a higher frequency of enterovirus RNA in the serum/blood of type 1 diabetic patients at diagnosis. Advances in molecular biology have improved our understanding of enteroviral biology and the potential alternative pathogenic mechanisms through which enteroviruses may cause diabetes.

Although there exist a number of excellent books on diabetes in the global scene, there are few reflecting the putative etiologic association between enterovirus infection and type 1 diabetes. We recognise that this is an area of controversy, since there are studies that fail to find associations, although methodological reasons may account for these discrepancies. The literature, upon which we are so dependent, is influenced by the history of this controversy. We will not comment on this further here, except to acknowledge it as now part of the problem. Dogmatism is the enemy of science.

The book which covers the fundamental issues of diabetes and enterovirus is divided in 4 chapters. The first and second chapter deals with general aspects of type 1 diabetes and enterovirus infections. The third and and fourth chapter is devoted to discuss literature data concerning the viral etiology of the autoimmune type 1 diabetes as well as present our own experience in this field. We have reviewed much of the published literature on such studies, using manual searching of relevant journal, reference list of publications and computer-based searches of the Medline references database (1969-2006). The review is probably not exhaustive, in particular having missed non-English and non-Spanish language publications, but should not be otherwise biased. We hope will provide the reader with the fullest possible perspective on enterovirus infections and their relationship to type 1 diabetes.

Although the emphasis is on the potential association of enterovirus infection with type 1 diabetes, basic science information has been elaborated in the chapters which will be a great help to many beginners in the field of diabetology and virology. Within this single volume is compiled a wealth of new and historical information essential for those persons who deals with the research surrounding human enterovirus infections and diabetes. Our goal in preparation of this monograph is that it be a definitive and current resource for diabetes - oriented professionals, scientists wanting clinical correlates and clinicians seeking explanations. The book represents a compilation and assessment of the most valid, accurate and useful data on enterovirus and type 1 diabetes mellitus. It should serve as a useful reference to clinicians and investigators in virology and diabetes research.

Chapter I

TYPE 1 DIABETES

Eduardo Cabrera - Rode *

Department of Immunology of Diabetes, National Institute of Endocrinology, Havana, Cuba.

ABSTRACT

Diabetes Mellitus is a group of heterogenous metabolic diseases characterized by chronic hyperglycemia resulting from numerous defects in insulin secretion, insulin action, or both. The achievements in molecular biology, genetics and immunology have helped to clarify the etiology and pathogenesis of several types of diabetes. This chapter on type 1 diabetes provides an overview of classification, epidemiology, genetic and immunologic aspects on this disease and discusses the latest research in this rapidly developing field.

Keywords: diabetes mellitus, type 1 diabetes, classification, epidemiology, genetic, immunology, autoantibodies.

I. CLASSIFICATION OF DIABETES MELLITUS

The current classification of diabetes is carried out on the basis of the etiology. We believe that the basis of classification should be on the presence or absence of β-cell autoimmune process, quantitative differences of the function of such cells and the resistance to their peripheral action. As these variables influence in the clinical characteristics of the diabetic patients, within which are found with rising levels of glucose concentration in blood and the need or not of insulin. One of the aims of the diabetes classification is the chance to study its epidemiology, etiology and pathogenesis which provide effective interventions in its prevention and treatment.

Description of Diabetes Mellitus

Diabetes mellitus is a group of metabolic diseases characterized by chronic hyperglycemia resulting from defects in insulin secretion insulin action or both. The abnormalities in carbohydrate, fat, and protein metabolism that are found in diabetes are due to deficient action of insulin on target tissues. This chronic hyperglycemia of diabetes mellitus is associated with long-term damages, dysfunction, and failure of various organs, especially the eyes, kidneys, nerves, heart, and blood vessels [1,2].

Several pathogenic processes are involved in the development of diabetes. These range from autoimmune destruction of the β-cells of the pancreas with consequent insulin deficiency to an amount of abnormalities that result in resistance to insulin action. Insufficient insulin action results from an inadequate insulin secretion and/or diminished tissue response to insulin at one or more points in the complex pathways of hornmone action. Impairment of insulin secretion and defects in insulin action frequently coexist in the same patient, and it is often unclear which abnormality, if either alone, is the primary cause of hyperglycemia [1,2].

Hyperglycemia symptoms include polyuria, polydypsia, and weight loss, sometimes with polyphagia, and blurred vision. Impairment of growth and susceptibility to certain infections may also accompany chronic hyperglycemia. Acute, life-threatening consecuences of uncontrolled diabetes are hyperglycemia with ketoacidosis or the nonketotic hyperosmolar syndrome. During the treatment of hyperglycemia, episodes of hypoglycemia can be produced, which can cause convulsions and loss of conscience [1,2].

Long-term complications of diabetes include retinopathy with potential loss of vision; nephropathy leading to renal failure; peripheral neuropathy with risk of foot ulcers, amputations, Charcot joints; and autonomic neuropathy causing gastrointestinal, genitourinary, and cardiovascular symptoms and sexual dysfunction. Patients with diabetes have an increased incidence of atherosclerotic cardiovascular; peripheral arterial, and cerebrovascular disease. Hypertension and abnormalities of lipoprotein metabolism are often found in people with diabetes [1,2].

Most of diabetes cases fall into two broad etiopathogenetic categories (discussed in greater detail below) In one category, type 1 diabetes, the cause is an absolute insulin deficiency. Individuals at increased risk of developing this type of diabetes can often be identified by serological evidence of an autoimmune pathologic process occurring in the pancreatic islets and by genetic markers. In the other, which is much more frequent category, type 2 diabetes, the cause is a combination of resistance to insulin action and an inadequate compensatory insulin secretory response. On this type of diabetes, a degree of hyperglycemia sufficient to cause pathologic and functional changes in various target tissues, but without

* Correspondence concerning this article should be addressed to Eduardo Cabrera-Rode. Department of Immunology of Diabetes, National Institute of Endocrinology, Zapata and D, Havana 10 400, Cuba; fax: 53-7-333417; email: diabetes@infomed.sld.cu.

clinical symptoms, may be present for a long period of time before diabetes is detected. During this asymptomatic period, it is possible to demonstrate an abnormality in carbohydrate metabolism by measurement of plasma glucose in the fasting state or after a challenge with an oral glucose load [1,2], and an abnormality in insulin secretion by measurement of plasma insulin in the fasting state or after a challenge with an oral glucose load, as well as insulin resistance measurement by hyperinsulinemic-euglycemic clamp techniquee or homeostasis model assessment (HOMA IR). At the same time, in this asymptomatic period it is possible to find some early manifestations associated with type 2 diabetes such as obesity, hypertension and irregularities in the lipid levels even without observing disorders in carbohydrates metabolism [1,2].

Classification of Diabetes Mellitus

The identification of the type of diabetes in an individual often depends on the circumstances present at the time of diagnosis and it turns difficult to include many subjects with diabetes into a particular group [1,2,11]. For example, a person with gestational diabetes mellitus may continue to be hyperglycemic after delivery and may be determined to have, in fact, type 2 diabetes. Alternatively, a person who acquires diabetes after a treatment with large doses of steroids or other diabetogenic drugs and may become normoglycemic once the treatment is discontinued [1,2,11]. Other subjects develop diabetes after diseases of the exocrine pancreas, infections, endocrinopathies, intake of chemical products and some genetic syndromes [1,2,11]. Thus, for the clinician and patient, it is less important to label the particular type of diabetes than it is to understand the pathogenesis of the hyperglycemia and to treat it effectively [2].

Currently, a new knowledge has appeared in which defects at cell level, tissue or functions related to the expression of the disease have been identified. This has given rise to the appearing of new proposal in order to classify diabetes mellitus.

There are reports from the Experts Committee of the Diabetes American Association (ADA) [1,2], from the World Health Organization (WHO) [11] and other reports [52,53,176,195,280] which suggest different classifications of diabetes mellitus.

Next, we will start to describe the classification suggested by ADA [1,2] and WHO [11] which is currently used. This classification is based on the pathogenesis rather than on the insulin requirements.

A- Type 1 Diabetes

It includes all forms of diabetes which are due to a primary failure by destruction of pancreatic β-cells with consequent loss of insulin secretion until an absolute deficiency is reached.

Immune-Mediated Diabetes (Common Form of Diabetes Mellitus)

This form of diabetes previously referred to as insulin dependent diabetes, type 1 diabetes, or juvenile diabetes, account for only 5-10% of subjects with diabetes. It is caused by cellular–mediated autoimmune destruction of the β-cells of the pancreas that result in a failure in insulin secretion and an absolute insulin deficiency. As a consequence of this immune destruction process of the β-cells, autoantibodies are originated against the islet cells (ICA), insulin (IAA), the glutamic acid decarboxylase (GADA) and the tyrosine phosphatases IA-2 and IA-2β (IA-2A and IA-2βA). One and usually more of these autoantibodies are present in 85 to 90% of individuals when fasting hyperglycemia is initially detected. Also, the disease has strong HLA associations, with linkage to the DQA and DQB genes, and it is influenced by the DRB genes. The combination of HLA-DR/DQ alleles can be either predisposing or protective [1,2].

In this form of diabetes, the rate of β-cell destruction is quite variable, being rapid in infants and children and slow in adults. Some patients, particularly children and adolescents, may present with ketoacidosis as the first manifestation of the disease. Others have modest fasting hyperglycemia that can rapidly change to severe hyperglycemia and/or ketoacidosis in the presence of infection or other stress. However, other subjects, particularly adults, may retain residual β-cell function sufficient to prevent ketoacidosis for many years; such individuals eventually become dependent on insulin for survival and are at risk for ketoacidosis. At this latter stages of the disease, there is very little or no insulin secretion, as manifested by low or undetectable levels of plasma C-peptide. This type of diabetes usually occurs in childhood and adolescence, but it can occur at any age, even in old age [1,2].

In adults, type 1 diabetes is incorrectly classified frequently, because it is less dramatic and it is considered as a type 2 diabetes [47,49,237,252]. When this wrong classification is made, there is a big mistake of not using insulin treatment in these subjects with autoimmune diabetes, that is, adults that have autoantibodies associated with type 1 diabetes [47,49,202,237]. These type of diabetes is frequently named "latent autoimmune diabetes in adults (LADA)", type 2 diabetes ICA+, "diabetes 1,5" or "slowly progressing type 1 diabetes [47,49,202,237,252]. Slowly progressing type 1 diabetes in adults show a pathogenesis, genetics and antigenic recognition of ICA different from classical type 1 diabetes [47,49,252,297].

Autoimmune destruction of β-cells has multiple genetic predispositions and is also related to environmental factors that are still not well defined [2]. Although most of the persons with this type of diabetes are not obese, the presence of obesity is not incompatible with the diagnosis. These patients are also prone to other autoimmune disorders such as Graves´s disease, Hashimoto´s thyroiditis, Addison´s disease, celiac disease, vitiligo, myasthenia gravis, autoimmune hepatitis and pernicious anemia [2].

Idiopathic Diabetes (Not Autoimmune)

Several forms of type 1 diabetes has unknown etiologies. Some of these forms of diabetes have a permanent insulinopenia and are prone to ketoacidosis, but have no evidence of autoimmunity. Although only a minority of patients with type 1 diabetes fall into this category, of those who do, most are of African or Asian ancestry. Those with this form of diabetes suffer from episodic ketoacidosis and exhibit varying degrees of insulin deficiency between episodes. This form of diabetes is strongly inherited, lacks immunological evidence for β-cell autoimmunity, and is not HLA associated. An absolute requirement for insulin replacement therapy in affected patients may come and go [2].

B- Type 2 Diabetes

It includes all forms of diabetes which have an insulin resistance with a relative insulin deficiency and/or a secreting defect. This form of diabetes previously referred to as non-insulin-dependent diabetes, type II diabetes, or adult-onset diabetes account for ~90% of all diabetes. It includes individuals who have insulin resistance and usually have relative (rather than absolute) insulin deficiency. At the beginning of this disease, and often throughout their lifetime, these individuals do not need insulin treatment to survive. There are probably many causes of this form of diabetes [2]. Although the specific etiologies are not known, autoimmune destruction of β-cells does not occur, and patients do not have any of the other causes of diabetes listed above or below [2].

Most patients with this form of diabetes are obese, and obesity itself causes some degree of insulin resistance. Patients who are not obese by traditional weigh criteria may have an increased percentage of body fat distributed mainly in the abdominal region. Ketoacidosis seldom occurs spontaneously in this type of diabetes; when seen, it usually arises in association with the stress of another illness such as infection [2]. This form of diabetes frequently goes undiagnosed for many years because the hyperglycemia develops gradually and at earlier stages is often not severe enough for the patient to notice any of the classic symptoms of diabetes. Nevertheless, such patients are at increased risk of developing macrovascular and microvascular complications. Whereas patients with this type of diabetes may have insulin concentrations that appear normal or elevated, the higher blood glucose concentrations in these diabetic patients would be expected to result in even higher insulin values had their β-cell finction been normal. Therefore, insulin secretion is defective in these patients and insufficient to compensate for insulin resistance. Insulin resistance may improve with weight reduction and/or pharmacological treatment of hyperglycemia but is seldom restored to normal. The risk of developing this form of diabetes increases with age, obesity and lack of physical activity. It occurs more frequently in women with prior gestational diabetes and in individuals with hypertension or dyslipidemia and its frequency varies in different racial or ethnic subgroups. It is often associated with a strong genetic predisposition, more so than is the autoimmune form of type 1 diabetes. However, the genetics of this form of diabetes are complex and not clearly defined [2].

C. Other Specific Type of Diabetes

It includes some specific forms of diabetes resulting from a primary failure of β-cell function, damage of β-cells, abnormalities in the insulin action and insulin secretion, as well as those associated with other genetic syndromes.

Genetic Defects of β-Cell

Several forms of diabetes are associated with a monogenetic defect in β-cell function [2]. These forms of diabetes are referred to as maturity-onset diabetes of th young (MODY) and are characterized by onset of hyperglycemia at an early age, mainly before age of 25 years and by impaired insulin secretion with minimal or no defects in insulin action. They are inherited in an autosomal dominant pattern. Abnormalities at six genetic loci on different chromosomes have been identified to date. The most common form is associated with mutations on chromosome 12 in a hepatic transcription factor referred to as hepatocyte nuclear factor (HNF)-1α (MODY 3). A second form is associated with mutations in the glucokinase gene on chromosome 7 (7p) and results in a defective glucokinase molecule (MODY 2). This enzyme converts glucose to glucose-6-phosphate, the metabolism of which, in turn, stimulates insulin secretion by the β-cell. Thus, glucokinase acts as the "glucose sensor" for the β-cell. Because of defects in the glucokinase gene, increased plasma levels of glucose are necessary to elicit normal levels of insulin secretion. Other mutations have been identified at the level of chromosome 20 (20q) referred to HNF-4α (MODY 1), chromosome 13 named (insulin promoter factor (IPF)-1, MODY 4), chromosome 17 (17q) named HNF-1β (MODY 5) and chromosome 2 (2q), named NeuroD1 (MODY 6). The mutations found in the transcription factors which comprise MODY 1, 4, 5 and 6 are less common forms [2].

Mutations in DNA mitochondrial (transmitted through maternal inheritance) have been found to be associated with diabetes mellitus and deafness. The most common mutations occur at position 3243 in the tRNA leucine gene, leading to an A-to-G transition. An identical lesion occurs in the MELAS syndrome (mitochondrial myopathy, encephalopathy, lactic acidosis, and stroke-like syndrome); however, diabetes is not part of this syndrome, suggesting different phenotypic expressions of this genetic lesion [2]. Mitochondrial diabetes and other mitochondrial mutations which occur in MELAS syndrome can be potentially prevented [54].

Genetic abnormalities that result in the inability to convert proinsulin to insulin have been identified in a few families, and such traits are inherited in an autosomal dominant pattern. The resultant glucose intolerance is mild. Also, the production of mutant insulin molecules with resultant impaired receptor binding has also been identified in a few families and is associated with an autosomal inheritance and only mildly impaired or even normal glucose metabolism [2].

Genetic Defects in Insulin Action

There are unusual causes of diabetes that result from genetically determined abnormalities of insulin action. The metabolic abnormalities associated with mutations of the insulin receptor may range from hyperinsulinemia and modest hyperglycemia to severe diabetes. Some individuals with these mutations may have acanthosis nigricans. Women may be virilized and have enlarged, cystic ovaries. In the past, this syndrome was termed type A insulin resistance. Leprechaunism and the Rabson-Mendenhall syndrome are two pediatric syndromes that have mutationS in the insulin receptor gene with subsequent alterations in insulin receptor function and extreme insulin resistance. The former has characteristic facial features and is usually fatal in infancy, while the latter is associated with abnormalities of teeth, nails and pineal gland hyperplasia.

Alterations in the structure and fuction of the insulin receptor cannot be demonstrated in patients with insulin-resistant lipoatrophic diabetes. Therefore, it is assumed that the lesion (s) must reside in the postreceptor signal transduction pathway [2].

Diseases of the Exocrine Pancreas

Any process that diffusely injures the pancreas can cause diabetes. Acquired processes include pancreatitis, trauma, infection, pancreatectomy, and pancreatic carcinoma. With the exception of that caused by cancer, damage to the pancreas must be extensive for diabetes to occur; adrenocarcinomas that involve only a small portion of the pancreas have been associated with diabetes. This implies a mechanism other than simple reduction in β-cell mass. If extensive enough, cystic fibrosis and hemochromatosis will also damage β-cells and impair insulin secretion. Fibrocalculous pancreatopathy may be accompanied by abdominal pain radiating to the back and pancreatic calcifications identified on X-ray examination. Pancreatic fibrosis and calcium stones in the exocrine ducts have been found at autopsy [2].

Endocrinopathies

Several hormones (e.g., growth hormone, cortisol, glucagón and epinephrine) antagonize insulin action. Excess amounts of these hormones (e.g., acromegaly, Cushing´s syndrome, glucagonoma, pheochromocytoma, respectively) can cause diabetes. This generally occurs in individuals with preexisting defects in insulin secretion, and hyperglycemia typically resolves when the hormone excess is resolved [2].

Somatostatinoma- and aldosteronoma-induced hypokalemia can cause diabetes, at least in part, by inhibiting insulin secretion. Hyperglycemia usually resolves after succesful removal of the tumor [2].

Drug- or Chemical-Induced Diabetes

Many drugs can impair insulin secretion. These drugs may not cause diabetes by themselves, but they may precipitate diabetes in individuals with insulin resistance. In such cases, the classification is unclear because the sequence or relative importance of β- cell dysfunction and insulin resistance is unknown. Certain toxins such as Vacor (a rat poison) and intravenous pentamidine can permanently destroy pancreatic β-cells. Such drug reactions fortunately are rare. There are also many drugs and hormones that can impair insulin action. Examples include nicotinic acid and glucocorticoids. Patients receiving α-interferon have been reported to develop diabetes associated with islet cell antibodies and, in certain instances, severe insulin deficiency. Other well-known drug and hormones that can impair insulin action are: Dilatin, thyroid hormone, diazoxide, β-adrenergic agonists, and thiazides, among others [2].

Infections

Certain viruses have been associated with β-cell destruction. Diabetes mellitus occurs in patients with congenital rubella, although most of these patients have HLA and immune markers characteristic of type 1 diabetes. In addition, enterovirus, other viruses such as cytomegalovirus, adenovirus, and mumps have been implicated in inducing certain cases of diabetes [2,50,142].

Uncommon Forms of Immune-Mediated Diabetes

In this category, there are two known conditions, and others are likely to occur. The stiff-man syndrome is an autoimmune disorder of the central nervous system characterized by stiffness of the axial muscles with painful spasms. Patients affected by this disease usually have high titers of the GAD autoantibodies, and approximately one-third of them develop diabetes [2].

Anti–insulin receptor antibodies can cause diabetes by binding to the insulin receptor, thereby blocking the binding of insulin to its receptor in target tissues. However, in some cases, these antibodies can act as an insulin agonist after binding to the receptor and can thereby cause hypoglycemia. Anti–insulin receptor antibodies are occasionally found in patients with systemic lupus erythematosus and other autoimmune diseases. As in other states of extreme insulin resistance, patients with anti–insulin receptor antibodies often have acanthosis nigricans. In the past, this syndrome was termed type B insulin resistance [2].

Other Genetic Syndromes Sometimes Associated with Diabetes

Several genetic syndromes are accompanied by an increased incidence of diabetes mellitus. These include the chromosomal abnormalities of Down's syndrome, Klinefelter's syndrome, and Turner's syndrome. Wolfram's syndrome is an autosomal recessive disorder characterized by insulin-deficient diabetes and the absence of β-cells at autopsy. Additional manifestations include diabetes insipidus, hypogonadism, optic atrophy, and neural deafness. Other syndromes such as Friedreich´s ataxy, Huntington´s chorea, Laurence-Moon-Biedl, myotonic dystrophy, porphyria, and Prader-Willi syndrome, among others, are also included in this category [2].

D. Gestational Diabetes Mellitus

Gestational diabetes mellitus is defined as any degree of glucose intolerance with onset or first recognition during pregnancy. The definition applies regardless of whether insulin or only diet modification is used or whether the condition persists after pregnancy. It does not exclude the possibility that unrecognized glucose intolerance may have antedated or begun concomitantly with the pregnancy. Deterioration of glucose tolerance occurs normally during pregnancy, particularly in the 3rd trimester [2].

Impaired Glucose Tolerance (IGT)

The Expert Committee recognized as an intermediate group of subjects whose glucose levels, although not meeting criteria for diabetes, are nevertheless too high to be considered normal. Most of these cases represent early diabetes stages [2].

Critic to the Classification of Diabetes Recommended by ADA and WHO

The classification suggested by ADA and WHO is the most recognized and widely spread currently. Nevertheless, we consider that it has some deficiencies. For instance, in type 1 diabetes are included the cases of diabetes caused by β-cell destruction, resulting from immunological alterations or unknown cause (idiopathic). Type 2 diabetes is described as those forms with insulin resistance mainly and usually has relative deficiency of insulin secretion. The cases whose cause is essentially unknown are also included in this category [1,2]. A third group called "Other specific types of diabetes" is created, in which cases whose basic defect is known and can be identified are included. Paradoxically, in this group are included types 1 and type 2 diabetic patients, due to known causes. For example, types of diabetes which has insulin deficiency because of β-cell destruction although not from autoimmune reason, are included, as well as type 2 patients who have insulin resistance by recognized genetic defects.

Gestational diabetes is defined simply due to the fact that it appears during pregnancy and no etiological link is established. However, at present its heterogeneity is known: It is known that many women with gestational diabetes recover tolerance to normal glucose after delivery, while others can develop other forms of diabetes [66,204,318]. Gestational diabetes is indeed a previous event to different forms of diabetes [66,204,318], however, it is preferred to keep it in an independent classification because of its importance in morbidity and childhood and mother mortality.

Other Classifications of Diabetes Mellitus

The initial proposal for classification published by our group [53] has been modified as we suggest now, it take into account not only secretion state or insulin action, but also the cause which originate it, including the existence of autoimmunity or not [52].

Physiopathological Classification of Diabetes Mellitus [52]

1. Type 1 Diabetes

Primarily failure due to destruction or absence of β-cell (treatment: Insulin)

Autoimmune

Common form

Latent autoimmune diabetes of adult (LADA)

"Stiff-man" syndrome

Pluriglandular autoimmune syndrome (APS I and II)

Not Autoimmune

Idiopathic

Infections: congenital rubella, cytomegalovirus, adenovirus, enterovirus, and others

Drug- or chemical-induced diabetes: vacor, streptozotocin, pentamidine, alloxan, α-interferon

Diseases of exocrine pancreas: pancreatitis, trauma/pancreatectomy, cystic fibrosis, hemochromatosis, fibrocalculous pancreatopathy, etc.

Genetic syndromes: Wolfram's syndrome (DIDMOAD), congenital absence of pancreas, congenital absence of islets, epiphysis displasia and diabetes, as well as others [146,300].

2. Type 2 Diabetes

A. Insulin resistance and/or hyperinsulinism (initial treatment: biguanides/thiazolidinediones)

Autoimmune
Anti-insulin receptor antibodies
Type B insulin resistance (B-IgG antibodies)
Ataxia telangiectasia (IgG antibodies)

Not Autoimmune
Obese, common form
Genetic defects in insulin action: type A insulin resistance, leprechaunism and Rabson-Mendenhall syndrome, lipoatrophic diabetes syndromes and others [146,300].
Drug- or chemical-induced diabetes: nicotinic acid, glucocorticoids, thyroid hormones, β-adrenergic agonist and others
Endocrinopathies: Cushing´s syndrome, acromegaly, glucagonoma, hyperthyroidism and others
Genetic syndromes: Prader-Willi syndrome, Klinefelter syndrome and others.

B. Decrease of insulin secretion due to failure in β-cells function. (Initial treatment: Insulin secretagogues, sulphonilureas, and eventually, insulin).

Not Autoimmune
Not obese (with physiopathological disorders to be established)
Genetic defects in β-cells function: mitochondrial diabetes, insulinopathies, (proinsulin anomalies and insulin mutations), MODY 1, Hepatocyte Nuclear Factor (HNF-4), locus in chromosome 20q, MODY 2, Glucokinase, locus in chromosome 7p, MODY 3, HNF-1β locus in chromosome 12q, MODY 4, Insulin Promoter Factor 1 (IPF-1), locus in chromosome 13q, MODY 5, HNF-1ß, locus in chromosome 17q, MODY 6, NeuroD1, locus in chromosome 2q and others
Drug- or chemicals-induced diabetes: diazoxide, thiazides, dilantin, β-adrenergic agonist and others
Endocrinopathies: Somatostatinoma and aldosteronoma
Genetic syndrome: Down's syndrome, Laron nanism, etc [146,300].

3. Gestational Diabetes

It appears during pregnancy and can disappear or not after this stage is concluded. Some women suffering from gestational diabetes can develop other forms of diabetes after pregnancy [66,204,318].

In this physiopathological classification of diabetes mellitus [52] we consider more reasonable to distribute the so-called groups "Other specific types of diabetes" in type 1 and 2 diabetes, as they have all criteria mentioned in the classification. It would help clinicians to determine a more rational treatment and besides, in a way, to try to identify the etiology of each form of diabetes.

The class "tolerance to altered glucose" is kept the same as the previous classification by WHO and ADA [1,2,11], as it can constitute a transitional stage, for different forms of diabetes [1,2,52,53].

In our opinion, the several types of diabetes with different etiologies can present a similar degree of insulin deficiency or abnormalities in insulin action that is why diabetes should be classified according to the result that etiology produces in insulin secretion.

Kuzaya and Matsuka [176] suggest that the etiology and the degree of deficiency of insulin and/or insulin action should be examined separately, with both incorporated in the classification of diabetes. Each of the various etiologies (autoimmune process, defective in insulin secretion, decreased insulin sensitivity, several mutations) results in a stage of relative deficiency of insulin or insulin action. When deficiency turns sufficiently severe, the patient will be insulin dependent. Severe insulin deficiency of insulin or insulin action usually occurs as a result of the absolute lack of insulin. The patient would remain type 2 diabetes when the deficiency is mild or moderate.

The degree of deficiency of insulin or in insulin action is a characteristic to be determined as one dimension, but the etiologies of diabetes can be multiple [176]. Therefore, it is necessary to differentiate the basic etiology and grading of severity in the classification of diabetes [176].

In most situations, the degree of insulin deficiency can be evaluated by determining C-peptide (molecule which is simultaneously segregated with insulin production) without regard to etiology. Through the use of two dimensional criteria, diabetic patients would be classified as type 2 with etiology of type 1 diabetes; type 1 diabetes caused by chronic pancreatitis; insulin requiring diabetes of mixed etiologies; or type 1 diabetes (type 1 and type 2 etiologies), for example.

In the case of subjects with slowly progressing type 1 diabetes in which the process of β-cells damage is slow, patients with insulin reserve could be found and they could seem to be a type 2 phenotype. In subjects who develop type 1 diabetes after pancreatitis could be also classified as type 2, if the degree of the disease is not severe yet in order to find an insulin deficiency, and in type 2 diabetic patients with different etiological causes and deficiency of insulin secretion (who require insulin treatment) could be considered as type 1 diabetes. By using this method, much of the difficulty in fitting an individual patient into subclasses seems to be avoided [176].

Service et al [280] suggest that clinical criteria for the classification of diabetes are highly correlated with the evaluation of insulin secretory reserve. A small number of individuals considered to have type 2 diabetes clinically or by C-peptide have or develop a type 1 diabetes peptide response. The authors propose the following conclusions:

1) The clinical criteria for the classification of diabetes, although arbitrary and sometimes difficult to apply, however show a high degree of correlation with the evaluation of insulin secretory reserve.
2) The clinical criteria for the classification of diabetes seem to be better at predicting type 1 diabetes (once it is classified as type 1 diabetes, it can be confirmed inmediatly or later by the assessment of insulin secretory reserve).
3) The clinical criteria for type 2 diabetes are good, but one should allow for the inclusion of some patients with type 1 diabetes (approximately 10%), which is consisitent with the studies that show 10 to 15% ICA-positivity in persons clinically considered as type 2 diabetes [47,49,237,252].

The classification proposed by Service et al, considerably favors the categorization of the two most important forms of diabetes (type 1 and 2).

Recently, Maldonado et al., [195] classified patients with diabetes and ketoacidosis in four groups. This classification is based on positive or negative β-cell insulin function (B^+ or B^-), as well as the positive or negative autoimmune markers for type 1 diabetes (A^+ or A^-). Based on these criteria, they identify four groups: Group 1, patients with autoimmune markers for type 1 diabetes and low β-cell functional reserve ($A^+ B^-$), Group 2, patients with absence of autoimmune markers for type 1 diabetes and low β-cell function ($A^- B^-$). Group 3, patients with presence of autoimmune markers for type 1 diabetes and good β-cells functional reserve ($A^+ B^+$) and Group 4, patients with absence of autoimmune markers for type 1 diabetes and good β-cell function ($A^- B^+$).

This study shows heterogeneity associated with diabetes ketoacidosis and stimulates also the discussion about the development of standardized nomenclature and a global database to establish a better classification of ketosis-prone diabetes. In our criterion we believe that this classification can be also valid for diabetes mellitus without ketoacidosis. This proposal of diabetes with ketoacidosis in four groups offers us information about treatment and evolution of patients with diabetes according to the presence or not of autoimmune markers against β-cells and the β-cell functional reserve [195]. This way it is important in order to be able to distinguish type 1 diabetes from type 2 diabetes. On the other hand, this classification makes us aware of the current situation of onset-diagnosis of diabetic patients and the disease's stage. The classification of diabetes described by Maldonado et al., takes into account the same aspects as the classification proposed by our group [52,53].

According to the consensus report of the Expert Committee on Diagnosis and Classification of Diabetes Mellitus [1,2] and the World Health Organization (WHO) [11], group $A^+ B^-$ described by Maldonado and co-workers [195] corresponds to the form of classical type 1 diabetes (autoimmune type 1 diabetes), where as $A^- B^-$ would be considered as idiopathic type 1 diabetes (not autoimmune type 1 diabetes), because this group is non obese with negative autoimmue markers and requires insulin for prevention of recurrence of diabetes ketoacidosis. In this group some other specific forms of diabetes with deficiency in insulin secretion can be also included. The patients from group ($A^+ B^+$) perhaps represent those patients with diabetes recognized with the term type 2 diabetes positive for islet associated autoantibodies or latent autoimmune diabetes of adult (type 1 diabetes autoimmune). Finally, group ($A^- B^+$) consist of a heterogeneous group of type 2 diabetes subjects with several degrees of insulin resistance and varying degrees of insulin secretory capacity, in this group some other specific forms of diabetes can be included too, with the same characteristics in β-cell function, described for this group.

Maldonado et al., [195] by using a heterogeneous group and with ethnic diversity of diabetic patients who have ketoacidosis, prove that they can be included at least in four different diabetes syndromes which are separable by the status of islet associated autoantibodies, HLA genotype and quantitative assessment of β-cell insulin function.

Summarizing, with the previously reported data, it is necessary to carry out a consensus about the classification of diabetes mellitus which comprises β-cell function and the presence or not of autoimmune markers against β-cells, despite knowing or not the etiology of diabetes.

This classification should rebound in a better and precise categorization which exerts influence on the application of the right treatment for each diabetic patient, in order to avoid the appearing of future complications due to a wrong metabolic control.

II. Epidemiology of Type 1 Diabetes

Geographical variation in worldwide incidence of type 1 diabetes appears to reflect the global distribution of major ethnic populations, which demonstrates a different degree of genetic susceptibility to diabetes among populations.

The pathogenesis of type 1 diabetes is a multifactorial disease and it is characterized by the interaction of environmental factors with the genes predisposition to type 1 diabetes, as the susceptibility genes are necessary but not enough for the development of the disease. The genetic differences among the populations do not explain by itself, the wide variations in the incidence of this disease. The increase in the last years of worldwide incidence rates of type 1 diabetes has allowed us to compare the epidemiological results obtained in a great part of the world. The migration studies from a low to high incidence areas of type 1 diabetes or viceversa also reflect changes in the incidence of disease. For this reason, it is suggested that environmental factors considerably contribute to global variation in the incidence of type 1 diabetes among different ethnic groups. However, much about the environmental factors involved in the development of type 1 diabetes is still unknown.

In this chapter, some information about epidemiological features of type 1 diabetes at worldwide will be offered.

Incidence of Type 1 Diabetes

Geographical Localization

The incidence of type 1 diabetes worldwide varies greatly among different regions (from 0.1 to 37.4 x 100.000 children <15 years of age per year) [145,155]. The highest incidence rates of type 1 diabetes have been found in Finland (37.4/100.000 per year) [145] and Sardinia (36.8/100.000 per year) [155] and the lowest in Venezuela and China (Zunyi), (0.1/100.000) [155].

Type 1 diabetes mellitus is an autoimmune disease which is the result of an interaction between the genetic susceptibility and unknown environmental factors. Genetic studies show a clear association between HLA haplotypes (contributing in more than 50% of the total genetic risk) and the appearing of the disease. However, the susceptibility genes are necessary but not enough for the development of this pathology and it is possible that one of the factors which determine the variations in the incidence previously mentioned is the differences in the frequencies of HLA genotypes among the different populations. Currently, it is known that environmental factors (dietetic, infections, toxins) as well as psychosocial factors are of a great importance. Although it is not known the way they act, it has been hypothesized that they could be the triggers, accelerators or precipitators of the disease.

The records of type 1 diabetic patients in different countries have provided reliable data to compare the geographical differences, despite the fact that still exist some regions in Africa and South America where there are no accurate epidemiological data. A greater variation of > 350-fold in the incidence of type 1 diabetes before 15 years of age has been verified among different countries [145,155].

Next, the differences of type 1 diabetes are shown in children <15 years of age in different regions and countries [155].

The populations from Northern Africa show an intermediate incidence rate of type 1 diabetes (Table 1). Mauritius, an island on the east coast of the continent had a low incidence. Most of the populations in the Asian continent (26 out of 29) had a very low or low incidence. Exceptions were Israel and Kuwait with a high incidence, which represent Caucasoid populations (Table 2) [155]. The variation in the type 1 diabetes incidence in most of the Asian populations in comparison with Kuwait and Israel could be as a consequence of the interaction between the environmental factors and the high frequency of HLADQ-genotypes which confer a high risk of type 1 diabetes, found in these last ones [124,281,313].

Of the European populations, one-half (18 out of 39) had an intermediate incidence rates and the rest (21 out of 39) present high or very high rates (Table 3). Particularly, the highest incidence rates occur in Sardinia and Finland (~37/100.000 per year). Other populations with very high incidence rates in Europe were in Sweden and Norway. Despite the small total number of cases in Portalegre, Portugal, the incidence of type 1 diabetes was consistently high [155].

Table 1. Age standardized incidence of type 1 diabetes in children < 15 years of age (per 100.000 per year). African Region

Region (country and area)	Study period	Estimate of ascertainment (%)	Incidence (95% CI)	Cases
Africa				
Algeria				
Oran*	1990		5.7 (3.62-8.52)	23
Tunisia				
Beja*	1990-1994		7.8 (5.47-10.68)	38
Gafsa*	1990-1994		8.8 (6.59-11.51)	53
Kairoan*	1991-1993		5.7 (3.95-7.89)	46
Monastir*	1990-1994		4.9(3.35-6.96)	31
Sudan				
Gezira	1990	100	5.0 (3.74-6.54)	29
Mauritius	1990-1994	35-100	1.4 (0.83-2.07)	21

Data are incidence rates or incidence rates (95 % CI) unless otherwise indicated.
* Primary source only. Data are from reference [155].

Table 2. Age standardized incidence of type 1 diabetes in children < 15 years of age (per 100.000 per year). Asian Region

Region (country and area)	Study period	Estimate of ascertainment (%)	Incidence (95% CI)	Cases
Asia				
China				
Wuhan	1990-1994	100	4.6 (2.81-6.96)	22
Sichuan	1990-1994	80-100	2.3 (1.45-3.34)	22
Huhehor	1990-1994	100	0.9 (0.54-1.53)	16
Dalian	1990-1994	100	1.2 (0.75-1.76)	21
Guilin	1991-1994	100	0.8 (0.22-2.01)	5
Beijing*	1990-1994		0.9 (0.72-1.09)	90
Shanghai	1990-1994	69-100	0.7 (0.51-0.91)	47
Chang Chun	1990-1994	86-100	0.8 (0.49-1.30)	18
Nanjing	1990-1994	100	0.8 (0.51-1.29)	20
Jinan	1990-1994	100	0.4 (0.25-0.59)	23
Jilin	1990-1994	100	0.6 (0.38-0.90)	22
Shenyang	1990-1994	100	0.5 (0.29-0.67)	25
Lanzhou	1991-1994	100	0.4 (0.15-0.68)	8
Harbin	1990-1994	100	0.3 (0.19-0.38)	35
Nanning	1990-1994	100	0.5 (0.25-0.78)	14
Changsha	1990-1994	100	0.3 (0.16-0.42)	17
Zhengzhou	1991-1994	86-100	0.6 (0.38-1.10)	10

Table 2. (Continued)

Region (country and area)	Study period	Estimate of ascertainment (%)	Incidence (95% CI)	Cases
Hainan	1990-1994	100	0.2 (0.09-0.25)	17
Tie Ling	1990-1994	100	0.2 (0.13-0.26)	8
Zunyi	1990-1994	100	0.1 (0.00-0.37)	3
Wulumugi	1990-1994	100	0.8 (0.34-1.71)	9
Hong Kong*	1990-1994		1.3 (0.77-2.17)	17
Kuwait	1992-1994	91-100	**18.3** (15.52-21.35)	153
Israel	1990-1994	100	**6.0** (5.42-6.67)	361
Japan				
Chiba*	1990-1993		1.4 (1.07-1.81)	61
Hokkaido	1990-1993	100	2.2 (1.71-2.65)	89
Okinawa	1990-1993	77-100	1.4 (0.81-2.24)	17
Pakistan				
Karachi	1990	51	0.7 (0.44-0.99)	25
Russia				
Novosibirsk	1990-1994	87-100	**6.0** (5.18-6.94)	191

Data are incidence rates or incidence rates (95 % CI) unless otherwise indicated.

* Primary source only. Data are from reference [155].

Table 3. Age standardized incidence of type 1 diabetes in children < 15 years of age (per 100.000 per year). European region

Region (country and area)	Study period	Estimate of ascertainment (%)	Incidence (95% CI)	Cases
Austria†	1990-1994	99-100	9.6 (8.84-10.31)	660
Belgium (Antwerpen)†	1990-1994	90-100	**11.6** (9.40-14.21)	95
Bulgaria				
Varna	1990-1994	100	6.8 (5.80-7.83)	182
West Bulgaria	1991-1994	99-100	9.9 (8.71-11.21)	256
Denmark (4 counties)†	1990-1994	83-100	**15.5** (13.28-17.95)	177
Estonia*	1990-1994		**10.5** (9.05-12.20)	178
Finland*	1990-1994		**36.5** (34.83-38.26)	1,768
France (4 regions)†	1990-1994	95-99	8.5 (7.86-9.12)	709
Germany				
(Baden-Württemberg)†	1990-1994	91-100	**11.0** (10.25-11.69)	903
Greece (Attica)†	1990-1994	100	9.7 (8.55-10.92)	273
Hungary (18 counties)†	1990-1994	99-100	9.1 (8.43-9.81)	697
Italy				
Sardinia†	1990-1994	37-85	**36.8** (33.72-39.98)	548
Eastern of Sicily†	1990-1994	96-100	**11.7** (9.78-13.93)	128
Pavia	1990-1994	100	**11.7** (8.08-16.44)	34
Marche	1991-1994	100	9.7 (7.90-11.84)	99
Turín	1990-1994	97-100	**11.0** (9.32-12.15)	155
Lazio*†	1990-1994		8.1 (7.28-9.07)	326
Lombardia†	1990-1994	100	7.2 (6.55-7.92)	443
Latvia	1990-1992		5.9 (5.06-6.98)	106

Table 3. (Continued)

Region (country and area)	Study period	Estimate of ascertainment (%)	Incidence (95% CI)	Cases
Lithuania	1990-1994	100	7.4 (6.57-8.25)	307
Luxemburg†	1992-1994	100	**11.4** (8.14-15.59)	39
The Netherlands†				
5 regions	1990-1994	87-98	**13.0** (11.69-14.42)	353
Norway (8 counties)†	1990-1994	91-100	**21.2** (19.18-23.29)	409
Poland				
Krakow*	1990-1994		6.1 (5.38-6.92)	260
Wielkopolska	1990	100	5.0 (3.88-6.36)	68
Portugal				
Algarve†	1990-1994	74-100	**14.6** (10.62-19.64)	45
Coimbra	1990-1994	100	9.7 (6.76-13.36)	38
Madeira Island†	1990-1994	100	7.2 (4.46-11.05)	21
Portalegre†	1990-1994	86-100	**21.1** (13.29-31.86)	23
Romania (Bucharest)†	1990-1994	100	5.0 (4.14-6.05)	117
Slovenia†	1990-1994	100	7.9 (6.68-9.23)	158
Slovakia	1990-1994	100	8.5 (7.81-9.25)	550
Spain (Catalonia)	1990-1994	81-100	**12.5** (11.55-13.50)	696
Sweden*	1990-1994	100	**27.5** (26.36-28.67)	2,166
UK				
Aberdeen	1990	51	**24.0** (15.22-36.01)	23
Leicestershire†	1991-1994	97-100	**15.3** (12.85-18.07)	136
Northern Ireland†	1990-1994	95-100	**19.7** (17.81-21.79)	387
Oxford*†	1990-1994		**17.8** (16.18-19.46)	457
Plymouth	1990-1994	96-100	**17.3** (14.41-20.53)	128

Data are incidence rates or incidence rates (95 % CI) unless otherwise indicated.
* Primary source only. † EURODIAB ACE Study. Data are from reference [155].

Ronningen et al in 2001 [266], reported a correlation between the incidence of type 1 diabetes in children <15 years of age in Europe and HLA genotypes. This study suggests that a substantial part of the transnational variation in the incidence of childhood-onset type 1 diabetes in Europe is explain by variations between populations in the distribution of particular HLA-DQ haplotypes which confer a high risk of type 1 diabetes in the general population. The presence of a strong positive correlation between population frequency of genetic susceptibility markers and population diabetes risk by itself does not exclude the importance of non-genetic factors (or genetic factors not accounted in this study). These findings suggests that non-genetic causes interact with genetic susceptibility factors in type 1 diabetes and that such an interaction has been enhanced over the past decades in subjects carrying specific high-risk genotypes [313]. Therefore, the distribution of HLA-genotypes in newly diagnosed type 1 patients should change over time in populations who have changing incidences of type 1 diabetes [131,266]. The hypothesis could be supported by the rapid increase of type 1 diabetes incidence in children in the age group 0-4 years, observed in high incidence populations such as Finland and UK [266]. Recently in Finland [131], it was found that the frequencies of HLA-DR/DQ risk haplotypes and the high risk (DR3)-DQA1*05-DQB1*02/DRB1*0401-DQB1*0302 genotype were higher while proportion of patients carrying protective haplotypes (DR15)-DQB1*0602 and (DR1301)-DQB1*0603 or protective genotypes was lower in patients diagnosed before 1965 as compared to those who developed disease after 1990. These data suggest that the need for genetic susceptibility to develop type 1 diabetes has decreased over time due to an increasing environmental pressure and this result in a higher disease progression rate especially in subjects with protective HLA genotypes [131]. Another research carried out in Europe [243], suggests that the wide variation in childhood type 1 diabetes incidence rates in Europe could be partially explained by the indicators of national prosperity. These indicators could reflect the differences in environmental risk factors such as nutrition or lifestyle that are important in determining a country's incidence rate [243].

Table 4. Age standardized incidence of type 1 diabetes in children < 15 years of age (per 100.000 per year). North American Region

Region (country and area)	Study period	Estimate of ascertainment (%)	Incidence (95% CI)	Cases
North America				
Canada				
Alberta	1990-1994	75-96	**24.0** (20.62-27.82)	175
Prince Edward Island*	1990-1993	100	**24.5** (16.38-35.16)	29
U.S				
Allegheny, PA	1990-1994	87-100	**17.8** (15.45-20.33)	206
Jefferson, AL*	1991-1993		**15.0** (12.21-18.22)	101
Chicago, IL §	1990-1994	51-100	**11.7** (10.47-13.12)	300

Data are incidence rates or incidence rates (95 % CI) unless otherwise indicated.
* Primary source only; § African-American and Hispanic. Data are from reference [155].

In all populations from North America, incidence rates were high (Table 4). Particularly in the two regions studied from Canada, the incidence was particularly high (Table 4) [155]. The presence of HLA-DQ genotypes which confer a high risk of type 1 diabetes, is also increased in the Caucasoid white U.S. citizens [80], due to this data, it is suggested that the high frequency of these genotypes could explain the high incidence of type 1 diabetes in the North American populations.

Table 5. Age standardized incidence of type 1 diabetes in children < 15 years of age (per 100.000 per year). South, Central America and the Caribbean Region

Region (country and area)	Study period	Estimate of ascertainment (%)	Incidence (95% CI)	Cases
South America				
Argentina				
Avellaneda	1990-1994	88-97	6.5 (4.31-9.51)	26
Cordoba	1991-1992	88-92	7.0 (5.20-9.26)	47
Corrientes	1992-1994	90-100	4.3 (2.21-7.51)	12
Tierra del fuego	1993-1994	100	8.0 (2.18-17.60)	4
Brazil (Sao Paulo)	1990-1992	70-95	8.0 (5.53-11.14)	34
Chile (Santiago)	1990-1992	100	1.6 (1.28-2.04)	122
Colombia				
Santa Fe de Bogotá	1990	97	3.8 (2.88-4.93)	56
Paraguay*	1990-1994		0.9 (0.71-1.11)	79
Peru (Lima)	1990-1991	88	0.4 (0.22-0.61)	16
Uruguay (Montevideo)	1992	97	8.3 (5.38-12.10)	26
Venezuela				
Caracas (second center)*	1992		0.1 (0.09-0.18)	43
Central America and Caribbean				
Barbados*	1990-1993		2.0 (0.32-6.36)	5
Cuba	1990-1994	75-100	2.9 (2.63-3.24)	349
Dominica	1990-1993		5.7 (1.53-14.65)	5
México (Veracruz)	1990-1993	100	1.5 (0.70-2.94)	9
Puerto Rico	1990-1994	90-97	**17.4** (16.25-18.63)	844
Virgin Islands*	1990-1994		**13.1** (7.64-21.01)	16

Data are incidence rates or incidence rates (95 % CI) unless otherwise indicated.
* Primary source only. Data are from reference [155].

The incidence of type 1 diabetes among populations in South America ranged from intermediate (5 out of 11) to very low (3 out of 11) (Table 5) [155]. In Central America and the Caribbean, the populations in Puerto Rico and Virgin Islands shown high incidence rates, and the rest of the populations have intermediate or low incidence [155]. It is known that the presence of high risk HLA genotypes of type 1 diabetes is decreased in the population from Mexico, Colombia, Venezuela, Chile and Uruguay [73,279]. Therefore, the difference in type 1 diabetes incidence between Puerto Rico and Virgin Islands with the rest of the nations from South, Central America and the Caribbean, could be explained by the non-genetic factors intervention (environment) and due to the influence of non-HLA genes.

In Oceania, the incidence rates of type 1 diabetes were high in Australia and New Zealand, particularly in the Canterbury region in New Zealand (Table 6) [155]. It is suggested that the high incidence in Canterbury is partly due to an increased HLA-conferred genetic predisposition to type 1 diabetes in this population [103].

Table 6. Age standardized incidence of type 1 diabetes in children < 15 years of age (per 100.000 per year). Oceania

Region (country and area)	Study period	Estimate of ascertainment (%)	Incidence (95% CI)	Cases
Oceania				
Australia				
New South Wales	1990-1993	89-100	**14.5** (13.42-15.55)	722
New Zealand				
Auckland	1990-1994	100	**12.9** (10.87-15.28)	135
Canterbury	1990-1994	100	**21.9**_(17.33-27.32)	78

Data are incidence rates or incidence rates (95 % CI) unless otherwise indicated.
* Primary source only. Data are from reference [155].

The most recent data (2003) about the incidence and estimate of the prevalence of type 1 diabetes in children aged 0 - 14 years are shown in Table 7 [145].

The comparison of the incidence of type 1 diabetes within the most recent data from 2003 [145], and those from the decade of the 90´s (Table 7) show us that in 42% (21/50) of the countries, the incidence of type 1 diabetes has increased, however, in 8% (4/50) it has decreased. These data suggest to us that the incidence of type 1 diabetes among children < 15 years of age is increasing in most of the countries, in those of a high incidence, or an intermediate or low one.

In the last years, the worldwide incidence of type 1 diabetes before 15 years of age appears to be increasing in almost all populations, and the increase is particularly high in populations with a low incidence [145,155,232]. However, the incidence has increased in general in the populations with previous high incidence [108,145]. Therefore, it is suggested that this increase result from changing environmental (not genetic) or lifestyle factors in the populations, although in the countries with low incidence previous to the increase, it could be obey simply to an improvement in case ascertainment [155,216,243,250].

Pitkaniemi et al [250] state that probably environmental factors modifying the disease incidence. Environmental factors could either modify the penetrance of susceptibility gene(s) or as triggering factors, could contribute directly to the incidence [250].

Table 7. Age standardized incidence of type 1 diabetes in children < 15 years of age (per 100.000 per year) in 50 countries (IDF diabetes Atlas, 2003) in comparison to 90 decade

Countries	Population size (000´s) 0-14 yrs	Estimated no. of prevalent cases (000´s)	Incidence rates (145)	Incidence rates (155) (~90-94)
Finland	899	2.5	**37.4**	36.5
Sweden	1.498	3.1	**28.0**	27.5
Canada	5.759	9.1	24.1	24.2*
Norway	876	1.3	**22.5**	21.2
Kuwait	540	0.8	**20.9**	18.3
Denmark	982	1.2	**19.4**	15.5
United Kingdom	10.923	13.7	18.9	18.8*
Australia	3.931	4.4	**17.8**	14.5
Puerto Rico	934	1.1	17.4	17.4
New Zealand	864	0.9	15.2	17.4*
U.S	61.383	49.2	13.8	14.8*
Netherlands	2.864	2.5	13.0	13.0
Spain	5.664	4.4	**12.8**	12.5
Germany	12.028	10.1	**12.2**	11.0
Luxemburg	84	0.1	**11.9**	11.4
Belgium	1.713	1.3	11.8	11.6
Portugal	1.674	1.3	**11.5**	10.5*
Estonia	210	0.2	**11.4**	10.5
Hungary	1.581	1.1	**9.6**	9.1
Austria	1.275	0.8	9.5	9.6
Italy	8.633	5.6	9.5	9.9*
Slovakia	970	0.6	**9.2**	8.5
Greece	1.537	0.9	9.1	9.7
Bulgaria	1.108	0.7	**8.8**	8.3*
Slovenia	288	0.2	**8.5**	7.9
France	10.970	5.6	8.3	8.5
Uruguay	837	0.4	8.3	8.3
Brazil	48.424	23.8	8.0	8.0
Sudan	13.182	6.5	**8.0**	5.0
Lithuania	641	0.3	**7.8**	7.4
Latvia	359	0.2	**7.1**	5.9
Poland	6.662	3.0	**6.7**	5.5*
Tunisia	2.693	1.1	6.6	6.8*
Argentina	10.408	4.1	6.4	6.4*
Israel	1.783	0.6	5.9	6.0
Dominica	20	0.0	5.7	5.7
Algeria	10.530	3.9	5.7	5.7
Romania	3.694	1.2	5.0	5.0
Chile	4.322	1.1	**4.1**	1.6
Colombia	14.048	3.3	3.8	3.8
Cuba	2.240	0.4	2.9	2.9
Barbados	53	0.0	2.0	2.0
Japan	18.228	1.9	1.7	1.6*
Mexico	32.799	2.6	1.5	1.5
Mauritius	296	0.0	1.4	1.4
Pakistan	62.839	3.4	**1.0**	0.7
Paraguay	2.266	0.1	0.9	0.9
China, Republic	299.371	9.3	0.6	0.8*
Peru	8.578	0.2	0.4	0.4
Venezuela	8.32	0.1	0.1	0.1

Data are from reference [145, 155]. * Average value.

Different epidemiological studies have increased the knowledge about the incidence of type 1 diabetes rates with regards to the genetic factors [80,266,279] and environmental ones [216,243,250,279,312]. Several studies have shown that variation in the incidence of type 1 diabetes around the world is associated with the influence of different ecologic, socio-economic, geographic, infectious, viral and nutritional variables in the different populations [216,243,250,312]. For all aforementioned described, the differences in the incidences of type 1 diabetes between the countries are mostly due to the interaction of the susceptibility genes with the supposed environmental factors involved in the pathogenesis of type 1 diabetes [10,73,80,103,108,131,142,155,216,232,243,250,261,266,279, 312,313].

Latitude and Temperature

It is mentioned that probably there is one or several environmental factors which depend on the latitude and these are related to the high risk to develop type 1 diabetes. It has been initially proposed that the incidence of type 1 diabetes increase when there is a bigger distance from the equators [155,261], although some data contradict this hypothesis. In fact, Sardinia, Italy, Puerto Rico and Kuwait are regions with warm climates and present similar incidences to the one of the countries from Northern Europe, despite the fact that they are closer to the Equator [155,261].

Ecologic studies suggest an association between the incidence of type 1 diabetes with latitude and temperature [9,80,243]. In a European ecologic study, the temperature did not appear associated with the increase of incidence [243]. Recently, another ecologic study performed in Australia found a strong positive association between the latitude and prevalence of type 1 diabetes, on the contrary, a new inverse association between ultraviolet radiation and disease prevalence [283].

In the general population, the prevalence of β-cell autoimmunity appears to be roughly proportional to the incidence of type 1 diabetes in the populations [261]. In contrast, the frequency of β-cell autoimmunity in first-degree relatives of type 1 diabetic subjects does not differ dramatically among countries with high and low risk [261]. Another group of researchers found that frequency of type 1 diabetes associated antibodies (ICA, GADA, IA-2A, IAA) was similar to the first-degree relatives of subjects with type 1 diabetes from different European countries, in spite of the wide variation in the background incidence of childhood diabetes in those populations [315].

Age

Age-specific incidence of type 1 diabetes is generally calculated in 5-year age- groups (0-4, 5-9 and 10-14 years). In most populations, the incidence rates increased with age and were the highest among children 10-14 years of age. Although there is no proof in such sense, this suggests a likely relation with hormonal factors during puberty, for this reason, puberty is considered as a stage of higher incidence of diabetes [60,155]. In other countries (Finland, Sardinia, Puerto Rico and Spain) the incidence peaks of type 1 diabetes are also high in the ages of 5 - 9 and in others only in this last group of age, which may be due to alterations in the infections pattern [60,155,261]. The age-distribution of type 1 diabetes onset is similar across geographical areas and ethnic groups [145,155].

There are few studies that have analyzed the incidence of type 1 diabetes in adults, mainly because of difficulty of distinguish type 1 diabetes from insulin-requiring type 2 diabetes in older individuals. The incidence decreases in the third decade of life [261] and it is suggested that probably it is increased again in the fifth and seventh decades of life [261]. It is not very well known whether these differences in the incidences of type 1 diabetes are due to etiologic differences between childhood- and adult-onset type 1 diabetes [261]. At present, it is suggested that probably these divergences are due to a different contribution of HLA haplotypes [218].

Recently a study in eight European countries or nine areas found that incidence of type 1 diabetes in adults is lower than in children, and the range of incidence is also reduced, with a less than threefold variation in adults, against an eightfold variation in children [177].

The incidence of β-cell autoimmunity is higher in relatives younger than 5 years, compared to those 5-9 years old or older than 10 [261]. However, in a study of 8 European countries, relatives have similar rates of islet autoimmunity (in the same previous ages-group) despite wide variation in the background incidence of chilhood diabetes [315]. This same study showed that the frequency of ICA together with other additional antibodies (GADA and/or IA-2A) were more prevalent in relatives under 20 years of age in comparison with those over 20 [315]. Therefore, the relatives less than 20 years of age with multiple antibodies the risk of progression to type 1 diabetes is higher.

Races and Etnics

There is a remarkable racial difference in type 1 diabetes risk in multiracial populations, although not of the same magnitude as the geographical differences [261,279,313]. In the United States the non-Hispanic whites are about one and a half times as likely to develop type 1 diabetes as African americans or Hispanics [261]. This is similar to the differences reported in Montreal, where children of British descent had about one and a half the risk of type 1 diabetes in children of French descent [261].

In an ecologic study carried out in Latin America a strong negative correlation was found between the proportion of Amerindians in a country´s population and both incidence and estimated prevalence of childhood type 1 diabetes, suggesting that the presence of Amerindian component of the population in Latin America supplies protection against childhood-onset type 1 diabetes [67]. In Israel also exists a great difference in the incidence of type 1 diabetes among the three ethnic Jewish groups (Ashkenazi, non-Ashkenazi and Yemenites), as well as Arabs [279,313].

There is few data concerning β-cell autoimmunity is available for non-Caucasian populations [261]. During the screening of first-degree relatives of subjects with type 1 diabetes for the DPT-1 trial (Diabetes Prevention Trail-Type 1), lower prevalence of ICA was observed in Asian Americans and in Hispanics, compared to African Americans or non-Hispanic whites [261]. However, the pancreatic autoimmunity in first-degree family members of Mexican-American type 1 diabetes ocurrs in similar frequencies to that of non-hispanic and Caucasian families [321]. Therefore, it is difficult to elucidate that the frequency of β-cell autoimmunity is higher in some ethnic group in particular. It is suggested to carry out a large scale study with different ethnic groups to clarify whether there is a difference in the presence of pancreatic autoimmunity in the diverse ethnic populatons.

Gender

In general, the risk of type 1 diabetes before 15 years of age between female and male is similar [155,261], with the pubertal peak of incidence in females preceding that in males by 1-2 years. A male excess in incidence rate have been found in Sardinia (Italy), Oxford (UK) and Santa Fe de Bogota (Colombia) [155]. No population had a statiscally significant female excess in incidence rates [155]. Although in some populations (the Baltic countries, Macedonia, Yugoslavia, Rumania, etc) where the incidence of disease is below 4.5/100.000, an excess has been seen in female [261].

Type 1 diabetes diagnosed in adulthood seems to be associated with male excess in most populations of European Origin [177,261]. Recently, a study carried out in Europe found a male excess in incidence of type 1 diabetes, especially in the age group 25 to 29 years [177]. The differences in incidence rates between the sexes could be due to factors operating in males, in females or in both. One possible explanation of the sex-difference in incidences is under-acertainment of women with type 1 diabetes who are diagnosed with gestational diabetes, because these were excluded from the insulin-dependent diabetes in young adults study, although primary ascertainment source in each locality would be expected to register those with type 1 diabetes after delay [177].

DPT-1 screening data have suggested higher prevalence of ICA in male first degree relatives that in females [261]. Similar results were also found in the European study [315]. These antecedents could back the evidence of the high incidence of type 1 diabetes in male in most of the populations.

Seasons

The diagnosis of type 1 diabetes in children <15 years of age presents season fluctuations in all age-group, although this effect is much more remarkable in the age-group between 10-14 years [119,261], with a lower incidence during the warm months (summer) and a higher one in autumn and winter, implcating a climatic factor. This seasonal pattern appears to occur only in older children, suggesting that factors triggering diabetes possibly related to school attendance [261]. A similar behaviour has been observed in Cuba [78]. However, in the last year, this season variation has not been found in our country [68]. Although we cannot rule out that these season fluctuations could be related to similar changes in the environmental circulation of other factors with this feature, as it happens in the case of certain viral infections (enterovirus) [142,261,312]. No consistent information is available concerning potential seasonal or annual variation in the incidence of β-cell autoimmunity [261]. By contrast, Kimpimaki et al found that the first sign of β-cell autoimmunity in subjects with high-risk-genotype (HLA-DQB1*02/*0302) appear with higher proportion during autumn and winter than in spring or summer. The authors suggest that infections may play a role in the induction of the first signs of β-cell autoimmunity in some individuals [164].

Migrations

An increase in the incidence of type 1 diabetes has been reported in populations with a low primary incidence rate who have migrated to regions of high incidence and viceversa [102,279]. This suggests a strong contribution to the environment in the pathogenesis of type 1 diabetes. Parslow et al [242] found in Yorkshire (UK) that the incidence of childhood type

1 diabetes is highest in areas where limited childhood population mixing occurs and the diversity of origins of incoming children is low; those over 4 years are at greatest risk. This is consistent with an infectious hypothesis where absence of stimulation to the developing immune system increases vulnerability to late infectious exposure, which may precipitate diabetes [242].

In general, these data suggest wide differences of incidence of type 1 diabetes among populations from different countries and regions, and the genetic diversity could be important but they do not explain such situation completely.

Environmental Factors

The results from different studies indicate that there are several environmental factors that could initiate, accelerate and/or precipitate the process of β-cell destruction, years before the clinical manifestation of type 1 diabetes. These environmental factors include: nutritional factors, infections (virus, bacteria and parasites), vaccinations and level of hygiene, chemical products and toxins, psychosocial factors, latitude and temperature, prenatal and perinatal risk factors. Most of these environmental factors affect pancreatic β-cell through autoimmune mechanism, some of them do it directly and others it is not known how they act [9,129,134,142,167,179,216,309,312].

The environmental factors previously described act in the same or different stages of the development of the disease. It is possible to consider that the occurrence of several of these environmental factors lead to type 1 diabetes. Haverkos postulated the idea that the destruction of the islet cells is due to an interaction or combination of different environmental factors, where the interaction between enteroviral infections and nutritional factors (particularly animal protein and/or nitrosamine/nitrosamide content in the diet) in susceptible hosts could initiate an immuologic reaction against the pancreas. Finally, the stress, acting as a terminal injury triggers the development of the disease [9,129].

Nutritional Factors

The mechanisms of action of different nutritional constituents that may play a role in the development of β-cell autoimmunity are largely unknown. It also remains to be defined whether these exposures or lack thereof initiate β-cell autoimmunity, or promote or accelerate an ongoing process. The effects of nutritional risk predictors may be different in the fetal period, in early infancy, and later in childhood. The effects may be specific or non-specific, eg, a dietary protein might induce immunity cross-reacting with a specific β-cell antigen, or obesity could modify the natural course of β-cell autoimmunity through general effects on the immune system. Individual characteristics such as the HLA genotype most probably modify the effect of environmental factors [309].

Cow Milk

Cow`s milk or introduced at weaning trigger insulitis and diabetes in animal models perhaps through a molecular mimicry [261]. The data in humans are conflicting but predominantly negative [261,283]. Several ecologic or case-control studies, are controversial as to the association between decrease in breastfeeding and increase in type 1 diabetes incidence [9,67,216,241,243,261,309]. However, some studies suggest but not others a dose-response relationship between breastfeeding duration of less than 3 months and protection against type 1 diabetes [216,241,243,244,261,309]. Breastfeeding could be seen as a substitute for the delay in the introduction of diabetogenic substances present in formula or early childhood diet during the first years of life [261].

Several ecologic studies have found a positive correlation between the incidence of type 1 diabetes and the per capita intake of milk [67,216,217,241,243,309]. However, cases-controls and cohort studies in humans reported controversial findings on the relation between the introduction of cow milk in the infant diet and the development of type 1 diabetes, because some studies found a positive association, whereas in others no association was observed [9,167,241,244,261,309,310].

An abnormal and intense humoral immune response (IgA and IgG) against cow milk proteins and β-lactoglobulin as well as against bovine seroalbumine (BSA) have been detected repeatedly in children with newly diagnosed type 1 diabetes [9,167,244,261,309]. It has been described that it contains a sequence of 17 aminoacids, which they call ABBOS, towards which the major part of anti-BSA (IgG) antibodies are directed [9,167].

The antibody reaction in sera from diabetic patients has been reported against an interferon-inducible autoantigen from islet cells which present a molecular weight of 69KD (p69). There is a hypothesis that, due to an antigenic simulation mechanism or molecular mimicry, β-cell autoimmunity is triggered through similarity between protein p69 (auto antigen) and the BSA (foreign antigen containing a sequence homology with p69) from cow milk. This phenomenon occurs especially in genetically susceptible children after viral infections which induce the increase of interferon gamma levels [9,167].

These studies, along with the findings of anti-BSA antibodies in patients with type 1 diabetes, have originated the hypothesis that cow milk-specific proteins play a central role in the aetiology of the disease. The cow milk consumption in neonatal periods and in the first two or three months of life lead to the entrance in blood circulation of intact foreign proteins or partially degraded ones, due to the insufficient gastric acidity common at this age, and this permeability can even increase temporally in later months, due to diarrhoeas or after an episode of acute gastroenteritis.

Therefore, the exposition to BSA leads to an immunological sensitization, cellular or humoral, which, along with the later generation of interferon gamma provoked by some viral infection induces the transitional expression of protein p69 (with structural similarities to BSA) on β-cell and therefore the auto-destruction of these cells, mediated by effectors of the immune system previously sensitized [9].

In the year 2000, a group of Finnish researchers found that the first immunization to insulin occurs due to the exposition to bovine insulin present in cow milk formula in first degree relatives with type 1 diabetes and increased genetic risk for the diseases. The same authors found at the age of 3 months, both cellular and humoral reponses to bovine insulin were higher in infants exposed to cow milk formula than in infants fully brest-fed. IgG antibodies to bovine insulin were higher in infants who received cow milk formula than in infants who received hydrolyzed casein formula at 3 months of age, but no difference in T-cell responses was seen between groups. T cell responses to bovine insulin at 9 months of age and to human insulin at 12 and 24 months of age as well as IgG antibodies to bovine insulin at 24 months of age were lower in children with diabetic mother than in children with a diabetic father or a sibling, suggesting possible tolerization to insulin by maternal insulin therapy. The authors suggested that the priming of insulin-specific humoral and T-cell immunity occurs in early infancy by dietary insulin, and this phenomenon is influenced by maternal type 1 diabetes [241].

A follow-up study of initially non - diabetic siblings of children with type 1 diabetes showed that higher milk consumption is associated with.a greater risk of developing type 1 diabetes during the 10 year follow-up period [310]. The daily consumption of $\geq$ 0.5 liters milk was associated with a 3-fold risk of diabetes, and the risk increased to 5 times when the child's HLA genotype was taken into account [310]. This finding suggests an interaction between milk consumption and genetic risk [310].

In conclusion, in order to resolve this controversy about whether the cow milk is associated with the development of type 1 diabetes, a dietary intervention trial is being performed in Finland (TRIGR: Trial to reduce IDDM in the Genetically at Risk) to prevent type 1 diabetes with the elimination of cow milk in the infant diet for a short-term [261,309].

Other Nutritional Factors

Next, we will mention other nutritional factors which are associated with the increase of type 1 diabetes among them are found: cereals, nitrites and nitrates, fats, coffee and tea, zinc deficiency and vitamin D [9,167,309].

Cereals

Animal studies have linked wheat gluten with an increased risk of autoimmune diabetes [167,309]. A greater reactivity of T cells to gluten was detected among childrem with newly diagnosed type 1 diabetes than in control children [309]. In an ecologic comparison, per capita intake of cereal products was inversely related to the incidence of type 1 diabetes [216], whereas no relation was observed between cereal protein intake and the risk of diabetes in an Australian case-control study [309].

These events make us doubt about the certainty of the effect of cereal (gluten) in the development of type 1 diabetes in humans. Several studies in humans have shown that the exposition to cereals during the first stage of infancy (between ages 0 and 3 months) in children genetically susceptible had increased risk to develop islet-autoimmunity (autoantibodies) [228,323]. A long exposition to gluten (> 5 years) in patients with celiac disease is related to a high frequency of type 1 diabetes associated autoantibodies in comparison with those who were exposed for a short time or presented free gluten diet [305]. These results indicate that early exposition and a long consumption of gluten could be a risk for the induction of pancreatic autoimmunity and therefore the development of type 1 diabetes in persons with genetic susceptibility.

Fats

The intake of oils (not saturated fatty acids) from cod liver and fish such as salmon, mackerel and sardines (rich in vitamin D) prevent the development of type 1 diabetes in animal models [134,167,309]. A Norwegian case-control study in children found that use of oil from cod liver during infancy was associated, considerably, with a reduction of the risk to develop type 1 diabetes [287]. However, the high incidence of type 1 diabetes in children and adolescents between the ages of 10 and 16 years was correlated to the high consumption of saturated fatty acids [292].

N- Nitroso Compounds, Nitrites and Nitrates

Ecologic, animal, and human case-control studies have implicated that dietary N-nitroso compounds, nitrate, or a combination thereof may play a role in the etiology of type 1 diabetes [129,134,167,261,309]. The most important exogenous source of N-nitroso compounds is food. In addition, they may originate from cigarettes, car interiors, and cosmetics. Processed meat and fish product and beer are the most important food sources. Nitrate and nitrite are used as food additives in the processing of meat product because of their antimicrobial action and their ability to improve colour and taste. Other important natural sources of nitrates are potatoes, cabbages, carrots and beet roots [309].

Circumstantial evidences suggest a connection between type 1 diabetes and the intake of food and water which contain nitrates, nitrites or nitrosamines [9,129,261,309]. Several case-control studies have assessed the significance of dietary N-nitroso compounds, nitrate, nitrite, or a combination thereof in the development of type 1 diabetes [309]. A Canadian study compared the consumption frequencies of 6 meat products high in nitrosamines, but did not find a difference between cases with diabetes and controls [309]. The Swedish study reported that the high frequency of the use of foods containing nitrosamines (eg, smoked fish, bacon, and smoked sausage) was associated with 2.5-fold risk of diabetes [309]. In the Australian study, no relation between the increase risk of diabetes and the higher intake of food rich in nitrosamine was found. In Finland, the children´s nitrate intake was not related to the risk of type 1 diabetes [309]. Animal data suggest that nitrosamines increase the diabetogenic effect of certain viruses [261,309]. There are still some controversies about the relationship of these compounds in the diet and type 1 diabetes [9,129,309].

Coffee and Tea

A Finnish case-control study found an enhanced risk of type 1 diabetes was seen in the children who consumed coffee or tea daily, independently of putative confounding sociodemographic factors [309,311]. An ecological study observed an association between the coffee consumption and the incidence rates in 34 European countries [243].

Zinc Deficiency

The consumption of drinking water enriched with zinc prevents diabetes in the experimental model of diabetes mice [274]. Zinc concentrations in drinking water were also observed to be inversely related to the risk of type 1 diabetes in a Swedish case-control study [167,309]. Recently, in a Finland study, no significant effect was found between the concentration of zinc in drinking water and the variation in incidence of childhood Type 1 diabetes [211].

Vitamin D

Lower serum concentrations of active vitamin D (1,25 dihidroxy D_3) were observed in adolescents and adults with newly diagnosed type 1 diabetes than in controls of a similar ages [309]. In mice models, type 1 diabetes was prevented by treatment with $1.25(OH)_2D_3$ early in life. When nonobese diabetic mice, who typically develop type 1 diabetes, received $1.25(OH)_2D_3$ throughout their life, their risk of developing type 1 diabetes was reduced by 80% [134]. This is in good agreement with the observation by Hypponen et al., that children who received 2000 IU of vitamin D from the first year of life, the risk of type 1 diabetes decreased in 80 % of them [134,143].

Total Energy and Energy Produced by Nutrients

A high consumption frequency of solid foods rich in protein and carbohydrate was related to an increased risk of type 1 diabetes in a Swedish case-control study [167,309]. This result may simply reflect a higher consumption of energy in cases than in controls, which suggests that either an increased energy intake could be a risk predictor of type 1 diabetes, or that a higher intake of energy could be due to a metabolic dysregulation induced by the diabetic state [309].

In an ecologic study (which comprised 40 countries), average daily total energy intake was not related to the incidence of type 1 diabetes. On the contrary, the incidence of type 1 diabetes was directly correlated with average daily intake of energy of animal origin (meat) and inversely correlated with energy from vegetable food items (cereals). Intakes of fruit, vegetables and legumes were not correlated with diabetes incidence [216].

Evidence from experimental animal and human studies suggests that a high protein intake, particularly of animal protein, is involved in the pathogenesis of type 1 diabetes. The underlying mechanism of this association is not clear. However, beef or chicken proteins have been shown to elicit a strong insulinogenic response in humans [216]. As insulin is a specific antigen from β-cell, its augmented expression could increase the risk of developing type 1 diabetes [216]. Consequently with this theory, hyperinsulinism following overnutrition early in life was shown to predispose to type 1 diabetes [79,105,148,216]. On the contrary, type 1 diabetes incidence is reportedly low in countries with low average of protein intake [216] and among subjects born in periods of food shortage, when a greater proportion of daily energy consumption is from food items of vegetable origin [216].

Infected Tuberous

Bafilomycin A1, which is produced by *Streptomyces* species in soil, was recently shown to induce glucose intolerance and to reduce the pancreatic islet size in mice. *Streptomyces* species can infest tuberous vegetables such as potatoes and beet [179,216,220]. This toxic antibiotic from these microbes may induce damage to pancreatic β-cells and subsequent induction of type 1 diabetes. The role of bafilomycin A1 in the increasing of type 1 diabetes remains to be determined in the future studies [179,220].

The previous data suggest that it is necessary to carry out longitudinal studies starting during pregnancy, proceeding through the development of preclinical type 1 diabetes, and ending at the time that the disease is diagnosed in order to generate new reliable information on the possible contribution of dietary factors to progressive β-cells destruction [309]. Food consumption methods need to be developed for use in infants, children, and adolescents. Therefore, if a nutritional factor is confirmed to protect against or predispose to type 1 diabetes, the dietary exposition to that factor can be manipulated as an initial form of preventing the β-cells autoimmunity and disease [10, 309].

In spite of fact we still do not have all the elements which relate the different nutritional factors with the development of pancreatic autoimmunity and type 1 diabetes, we recommend the following strategies for prevention of type 1 diabetes: to encourage breastfeeding al least until the 4 months of age, decrease the cow milk consumption in newly-born and during infancy, avoid the consumption of food with gluten in the first three months of age, as well as its high consumption for a lifetime, to eliminate the consumption of smoked meat and sausages, to reduce the intake of animal source products (mainly all types of meats), to decrease the fats from animal source, to moderate coffee or tea intake or some product containing caffeine, to increase the consumption of products from vegetable source (vegetables, fruits and legumes, etc) avoiding the infected tuberous, and to increase the intake of fish and oil from blue fish (mainly salmon, mackerel, and sardines, etc).

Effects of Infections in Type 1 Diabetes

Among the environmental factors that may possibly play an important role in triggering autoimmunity there are numerous viruses of different genera, such as the viruses of mumps, rubella, herpes virus, cytomegalovirus, retrovirus, rotavirus [9,142,167,179] and enteroviruses [9,10,50,77,128,142,167,189,233,261,309,312]. The presence of at least one of the antibodies associated with type 1 diabetes (ICA, IAA, GADA, IA-2A) have been detected after infections by parotiditis (mumps) [42,51,55,99,261], rubella [142,261], measles [142,261], chickenpox [142,261], coxsackie [27,142,261] echovirus 4, 6, 16 and 30 [42,50,51,77,142,233,261], cytomegalovirus [142,179], retrovirus [142] and rotavirus [135,142,261].

The cases of diabetic patients due to viral infection-associated β-cells damage are rare. In patients with acute clinical diagnosis it has been impossible to detect RNA or specific antibodies against viruses whose relation with type 1 diabetes has been proved. However, several mechanisms have been proposed through which viruses related to type 1 diabetes could trigger autoimmune response. For example, it has been found that coxsackievirus protein P2C share a sequence homology with glutamic acid decarboxilase (an enzyme present in β cells), and by means of a mechanism of antigenic simulation, this or another viral protein could start an autoimmune process [9,77,142].

There are other proposed mechanisms which lead to β-cells damage caused by viruses. These mechanisms include the induction HLA class II molecular expression with its subsequent antigenic presentation or alteration in T lymphocytes receptors [9,77,142]. Besides, viral infections can act as a stress factor leading to clinical manifestation of disease. These can act either directly by cytolysis of β cells, or the viral induction of autoimmune response against β cells [9,77,142].

In chapter III, we will explain with further details, the possible role of enteroviruses in the development of β-cells autoimmunity and type 1 diabetes.

Hygiene Norms and Vaccinations

Part of the risk of type 1 diabetes could be due to the lack of early expositions and sustained expositions to protection factors. The so-called "hygiene hypothesis" proposes that the decrease of non-specific infections and microbes in many populations has caused the concomitant increase with atopic diseases in the past decade and this hypothesis has been recently extended to type 1 diabetes [9,115,135,179,242,261,309,312].

The incidence of autoimmune diabetes can be substantially reduced in rats BB and NOD mice due to expositions of rodents to high dosages of microbial antigens in the early stages of life [9,261]. Based on these observations and the unquestionable increase of hygiene conditions in the last two decades in industrialized countries with a higher incidence of type 1 diabetes, some authors suggest that the increase of type 1 diabetes in a large part of European countries may be due to decrease of infections, which are thought to be associated with improved hygiene and medical care, giving rise to a post-natal reduction of microbial antigens [9,242,261,289,309]. In these countries, also the diet has become more processed and sterile, and the ratio of fatty acids has increased. The exposure to microbes via foods and the intake of foods that affect gut microbes has altered considerably by the development of refrigeration, heating, and the food-processing technologies [309]. However, there are no direct evidences in favor of the associations between the hygiene norms and the incidence of type 1 diabetes in humans [9]. A protective effect of common infections in children and pregnant mothers has also been suggested in some studies [101,115,242,257,289], but very few or no data are available in prospective studies.

The vaccination programs have almost eradicated completely a group of pediatric infectious disease in the last decades in many countries, as well as in Cuba. Some authors have proposed that vaccinations could modify the type 1 diabetes incidence and are hypothesis that this could be related to the stimulus of immunological memory. The BCG vaccine has reduced type 1 diabetes incidence in the countries which have applied it, except in Sweden [9]. None of the routine childhood immunization (vaccines) has been shown to increase the risk of type 1 diabetes [261,286].

Effect of Chemical Substances and Drugs in the Development of Type 1 Diabetes

It has been proved that rodenticide Vacor has been the cause of type 1 diabetes in humans who have accidentally taken this product. Alloxan and streptozotocin are the classical chemical agents which cause diabetes in rodents, very similar to type 1 diabetes in humans [9]. Streptozotocin or dietary nitrates and nitrosamines induce β-cell autoimmunity in animal models [261]. Multiple hits of dietary β-cell toxins may render genetically resistant individuals susceptible to diabetogenic viruses leading to type 1 diabetes [261].

The use of treatment in rats with cyproheptadine, anti-serotonin drugs and antihistamines in the last 8 days of gestation affects the selective function of β-cells in the children [9].

Toxins can be a cause for type 1 diabetes by several mechanisms [9]:

- Direct damage against pancreatic β-cells.
- In combination with viral infections.
- Through autoimmune mechanism against pancreatic β – cells.

Psychosocial Factors

The possible role of psychosocial factors in the development of type 1 diabetes is still in discussion, although some evidence has been gathered about some events which cause stress and precede the clinical diagnosis of type 1 diabetes. In Sweden, there are reports of a study in which psychological stress is implied in the development of type 1 diabetes. An example of stress was the loss of a family member years before the diagnosis of the disease and this was more frequent in diabetic children than in controls. In Italy, the lack of attention at family level is associated with the increase of frequency of ketoacidosis to type 1 diabetes diagnosis [9].

Psychosocial stress in families may affect children negatively due to a link to hormonal levels and nervous signals that in turn influence both insulin sensitivity/insulin need and the immune system [278]. In a large prospective population-based study it has been proved that psychological stress, measured as psychosocial tension in the family (high parenting stress, experiences of a serious life event, foreign origin of the mother and low paternal education) seems to be involved in the induction, or progression, of diabetes-related autoimmunity in the child during the first years of life [278].

The recognition of exogenous factors triggering and driving β-cell destruction offers potential means for intervention aimed at the prevention of type 1 diabetes. Consequently, it is important to pursue studies on the role of environmental factors in the pathogenesis of type 1 diabetes. Environmental modification is likely to offer the most powerful strategy for effective prevention of type 1 diabetes, since such an approach can target the whole population or at least that proportion of the population carrying increased genetic diseases susceptibility and would therefore prevent both sporadic and familial type 1 diabetes if successful.

Factors of Pre-Natal and Peri-Natal Risk

Evidences indicates that the pathogenic process that leads to type 1 diabetes may star to emerge early in infancy (in the uterus). Some of these evidences are described below:

-Enteroviral infections during pregnancy may be associated with the development of type 1 diabetes in the offspring [9,233,309].

- A study about the national records of diabetes in Sweden found an increase of some perinatal variables in children who developed diabetes, particularly in the ages of 0-4 years, as well as the maternal age > 35 years [9].

- A Yorkshire case and control study confirms that an increased risk of diabetes is associated with advanced maternal age and excessive weight gain during pregnancy [9]. Recently, another cohort study in UK proved that maternal and paternal age at delivery (≥ 35 years), birth order (from the third child on), high birth weight and gestational age was significantly associated with type 1 diabetes risk [57].

- In a Swedish population-based prospective study where pregnant mothers and their offspring were analyzed, suggests that it is possible to analyze the hypothesis that events during pregnancy (infections, blood incompatibility, birth weigh, mother's age and other prenatal or neonatal events) may trigger β-cell autoimmunity as a prerequisite for childhood type 1 diabetes [182].

- In United States a cohort study in newborns with high genetics risk for type 1 diabetes and offspring or siblings of persons with type 1 diabetes found that the increasing maternal age was related to risk of islet autoimmunity among first degree relatives of persons with type 1 diabetes [285]. The authors suggest that pregnancy in ages > 25 years, influences in utero or during delivery may affect the fetal immune system [285].

Twin Studies

Studies in monozygotic twins suggest that only 30-50% percent are concordant for the disease, which implies that there is either acquired postconceptional genetic discordance or differential exposure to putative environmental factors [39,125].

The knowledge of environmental factors which are implied in the pathogenesis of type 1 diabetes would allow creating strategies for an effective prevention of the disease, as in this way a primary prevention could be performed to all the population.

Genetic Factors

There is a great amount of evidences which show inheritance of genetic factors which influence on susceptibility or protection to type 1 diabetes. The main risk factor to develop type 1 diabetes is genetic susceptibility. The major genes predisposing of type 1 diabetes are located in the HLA-DR and DQ regions [39,146,255,259,261,266]. There are also other candidate genes out of the HLA region which have been identified as a risk to develop the disease [73,80,132,250,255,259,261,266,284].

The identification of all new genes associated with type 1 diabetes support that type 1 diabetes is a polygenic and multifactorial disease [146,255,259]. As we previously explained genetic predisposition alone, cannot explain the etiology of type 1 diabetes, therefore it is necessary the interaction of genetic factors with some of the supposed environmental agents. After the introduction of insulin, an increase in the proportion of genetically susceptible individuals has existed, for such a reason it has contributed to the increase of the incidence of diabetes worldwide [250].

The different combinations of HLA alleles and the other gene candidates contribute with a great susceptibility to develop type 1 diabetes, other combinations cause a moderate risk, while some protect the development of the disease [255,259]. Currently, it is important to determine the role of HLA genes and candidates of additional genes for type 1 diabetes in the initiation of autoimmunity and progression to diabetes in order to develop new strategies with the aim of counteract the activity of genes associated with type 1 diabetes. In the next section we will speak more widely about the genetics of type 1 diabetes.

III. Genetics of Type 1 Diabetes

The susceptibility to type 1 diabetes is determined by the interaction between environmental and genetic factors. Twin studies, family studies, and animal models have helped to elucidate the genetics of autoimmune diabetes. Although multiples genes are implied, human leukocyte antigen (HLA) class II gene, especially HLA-DR and DQ are the most important ones, and it is valued that they contribute with 50-60% of susceptibility to this disease. Typing of HLA class I and II offers us those haplotypes with higher risk for type 1 diabetes. The association of HLA genes to the disease varies, depending on the ethnic and geographical source. For this reason it is important the studies of HLA genotypes in the different populations in order to be able to identify the accurate polymorphism that can trigger type 1 diabetes and develop biological instruments for its protection. The monozygotic twins of patients with autoimmune type 1 diabetes have much more diabetes risk than HLA-identical ordinary siblings, which suggest the contribution of other non-HLA genes to type 1 diabetes risk. Other factors such as non-inheritable genes (somatic mutations and rearrangement of T cell receptors or immunoglobulin) and the environment can play a role in the progress to diabetes. This is suggested by the observation that the diabetes risk for monozygotic twins of patients with type 1 diabetes is not 100%. For all this, it is suggested that the genetic study of type 1 diabetes will offer us a better characterization of this disease and it will increase our capacity to identify the subjects with a high risk to diabetes progress, as well as to predict the risk to other autoimmune diseases associated to type 1 diabetes. Next, we will show some information about some of the genes associated to type 1 diabetes.

Twin Studies

Twin studies help define the role of genetic and environmental factors in the etiology of disease [200,259]. In a primarily genetic disorder, is essential to know the definition of concordance. Concordance is defined when both twins affected. It is higher in identical (monozygotic) than non-identical (dizygotic) twins. Differences between monozygotic twins must be due to environmental factors, to genetic factors not coded in the germ line (e.g., somatic mutations), or to genes that undergo random rearrangement (e.g., immunoglobulin, T-cell receptor genes) [259].

Several studies have been performed which analyzes twins identified through national registries and prospective studies of twins discordant for diabetes when recruited [144,245,259]. Concordance rates for type 1 diabetes have been reported among dizygotic twins of between zero and 13 percent [144,259]. The concordance rate among monozygotic twins has been reported between 21 and 70 percent [144,255,259]. It has been observed that monozygotic twins may become concordant many years after diagnosis in the index twin (the first twin to be diagnosed) [144,245,259]. The age for the diagnosis of type 1 diabetes in the index monozygotic twins, reduces the time become the other twin in a similar one, this is, the younger the age of the index case, the higher is the risk of the non-diabetic twin to develop type 1 diabetes in a few years [144].

Nondiabetic monozygotic twins of patients with type 1 diabetes show a high frequency of type 1 diabetes - associated antibodies, between 42 and 76 percent [245,259]. The appearance of multiple autoantibodies is followed in most instances by progression to type 1 diabetes [259]. Monozygotic twins show a much-higher risk of progressing to diabetes and expressing type 1 diabetes - associated antibodies than did dizygotic twins [259]. This data supports the hypothesis of an important role for genetic factors in the determination of anti-islet autoimmunity [259]. On the contrary, the risk of pancreatic autoimmunity (type 1 diabetes - associated antibodies) for nondiabetic dizygotic twins of patients with type 1 diabetes and siblings was similar. This latter observation suggests that environmental factors, shared by dizygotic twins more than by ordinary siblings, do not increase progression to anti-islet autoimmunity and diabetes [259,260]. There was also higher penetrance of anti-islet autoimmunity in monozygotic twins who were heterozygous for the two high-risk human leukocyte antigen (HLA) haplotypes (DR3/4 and DQ2/DQ8). Johnston et al [151] found a higher concordance for monozygotic twins with HLA-DR3/DR4, the alelles most-frequently found on the same haplotype with DQ2/DQ8. Therefore, this finding further supports the hypothesis that islet-cell autoimmunity may be predominantly genetically determined [144,259].

The observation that the concordance rate in monozygotic twins is not 100 percent indicates that nongermline (i.e., noninherited) genetic or environmental factors play a role [259].

In spite of the bound effect of the alleles associated to type 1 diabetes, the environmental risk factors may directly trigger the process leading to type 1 diabetes or may interact with diabetes susceptibility genes that modify the penetrance [144].

Family Studies

The observation of familial clustering of type 1 diabetes is a strong indication that genetic factors are involved in the etiology of autoimmune type 1 diabetes. The majority of newly diagnosed cases (80-85%) are sporadic; that is, the patients do not have a first-degree relative with type 1 diabetes [255,259,261]. In spite of this, first-degree relatives of patients with type 1 diabetes are at increased risk of developing islet associated autoantibodies and diabetes, compared to the general population [259]. The risk of type 1 diabetes in the general population is 0.4 percent, while the risk for siblings of affected individuals is approximately 3-10 percent [214,255,259,261,271]. The offspring of a mother with type 1 diabetes has a 1.4 - 4 percent risk of developing type 1 diabetes. The risk for the offspring of a father with type 1 diabetes is much higher (approximately six to nine percent). On the contrary, the risk for the parent of a subject with type 1 diabetic is 3% [259,261,271]. The familial clustering (λ_s) can be calculated as the ratio of the risk to siblings over the disease prevalence in the general population. Thus, $\lambda_s = 6/0.4 = 15$, means that the risk for siblings of affected individuals of developing type 1 diabetes is 15 times higher than in the general population [255,259].

This parent-of-origin difference in transmission of diabetes is observed also for expression of islet autoantibodies. The frequency and levels of type 1 islet associated autoantibodies is incresed in offspring of fathers with diabetes, compared to offspring from diabetic mothers [259].

The gender bias in transmission rate of diabetes has not been fully explained. It has been hypothesized that maternal sex hormones could modulate susceptibility *in utero*, immunologic tolerance to islet autoantigens, or selective fetal loss of potentially diabetic offspring [259].

Another possibility to decrease the incidence of type 1 diabetes in the offspring from diabetic parents could be the immunization of the mother to her offspring during a stable breast feeding which leads to a normal immunological tolerance, and this way avoids the early introduction of antigens to the diet (cow milk, gluten or bovine insulin, etc) to her offspring when there is still no adequate maturity of the intestinal immune response [309].

Major Histocompatibility Complex (MHC): Description and Nomenclature

The major susceptibility loci are within the HLA (Human Leukocyte Antigen) region on the short arm of chromosome 6. The HLA complex is able to present foreign peptide to immune system. Depending on the structure and function of the proteins produced by HLA genes, they are to termed HLA class I and class II molecules. The main function of these molecules is the link and presentation of antigens to the receptors of CD4+ and CD8+T lymphocytes [255,259]. Peptides bound to HLA class I molecules are recognized by CD8 T cells. Antigens bound to HLA class II molecules are recognized by CD4 T cells. HLA class I molecules are glycoproteins. Nearly all nucleated cells of human body express MHC class I molecules. HLA class II molecules (also glycoproteins) are expressed by B lymphocytes, macrophages, and other antigen-presenting cells, and, in humans, by activated T lymphocytes. In addition, most epithelial cells can be induced to express class II molecules [255,259].

The HLA genes are inherited together in Mendelian codominance, this is, each allele is expressed regardless the other alleles. These HLA genes are transmitted in the form of haplotypes, which are defined as a series of alleles with different genes in a chromosome segment. One of the features of HLA system is that certain alleles have a tendency to appear together in the same haplotype, much more frequently than what would be expected according to the random combination of breakings and chromosome recombinations during many generations. This phenomenon is termed "linkage disequilibrium". The MHC molecules (in humans, also called HLA) are highly polymorphic; multiple different peptides could be presented to T cells. MHC polymorphism results from different genes encoding families of MHC molecules, with each of these genes having multiple germline-encoded alleles. Both MHC class I and class II molecules are heterodimers which consist of two chains, alpha and beta. The alpha chain of MHC class I and both chains of MHC class II are encoded by genes within the MHC region on chromosome 6. However, the beta chain of MHC class I (beta-2-microglobulin), which is not polymorphic, is encoded by a gene on chromosome 15 [259].

The MHC region in humans contains more than 200 genes, including HLA genes, [255,259]. HLA class I molecules include several genes HLA-A, -B, -C, -D, -E, -F, -G, -H, -J, -K, –L. The alpha chains of three major MHC class I molecules are encoded by three different genes, HLA-A, HLA-B, and HLA-C. Each allele is identified by a unique number corresponding to a unique nucleotide sequence of the alpha chain (e.g., HLA-B0801) [255,259]. Locus HLA-A, B y C encode molecules (antigens) which express peptides from viral origin.

The class II molecules, also known as immune response genes, are termed DR, DP, and DQ. Only the beta chain in DR molecules is polymorphic. Thus, different DR molecules are identified by one number denoting the allele encoding the beta chain (e.g., DRBI *0401). Both beta and alpha chains in DQ molecules are polymorphic. The resulting DQ molecule is therefore identified by two numbers (e.g., DQAl*0301, DQBl*0302) [259]. Locus HLA-DR, DQ and DP produce antigens which normally present peptides which have been escinded and lumped together by the cells in order to be processed to specific antigens as part of the immunological surveillance process.

The terminology of alleles by serology is the following way HLA-A3, HLA-B5 and HLA-DR2; on the contrary, when the analysis of the alleles is carried out through molecular biology, it is represented this way HLA-DRB1*1301.

HLA: Prefix of the genes of HLA region; DRB1: Particular locus of the gene which codifies for the beta chain of a DR molecule, here is a first DR; 13: group of alleles which codify to a serological specificity, here antigens DR13; 01: number of the specific allele of an allelic series. The name of the alleles can be longer [199].

HLA-DRB1*1301N: indicates a null allele (not expressed).

HLA-DRB1*130102: indicates an allele which differs from HLA-DRB1*1301 through a synonyms mutation.

HLA-DRB1*13010102: indicates an allele which contains a mutation out of the region it codifies.

HLA-DRB1*13010102N: indicates a null allele which contains a mutation out of the region it codifies.

Additional genes within the MHC encode other molecules involved in the immune response, such as transporters associated with antigen processing (TAP-l and TAP-2) the DM molecule, and proteosome subunits. The MHC class III region encodes complement and other genes [255,259].

The study of HLA molecules has several uses; among them are the performance of transplants, association with diseases, legal medical studies, hemotherapies and designs for vaccination strategies.

Genetic Susceptibility and Resistance for Type 1 Diabetes Mellitus

Inherited Susceptibility Loci

Both association studies and linkage analysis using various analytical methods have been used to identify susceptibility loci, and these are conventionally noted using the abbreviation IDDM and a number, e.g., IDDM1, IDDM2, etc. The number usually reflecting the order in which such loci were reported.

Using the candidate gene approach allowed to know the diabetes associated genes. Association studies dating now to about two decades ago provided evidences for the first two susceptibility loci, the HLA region (IDDM1) and the insulin gene (INS) locus (IDDM2). These two loci only contribute a portion of the disease familial clustering, suggesting the existence of additional loci. Genome scans conducted by several groups confirmed linkage with IDDM1 and IDDM2 and provided evidence for the existence of at least 15 additional loci. A comprehensive list of the known susceptibility loci is shown in Table 8 [125,255,259].

Table 8. Defined and Putative Type 1 diabetes loci

Locus	Chromosome	Markers
IDDM1	6p21.31-21.32	IDDMHLA, HLA
IDDM2	11p15.5	5'INS-VNTR, TH
IDDM3	15q26.2	D15S107
IDDM4	11q12.1-13.2	FGF3, D11S1917, MDU1, ZFM1, RT6, ICE, CD3, LRP5
IDDM5	6q25.1	ESR, a046Xa9, MnSOD
IDDM6	18q12.2-21.1	D18S487, D18S64, JK
IDDM7	2q32.1	D2S152, D251391, GAD1
IDDM8	6q26-27	D6S281, D6S264, D6S446
IDDM9	3q22.3-26.2	D3S1303
IDDM10	10p11.1-12.1	D10S193, D10S208, GAD2
IDDM11	14q31.3-32.12	D14S67
IDDM12	2q33.2-33.3	CTLA-4, CD28
IDDM13	2q35	D2S137, D2S164, IGFBP2, IGFBP5
IDDM15	6q21	IDDMFYN, D6S283, D6S434, D6S1580
IDDM17	10q25.1-25.3	D10S554, D10S592
IDDM18	5q31.3	IDDMIL12B, IL12B

Data are from reference [125].

Analysis on the Genetic Component in Type 1 Diabetes

We have previously talked about evidence demonstrates that type 1 diabetes has a genetic component. As to this component, segregation analysis indicates that the disease cannot be classified according to a specific model of recessive, dominant or intermediate inheritance. There are three major differences with regards to Mendelian diseases [39]:

1) More than one gene is involved, therefore the disease is polygenic instead monogenic.
2) The genes responsible for the disease do not represent uncommon variants or a rare mutation, but are polymorphic genes presenting different allelic variants, each with a frequency greater than 1% of the general population and which can differ among each other in some functional characteristics, for instance the quantitative type.
3) Type 1 diabetes is caused by the interaction between different genes and environmental factors.

At least one of the genes involved maps in the HLA region, although non HLA genes play an important role in causing the disease [39]. In this section we present here updated evidence of the regions and genes associated with type 1 diabetes.

HLA Genes and Autoinmune Type 1 Diabetes

The association of type 1 diabetes with HLA antigens is known since many years ago [255]. It is stated that HLA genes offer from 40 to 60% of the risk to inherit type 1 diabetes [125,255]. The first HLA genes associated with diabetes were HLA class I antigens (B8, B15 and B18), which were determined through serology [255]. Other studies have found that HLA alleles class I A*2 and A*24 also predispose the development of type 1 diabetes [255].

With the development of new technologies and reagents for typing, HLA class II genes were shown to be even more strongly associated with the disease. However, other loci inside or near the HLA region seem to modulate diabetes risk, and add further complexity to the analysis of IDDM1-encoded susceptibility [255].

Locus IDDM1

The HLA Class II Region

The great majority (90-95%) of patients with type 1 diabetes mellitus of Caucasian origin carry the HLA-DR3 and/or -DR4, or both antigens (HLA-DR3/DR4), in comparison with control population (45-55%) [199]. Approximately 30% of patients are HLA-DR3/DR4 heterozygotes. The DR3/DR4 genotype confers the highest diabetes risk with a synergistic mode of action, followed by DR4 and DR3 homozygosity, respectively. Following the development of DNA-based sequencing and typing technology, the HLA-DQ locus was found to be the most strongly associated with diabetes susceptibility. This locus encodes for several variants of the HLA-DQ molecule [255]. In Caucasians, the HLA-DQ heterodimers (the alfa chains are labeled DQA1 and the beta chains DQB1) encoded by the alleles have the strongest association with diabetes (DQA1*0301, DQB1*0302 and DQA1*0501, DQB1*0201). These alleles are in linkage disequilibrium with the HLA-DR4 and DR3 alleles, respectively. Table 9 show HLA class II susceptibility-resistance genes in Caucasian population.

HLA-DR3 and DR4 are strongly associated with type 1 diabetes. However, this association is likely in part secondary to linkage disequilibrium (nonrandom association of alleles) between DR and DQ [259]. A haplotype is defined as a series of alleles of different genes on a chromosomal segment. HLA-DRB1*0401, *0402, and *0405 alleles with DQA1*0301-DQB1*0302 (also called DQ8) are associated with high risk for diabetes. HLA-DRBl*0301-DQA1*0501-DQB1*0201 (also called DQ2) is another high-risk haplotype [255,259]. Ninety percent of individuals with autoimmune type 1 diabetes have at least one of these two high-risk HLA haplotypes, compared to 20 percent of the general population [259]. The risk conferred by the DQ8 molecule is modified by the DRBl allele present on the same haplotype. The DRBl*0402, *0401, and *0405 alleles are associated with high susceptibility, the DRB1*0404 with moderate susceptibility, and the DRB1*0403 with "protection" against autoimmune type 1 diabetes [259].

Table 9. Risk of autoimmune type 1 diabetes associated with DR and DQ alleles

HLA-DR	DQA1	DQB1	DRB
		High Risk	
DR3	0501	0201	0301
DR4	0301	0302	0401
DR4	0301	0302	0405
		Moderate Risk	
DR2	0102	0502	1601
DR4	0301	0302	0402
DR4	0301	0302	0404
DR8	0401	0402	0801
DR9	0301	0303	0901
		Weak or Moderate Protection	
DR2	0103	0601	1502
DR4	0301	0302	0403
DR4	0301	0301	0401
DR4	0301	0303	0401
DR7	0201	0201	0701
		Strong Protection	
DR2	0102	0602	1501
DR6	0101	0503	1401
DR7	0201	0303	0701

Data are from reference [255,259].

The presence of the HLA-DR4/DQ8 haplotype in first-degree relatives of patients with type 1 diabetes is associated with anti-insulin and ICA512 autoantibodies, both in individuals who developed diabetes on follow-up and in those who did not [259,324]. Other study showed that the frequency of the high-risk haplotypes was higher among ICA-positive first-degree relatives, compared to autoantibody-negative relatives [255,259].

HLA alleles also confer protection from diabetes (256,259]. The best-known "protective" allele is DQBl*0602, usually found on "DR2" (DRB1*1501-DQA1*0102-DQB1*0602) haplotypes. Approximately 20 percent of Americans and Europeans have DQA1*0102-DQB1*0602, while less than one percent of children with type 1 diabetes carry these alleles in most populations studied, including those of Caucasian (both European and North-American), Asian, African-American, Mexican-American origin [255,259]. The protection conferred by the DQA1*0102-DQB1*0602 haplotype appears to be dominant, since it is protective even in the presence of a high-risk haplotype in the same individual [259]. The DQB1*0602 allele in particular is the only class II allele exclusively found on protective DR2 haplotypes while all the other alleles (DQA1*0102, DQA1*0103, DQB1*0601, DQB1*0502, DRB1*1501, DRB1*1502, DRB1*1601) can be found on neutral or moderately predisposing DR2 haplotypes [255,259]. It is well known that the frequency of the protective allele DQB1*0602 was similar among ICA-positive first degree relatives and first degree relatives who were autoantibody negative [256,259]. However, the progression to diabetes is not frequent in 0602 positive, even in the presence of positive autoantibodies [259]. Nevertheless, autoimmune type 1 diabetes can develop in persons who carrying the DQB1*0602 allele, indicating that the protective effect associated with this allele is not absolute [259].

The protective effect of DQB1*0602 may differ among ethnic groups [255,259]. Recently, we report of an adolescent of mixed origin (mulatto) that developed type 1 diabetes after meningitis infection by echovirus 30. The adolescent was found to carry the genotype DR2 (*1501)/DR7 and DQ2/DQ6 [50]. Craig and co-workers [72] also reported a subgroup of non-white type 1 diabetic patients, who are at low frequency HLA-DRB1*03-DQB1*02 (high risk haplotype), that is associated with enteroviral RNA. African American, ICA-positive relatives were more likely to carry the DQA1*0102-DQB1*0602 haplotype than other ethnic groups. Hispanic, ICA-positive relatives with DQB1*0602 were more likely to have positive insulin autoantibodies or to have low first-phase insulin release than other racial groups [120,259].

The DQB1*0602 allele is usually found on DR2-DRB1*1501-DQA1*0102-DQB1*0602 haplotypes. However, protection from diabetes by this haplotype seems to be an effect of the DQB1 molecule [255,259]. It has been described three siblings with type 1 diabetes who carried DR2 [93,259]. Utilizing sequence analysis, an unusual DQB1 allele was found on their DR2 haplotype, while the DRB1 alleles on these DR2 haplotypes was the conventional allele (*1501). DQA1*0102-DQB1*0602 haplotypes were infrequently transmitted to diabetic offspring (2/313), while rare DRB1*1501 haplotypes without DQA1*0102-DQB1*0602 were transmitted to affected offspring (5/11). This finding again supports the hypothesis that the protection associated with the DQA1*0102-DQB1*0602 haplotype is an effect of the DQ alleles rather than the DRB1*1501 in linkage disequilibrium [259]. Two additional strongly protective haplotypes are DR6 (DQA1*0101-DQB1*0503-DRB1*1401) and DR7 (DQA1*0201-DQB1*0303-DRB1*0701) [255,259].

It has been observed that susceptibility and protection to type 1 diabetes is particularly related to the aminoacid at position 57. It has been found too, a particular association of the genes from the DQ alpha and beta chain, in order to confer susceptibility to the development of type 1 diabetes. It is stated that the absence of aspartic acid (replaced by a neutral aminoacid: valine, serine and seldom alanine) in DQB region and the presence of arginine at position 52 of the DQ-alpha region, indicate the expression in the surface of β-cell of a heterodimer DQ alpha-beta, which seems to be critical for the bind and recognition of the peptide to present to CD8 T cells. Most of the haplotype that determine the high risk for type 1 diabetes do not have arginine at position 52 of the DQ region and present arginine at position 52 of the DQ-alpha region, however the neutral/protective or resistance haplotype for type 1 diabetes has an aspartic acid at position 57 (asp 57).

The protective DQ haplotype, DQA1*0102-DQB1*0602, has an aspartic acid at position 57 of the DQ beta chain. On the other hand, the two DQ haplotypes that determine the highest risk for diabetes, DQA1*0301-DQB1*0302 and DQA1*0501-DQB1*0201, do not have an aspartic acid residue at that position but rather alanine [255,259]. However, the DQA1*0401-DQB1*0402 haplotype is also associated with diabetes risk. Although it has arginine at position 52 of the DQ-alpha chain, it has aspartic acid at position 57 of the DQ-beta chain, as do DQB1*0301 and DQB1*0303 alleles associated with moderate risk [259].

The hypothesis of conformational structure influencing diabetogenicity of some HLA alleles or haplotypes is further supported by inter-ethnic group studies. For instance, among the Japanese, the DQBl*0401 allele (which differ only by one amino acid) is usually found on DR4-DQA1*0301-DQB1*0401 haplotypes and is associated with diabetes [15,259]. Among Norwegians, the heterozygous DQA1*0301-DQB1*0302/DQA1*0401-DQB1*0402 genotype appears to be associated with type 1 diabetes. A very similar molecule could be formed among Japanese in cis (DR4-DQA1*0301-DQB1*0401) and among Norwegians in trans (DQA1*0301- DQB1*0402) [259].

In Koreans, HLA DR and DQ alleles are the ones previously shown to have the highest association with type 1 diabetes. DQB1*0201 was the only DQB1 allele that is positevely associated, while DQB1*0602, *0601 and *0301 alleles were negatively associated with type 1 diabetes. Two DRB1 alleles (DR3 and DR9) were positively associated with type 1 diabetes, while four DR alleles (DR15, DR12, DR10 and DR14) were negatively associated with type 1 diabetes [239].

Analyses of Koreans genotypes revealed nine genotypes that confer increased risk to type 1 diabetes. Seven haplotypes were involved in these nine genotypes: DR1-DQB1*0501, DR3-DQB1*0201, DR4s-DQB1*0302 (DR4s: *0401, *0402, *0404, *0405 and *0407), DR7-DQB1*0201, DR8-DQB1*0302, DR9-DQB1*0303 and DR13-DQB1*0604. Although the frequency of HLA-DR4-DQB1*0302 haplotype did not differ in type 1 diabetic patients versus controls, the HLA-DR3/4-DQB1*0302 genotype had an increased risk indicating a synergistic effect [239]. This data confirm that the association of each HLA allele seems to be different within the populations. The ethnic differences among the associated alleles are due to the variety in linkage disequilibrium of DRB1 and DQB1 alleles [239]. Recently, an association of type 1 diabetes with the DPB1 locus has been found, especially with

DPB1*0202 and DPB1*0301 (predisposing) and for DPB1*0402 alleles (protective) [73,92,149,227].

The HLA Class III Region

A case control study analyzed other markers in the HLA region in type 1 diabetic patients fully matched for the highest risk DQA1*0501-DQB1*0201/HLA-DQA1*0301-DQB1*0302 (DR3/DR4) genotype. This study provided strong evidence that another critical region, approximately 200 kb in size, lies around the microsatellite locus D6S273 which is located between the TNF and HSP70 genes [210,255]. Another study has independently confirmed linkage with marker D6S273 showing evidence for non-random transmission from DQA1*0501-DQB1*0201 homozygous parents [255]. Linkage disequilibrium analysis suggested that "diabetogenic haplotypes" might have resulted from a recombination telomeric of D6S1014 in the region of D6S273 and TNF. The TNF gene is a strong candidate since polymorphisms of this gene may affect the production of TNF-α (Tumor Necrosis Factor), a potent cytokine, and in turn the magnitude of immune response. It has also been reported that TNF-α polymorphisms are associated with age-of onset may and influence the inflammatory process leading to the destruction of pancreatic β-cell and the development of type 1 diabetes [255]. In addition, the class I chain-related MIC-A and MIC-B genes, located between the HLA-B and the TNF-α genes, may also affect type 1 diabetes susceptibility [255]. In a case-control study of Italian patients, the frequency of the MIC-A5 allele was increased in patients while none of the TNF-α alleles was statitically significantly associated with the disease. In this study, the MIC-A5 allele was associated with type 1 diabetes independently of class II alleles, suggesting an independent contribution of this locus to diabetes risk [110,255].

Finally, HSP70-2 and HSP70-Hom genes are also located in the class III region although there is no evidence for an independent association with type 1 diabetes from studies that could not circumvent linkage disequilibrium [255].

Clinical Heterogeneity of Type 1 Diabetes in Relation to the IDDM1 Locus

Age dependent HLA heterogeneity has been observed in Caucasian type 1 diabetic patients, indicating that high risk HLA genotypes occur at a higher frequency among the younger age onset groups, whereas older age at diagnosis is associated with an increased heterogeneity of DRB1 and a decreased heterogeneity of DPB1 [255]. Several studies have found a decreased frequency of DR3 and DR4 haplotypes and of DR3/DR4 heterozygosity amongst patients who had developed diabetes after age 15 [56,255]. In individuals with type 1 diabetes onset after age 30 it has been found a significantly reduced frequency of HLA-DR3/DR4 heterozygotes. In the same group it has been also found an increased frequency of DR3 homozygosity, which seems to correlate with a slower rate of the disease progress [255].

The immunogenetic analysis of ICA positive first-degree relatives from a family study has confirmed that DR3 in the absence of DR4/DQB1*0302 is associated with a slower rate of progression to diabetes. This slower rate may be in part explained by a recessive lack of humoral response to insulin during the prediabetic period that it has been demonstrated in a subset of first degree relatives at increased type 1 diabetes risk. This lack of humoral anti-insulin autoimmunity is mostly associated with DR3 homozygosity, but could be observed it also in relatives with DR5 or DR8 haplotypes [255]. All these haplotypes carry DQA1 (*0401, *0501 and *0601) alleles. Therefore, lack of or reduced anti-insulin autoimmunity during the prediabetic period may be associated with this particular subset of DQA1 alleles rather than with DR3 itself [254,255]. The first-degree relatives homozygous for such DQA1 alleles were characterized by lack of or very low levels of insulin autoantibodies in contrast to relatives with DQA1 alleles (*0101, *0102, *0103, *0201 and *0301) who have shown high levels of these autoantibodies [254,255].

A study demonstrated a high correlation between the pairs of twins and siblings (not twins) for age at diagnosis of type 1 diabetes is genetically determined [98]. Recently, in a screening study of type 1 diabetes in newly born who carried HLA-DR/DQ genes, it was proved that HLA-DR3/4*0302 genotype was the most strongly associated with type 1 diabetes at a younger age. This observation suggests that these genes could be involved in a rapid progression to disease [91].

Non-HLA Genes and Autoimmune Type 1 Diabetes

Genes like the one of insulin in chromosome 11, IDDM2 locus, IDDM3-18 loci and other non-HLA genes spread through to genome have been identified. It has been suggested that these genes may contribute approximately with 10-20% of the genetic risk for type 1 diabetes [255,284]. Of note, in addition HLA loci, the non-HLA locus which contributes the most to the susceptibility to diabetes is IDDM2 (Table 8).

Insulin Gene (Locus IDDM2)

The IDDM2 locus has been mapped to a variable number of tandem repeats (VNTR) located in the ~0.5 kb upstream of the insulin gene (INS). This polymorphic repeat, also known as the insulin gene minisatellite or ILPR (insulin-linked polymorphic region), consist of a 14-15 base pair units consensus sequence (ACAGGGGTCTGGGG) with slight variation of the repeat sequence [255]. This gene is located on chromosome 11p15 and it provides approximately 10% of the type 1 diabetes susceptibility.

There are three main VNTR classes defined by VNTR size: class I (30-60 repeats), class II (approximately 80 repeats), and class III (120-170 repeats). Each of these classes may be further divided. Homozygosity for class I VNTR determines high risk for diabetes, while class III VNTRs confers dominant protection. Homozygosity for class I VNTR is found in 75-85% of the patients compared to a frequency of 50-60% in the general population, suggesting that it predispose to type 1 diabetes [255]. The VNTR class III allele is associated with higher expression of messenger RNA for insulin within the thymus [259]. Homozygosity for this allele confers protective effect [255]. One hypothesis is that expression of insulin within the thymus leads to negative selection (deletion) of autoreactive T cells and thus to development of tolerance. VNTR class I alleles, associated with low levels of proinsulin and insulin in the thymus during fetal life and childhood, may fail to shape the

T-cell repertoire and lead to the presence of anti-insulin autoreactive T cells [259]. Moreover, it has been postulated that homozygosity for the predisposing INS genotype increases the likelihood that identical twins will be concordant for type 1 diabetes [255]. A recent study confirms the association between INS and CTLA-4 loci (T-lymphocyte-associated antigen-4) with type 1 diabetes [284]. The rest of the non-HLA loci associated with type 1 diabetes (Table 1) present a lower genetic risk for type 1 diabetes in comparison with HLA, INS and CTLA-4 genes. For this reason we will not go deeps into them. [255].

As the knowledge of the function of susceptibility and resistant genes grows, the researcher that works in the field of genetic of type 1 diabetes will continue to gain new insights into the relationship between genetic risk and the autoimmunity that culminates in type 1 diabetes.

IV. Immunology of Type 1 Diabetes

Type 1 diabetes mellitus is known as a chronic immune-mediated disease with a subclinical prodromic period characterized by selective loss of insulin-producing β cells in the pancreatic islets in genetically susceptible persons.

During this asymptomatic period of variable duration, type 1 diabetes associated autoantibodies appear which represent the first detectable sign of emerging β-cell autoimmunity. There are four important disease-related autoantibodies that have been shown to predict overt type 1 diabetes. These autoantibodies include classical islet cell antibodies (ICA), insulin autoantibodies (IAA), autoantibodies to the 65kD isoform of glutamic acid decarboxylase (GADA), and the tyrosine phosphatase-related IA2 molecule (IA-2A). Studies carried out in relatives as well as in general population reveals that the number of detectable autoantibodies is definitely related to the risk progression to clinical type 1 diabetes. Positivity for three and four autoantibodies is associated with a risk of developing clinical type 1 diabetes in the range of 60-100% over the next 5-10 years. The presence of type 1 diabetes related antibodies can be also combined with genetic (HLA and non-HLA genes) and metabolic markers (first phase insulin response to the intravenous glucose tolerance test) in order to increase the identification of high risk individuals of progression to overt type 1 diabetes. Measurements of type 1 diabetes associated autoantibodies can assist in the diagnosis of autoimmune diabetes, either in children or in adults. The appearing of these antibodies in nondiabetic individuals indicates a significantly increased risk for the subsequent development of type 1 diabetes. When preventive therapies for type 1 diabetes become available, type 1 diabetes associated autoantibodies screening of the general paediatric population should be considered to identify at-risk individuals. The study of type 1 diabetes related autoantibodies profiles in large prospective follow up studies in children from their birth up to adolescence has enlarged and improved the knowledge about the variable natural history of autoimmune type 1 diabetes.

In this section we will describer the type 1 diabetes associated autoantibodies, as well as the usefulness they have in the diagnosis and prediction of autoimmune diabetes in high-risk individuals of progression to overt diabetes. We also will explain the knowledge, up to date, about the natural history of the prediabetic period.

Evidences which Classify Type 1 Diabetes as an Autoimmune Disease

The main evidences which allow the classification of type 1 diabetes as an autoimmune disease [9,23,88,162,275,302] can be synthesized as follow:

- Presence of autoantibodies against some components of the islet cells (ICA, IAA, GADA, ICA512/IA-2A).
- Cellular-mediated immunity targeted against islet cell antigens (lymphocytic infiltration, insulitis)
- Link to major histocompatibility complex class II molecules associated with autoimmune diseases.
- Coexistence of type 1 diabetes with endocrinology autoimmune diseases (graves' disease, Hashimoto's thyroiditis, Addison´s disease) and other organ-specific autoimmune disorders (pernicious anemia, miastenia gravis, vitiligo, etc)
- The pancreas from a non-diabetic monozygotic twin transplanted to his (her) diabetic siblings develops insulitis without graft rejection.
- With immunosuppressive therapy, remission of diabetes onset can be induced.

For these and other reasons, it is considered that type 1 diabetes is an autoimmune disease of multifactorial etiology which starts with the destruction of pancreatic β cells.

Natural History of Autoimmune Type 1 Diabetes

The natural history of type 1 diabetes consists of four distinct stages [261]:

1. Pre-clinical β-cell autoimmunity with a progressive defect of insulin secretion.
2. Onset of clinical diabetes.
3. Transient remission
4. Established diabetes associated with acute and chronic complications and premature death.

The first phase, the pre-diabetic one, presents its own natural history and makes progress towards diabetes in the following way [88,319].

1- Genetic susceptibility (HLA-DR/DQ).
2- Triggering events: Environmental factors (viruses, toxins, diet, nutrients, stress, etc).
3- Active autoimmunity (lymphocytic infiltration within islets and production of type 1 diabetes associated autoantibodies).
4- Gradual loss of insulin secretion stimulated by glucose.
5- Clinically manifested diabetes with some residual insulin secretion (depending if it occurs in childhood or adulthood the residual function might be smaller or bigger, respectively).
6- Total destruction of β cells.

In the first step, presumed environmental triggers (certain viruses, dietary factor, gain of weight, psychological stress, etc) cause the destruction of β-cells. It is assumed that pancreatic antigen-presenting cells engulf dead β-cells. The antigen-presenting cells are thought to migrate to lymph nodes that drain the pancreas and in which islet-β-cell–specific antigen presentation takes place. CD4+ T lymphocytes with T-cell receptors that recognize β-cell peptides lodged in a groove in the HLA class II molecule may then be activated, which initiates an islet autoimmune reaction [183].

As a result of this activation of T lymphocytes and stimulation of B lymphocytes, the type 1 diabetes associated autoantibodies start to be produced (ICA, IAA, GADA, IA-2A) followed by an eventual loss of the first-phase insulin response. Autoantibodies can be present in some patients for more than a decade before the onset of diabetes. It is well documented that combinations of islet autoantibodies enhance predictability of type 1 diabetes [183,319].

After autoantibodies have developed, there is a second step, in which genetic as well as environmental factors may aggravate the islet autoimmunity [183]. Perhaps CD8+ cytotoxic T cells are induced, leading to a rapid assault on β-cells [183]. Depending on the insulin sensitivity and the age of the patient, hyperglycemia proceed when 80 to 90 percent of β-cells have been destroyed. In the adult patient, the more residual beta cells appear to remain at the onset of hyperglycemia. Unfortunately, the disease process is more aggressive in young children, and type 1 diabetes is being diagnosed at progressively younger ages, even though the total incidence may not be increasing [183]. The progression to overt diabetes resulting in significant β-cell destruction is triggered by the development of a more aggressive T cell phenotype and a change in the Th1 to Th2 balance towards a more proinflammatory milieu. The expression of FasLigand on cytotoxic T cells also marks the progression to overt diabetes [75]. The observation of islet tissue obtained from a pancreatic biopsy from patients with recent onset type 1 diabetes confirms insulitis, with the presence of an infiltrate composed of CD4+ and CD8+T lymphocytes, B lymphocytes, and macrophages, suggesting that these cells have a role in destruction of the β-cells [75]. Examination of islet during insulitis suggests also that Fas mediated apoptosis occurs and therefore provides one possible mechanism of β-cell destruction [75]. The accurate mechanism and factors which initiate the immune response against β-cells still remain unexplainable.

Humoral Autoimmunity

The chronic lymphocyte infiltration of Langerhans islets (insulitis) is considered as an index of autoimmune diabetes and a cause of insulin deficiency [75,153]. This fact is followed by several immunological anomalies detected mainly at the onset of type 1 diabetes in genetically at-risk individuals [75,183,219,255,261,316,319].

Currently, the autoimmunity in type 1 diabetes is defined by the presence of autoantibodies, because their measurement is consistent and standardized across laboratories, in contrast with the cellular markers [59,219,261].

Many autoantibodies are detected at the onset of type 1 diabetes [316,319]. Islet cell (cytoplasmic) autoantibodies (ICAs) [36] and islet cell surface autoantibodies (ICSAs) [89,184,190,203,270,301] were initially described in the 1970s. In the 1980s, insulin autoantibodies (IAAs) [236], 64-kDa autoantibodies (64kAs) [113], insulin receptor autoantibodies [198], carboxypeptidase-H autoantibodies [58], and heat shock protein (HSP) autoantibodies [152] were recognized. In the very early 1990s, the nature of the 64kDa autoantigen was discovered as glutamic acid decarboxylase (GADs) leading to the recognition of glutamic acid decarboxylase autoantibodies (GADAs) [21]. Afterward, a cascade of various islet autoantibodies were identified including 51-kDa aromatic-L-amino-acid decarboxylase autoantibodies [267], chymotrypsinogen-related 30-kD pancreatic autoantibodies [163], DNA topoisomerase II autoantibodies [63], glima 38 autoantibodies [3], GLUT2 autoantibodies [150], glycolipid autoantibodies [41], GM2-1 islet ganglioside autoantibodies [82], Sulfatide autoantibodies [38,40,43], IA-2 autoantibodies (IA-2As) [180,258], IA-2β autoantibodies (IA-2βAs) [65], ICA69 autoantibodies [246], islet cell-specific 38-kD autoantibodies [235], proinsulin autoantibodies [29], and 52-kDa RIN (rat insulinoma) autoantibody (Rubella-related autoantibody) [154]. New autoantibodies associated with type 1 diabetes continue to be revealed as the SOX13 autoantibodies [156], autoantibodies to carbonic anhidrase II and lactoferrin autoantibodies [290]. From all type 1 diabetes associated autoantibodies previously mentioned, four autoantibodies have emerged as the most useful autoimmune markers of type 1 diabetes: ICAs, IAAs, GADAs and IA-2As (include ICA512 and IA-2c autoantibodies) because its measurement is reliable and standardized across laboratories. In addition measurements of these antibodies have shown a great specificity, sensitivity and a highly predictive of disease progression in otherwise healthy first-degree relatives [59,75,90,316,319]. On the other hand, the presence of these antibodies has been observed in the plasma of subjects during the pre-diabetic period [22,59,69,75,90,165,166,174,214,271,275,316,319].

Currently, it has been proved that combination of type 1 diabetes associated antibodies (GADA, ICA512A/IA-2A, IAA and ICA) allow us to identify almost all children at the time of diagnosis [22,166,231].

In table 10 the sensitivity, specificity and the positive predictive value of several antibodies and their combinations in healthy siblings of type 1 diabetic children is shown.

Table 10. Predictive characteristics of single autoantibody specificities and antibody combination in 755 initially unaffected siblings of children with type 1 diabetes observed up to diagnosis of type 1 diabetes or for a minimum of 7 years in the Childhood Diabetes in Finland (DiMe) study

Marker	Sensitivity %	Specificity %	Positive predictive value %
ICA	81	95	43
IAA	25	97	29
GADA	69	96	42
IA-2A	69	98	55
GAD and/or IA-2 antibodies	81	98	41
Three or four antibodies	72	98	66

ICA: Islet cell antibodies IAA: insulin autoantibodies

GADA: glutamic acid decarboxylase autoantibodies

IA-2A: tyrosine phosphatase autoantibodies (ICA 512bdc/IA-2)

Data are from reference [165].

The initial islet cell antibody assay, using immunofluorescence and pancreatic tissue have been notoriously difficult to standardize and have been replaced by a combination of specific β-cell autoantibodies (IAA, GADA and IA-2A). These tests have been shown to be rather sensitive and predictive in relatives of type 1 diabetes, adult type 1 diabetes and in general population [75,261,319]. The standard "biochemical" autoantibody assays measure antibodies reacting with insulin, GAD65, and IA-2 (also termed ICA512). It has been much easier to standardize assays for GAD65 and IA-2 as compared to insulin autoantibodies which probably relates to the much stronger signal for GAD65 and IA-2 autoantibodies [319]. The sensitivity of some biochemical characterized autoantigens is exposed below [319] (Table 11).

Table 11. Biochemically characterized autoantigens

Autoantígens	Sensitivity	Comment
Insulin	49-92%	Higher levels in young children
GAD	84%	Higher sensitivity in adult onset type 1 diabetes
ICA512/IA-2	74%	Higher frequency of IA-2A and IA-2βA in young children and adolescents at onset of disease, and low frequency in adult onset type 1 diabetes
IA-2beta/Phogrin	61%	

GAD: Glutamic Acid Decarboxylase
Data are from reference [319].

Islet Cell Antibodies (ICA)

The ICAs were discovered by Bottazzo, Christensen and Doniach in 1974, in a group of type 1 diabetic patients with autoimmune polyendocrine deficiencies which caused that diabetic autoimmune hypothesis turned important [36]. These antibodies are detected by indirect immunofluorescence using blood group O human pancreas as substrate. The ICA assay is labor intensive and non-automated and requires a very high level of quality assurance and quality control to produce accurate and precise results [316]. ICAs are polyclonal autoantibodies that react with all cells of the islet (e.g., α, β, γ, δ and PP cells). The ultrastructural studies carried out so far have not clarified if these antibodies also react with some component from the plasmatic membrane [262].

The antigens recognized by ICA on the sections of the frozen human pancreas continue being, so far, an enigma. Currently, some of them have described [316] and are presented now:

- Glycolipid. (glycolipids and ganglioside GM2-1) [43,69,84,225]
- Glutamic acid decarboxylase (GAD) [19,123,197,221]
- Tyrosine phosphatase (ICA512/IA-2, IA-2β) [32,197,221]
- Insulin [197,276]

The results of ICA absorption with diverse islet antigens (GADA, IA-2 and insulin) suggest that apart from these molecules (which partially inhibit the reactivity of ICA to the pancreatic islets) other antigens are related to the ICA reactivity [197], such as glycolipids [41] or other not known so far.

It seems that ICAs are the result of a secondary immune response to the phenomenon started by the exposition of antigens (cytoplasmic components) common in every islet cell. It is stated that these antigens are released in response to a cell damage produced by a primary destruction mechanism [183,262,319].

In the 1980´s, a subset of ICA that fixes complement identified as complement-fixing islet-cell antibodies (CF-ICA) has been revealed [35]. The CF-ICA had been found, which destroys the β cells "in vitro" [219,269]. The highest CF-ICA frequency (50-65%) seems to be found at the onset of type 1 diabetes, being, as a general rule, half of the ICA found [35,262]. However, the consensus is that the CF-ICA is simply ICA of high titer [262].

In 1992, two groups of investigators [112,114] independently reported the existence of two types of ICA. ICA minority type (termed "restricted" ICA or "selective" ICA, R-ICA) which reacts with human and rat pancreas but failed to react with islets of mouse [319]. This restricted ICA pattern reacting against glutamic acid decarboxylase (GAD) and showing a stain pattern specific to human β cells [112,319]. In contrast, non-restricted ICA pattern (NR-ICA) give a pattern of staining that involves all human islet cell types and does not go directly against GAD. The non-restricted ICA pattern reacts with islets of human pancreas, as well as rats and mouse pancreas. This pattern has a high predictive value in the development of type 1 diabetes. The NR-ICA frequency in patients with new-onset of type 1 diabetes ranges between 60–70% of the ICA-positive human pancreas and between 45–47% of the non-diabetic first-degree relatives of type 1 diabetic patients [61,62,114], in contrast to gestational diabetes which is 28% [71].

Different researchers have suggested that the detection of ICA in mouse pancreas (NR-ICA) carries increased risk for the progression of type 1 diabetes in the first-degree relatives of type 1 diabetic patients compared with NR-ICA-negative subjects [61,114,270]. Sai and coworkers observed that the increased NR-ICA titers during subject follow-up could be indicative of the worsening of the course during pre-diabetic phase [270].

Cabrera-Rode and coworkers identified three subtypes of NR-ICA-positive sera: sera with total, partial and null reactivity to glycolipid. NR-ICA positive sera totally and partially inhibited by pancreatic glycolipid extracts were found in all new-onset type 1 diabetic patients and in most of first-degree relatives of type 1 diabetic patients [46]. These data suggest that glycolipids are the major autoantigens of ICA on mouse pancreas [46]. Therefore, ICA reactivity on human and mouse pancreas are against pancreatic glycolipids [41,46]. Consequently, the reactivity of non-restrictive ICA pattern to human, rat and mouse pancreas is logical [114], due to the fact that ICA recognizing glycolipids antigen commonly present in human, rat and mouse islets [41,46,69,81,317].

Once ICA sub-specificities are analysed in blocking experiments not all ICA positive sera seem to react to the previously mentioned antigens, due to the fact that some ICA sera react specifically with human and not with mouse and rat pancreatic tissues, its reactivity to human pancreas cannot be inhibited when they are absorbed with GAD, IA2 or glycolipids.

Therefore, it is suggested that some ICA are directed to an uncharacterized target antigen [45, 277,319].

Conventional and Alternative Detection Methods of ICA

The first detection of islet cell antibodies was carried out independently by Botazzo et al. and MacCuish et al. by means of similar methods [36,192]. They determined ICA by indirect immmunofluorecence using unfixed frozen sections of human pancreas, incubating the pancreas section with serum, applying a second antibody labelled with fluorescein in order to reveal the ICA presence. The use of human pancreas from donors who have blood type O has been preferred because of the presence of isohemagglutinin antigens on the acinar tissue. The most important feature of the pancreas for use in the ICA assay is the state of the pancreas itself. The length of time form surgical removal of the pancreas to snap-freezing is critical and needs to be kept at a minimum. Because of the difficulties in obtaining fresh human pancreas, several other species have been used as substrates (i.e. rat, mice and monkey pancreas) despite some limitations. Non-specificity was apparent in one study. A modification in the duration of incubation (overnight) has been shown to increase the sensitivity of the assay. A protease inhibitor is mandatory for these prolonged incubation assays. Other conjugates such as peroxidase, glucose oxidase or other enzymes [262]. These modifications offer specific advantages: The use of non-human tissues eliminates the use of human tissues from cadaver. The length of incubation time for sera (using protease inhibitors) increasing the sensitivity detecting the low antibody levels. The advantages of enzymatic methods are the ability to store the slides indefinitely, the relative stability of the tissue staining for ICA, and the lack of need for a fluorescent microscope. However, despite all this beneficial modifications, most of the research laboratories remain using the conventional methodology [36,137,262]. Some researchers have obtained good results by using rat pancreatic tissue [62,270], although other has been associated with inability to determined lowers titers of ICA [114]. The prolonged incubation in the ICA determinations allows an increase of sensitivity without decreasing specificity [137,248]. The use of the second anti-IgG antibody labelled with golden chelates (Eu^{3+}) increases the specificity and sensitivity in the ICA determination [268].

There is a wide variation in the precision, sensitivity and specificity of the ICA test, which is extremely difficult to control [137,262]. Several modifications of this technique have been adopted over the years, but because they also used fresh human pancreas as substrate, these modifications suffer the same limitations as the parent technique, giving rise to the fact that the improved sensitivity and specificity of ICA determinations depend on the pancreas used [137,262].

Standardization of ICA Determination

Since the first description [36] of cytoplasmic islet cell autoantibodies in type 1 diabetic patients these humoral markers have been increasingly applied in clinical investigations. Thus, ICA determinations have been used to classify diabetes of autoimmune origin [1,2,11], as markers for identifying individuals at risk for developing type 1 diabetes [22,59,69,90,165, 166,174,231,316,319] and as a possible correlate of impaired β cell function [319], and to evaluate the therapeutic effects of several drugs [10,44,48,59,76,94,202,282,291,308], and to assess the result of the transplant (pancreas or β cells) [33], as well as an index for the future insulin deficiency in type 2 diabetic patients [47,49,122,237,297].

The importance of ICA measurements has prompted a number of international immunology of diabetes serum exchange workshops, in an attempt to improve the comparability of assays worldwide. After the first workshop showed wide variations in results, standard curves constructed from a reference serum (JDF standard) were used, and improved concordance was seen between laboratories in the second workshop. The third workshop indicated that the interlaboratory variation decreased when participating laboratories had access to the JDF standard. However, also few control sera were used in the third workshop to determine the specificity (negatively in health) of assays. In the fourth ICA workshop demonstrated excellent specificity and good concordance among control sera was seen among participating laboratories. In addition, all of the laboratories could distinguish controls from positive sera among group's newly diagnosed type 1 diabetic patients, healthy individuals who later developed type 1 diabetes, and first-degree relatives of type 1 patients [121,307].

Due to the appropriate and more frequent use of the ICA determination, it was necessary to quantify the ICA results. Thus, since 1986 up to now periodical workshops are organized by several international Immunology of Diabetes Workshops (IDW). The IDW and later the Immunology of Diabetes Society (IDS) carry out serum exchanges to standardize ICA and a proficiency testing programme to monitor assay performance in different laboratories and a uniformity in their interpretation is tried to be established [121,137,206,307]. With the use of ICA-positive international reference sera, each laboratory performs its standard curve and the results are informed in JDF units [137]. At the end of the decade of 1990, the strategy to produce an international standard sample for the standardization and uniformity of ICA concentration for the diagnosis of islet autoimmunity is approved [185,206]. On the basis of the ICA standardization results and with the agreement among the participants, the preparation 97/550 has been established by the World Health Organization Expert Committee on Biological Standards for establishment as the first international standard for islet cell antibodies with an assigned potency of 20 international units. In addition, 97/550 can serve as an international reference reagent for specific GAD65 and IA-2 autoantibodies. The serum itself also reduces the variability among laboratories for the measurement of islet cell antibodies (ICA, GADA and IA-2A) [207]. The production of available international standard serum turns very difficult from an antibody which is produced as a consequence of a polyclonal immune response as in the case of ICA, which can vary by affinity and avidity [208]. The results of this international workshops and the use of the WHO's international standard have shown a high degree of concordance for the positive and negative samples among the different laboratories (approximately 90%).

The standardization of the ICA determination reduces the disagreements among laboratories and therefore also favours that the epidemiological researches about the frequency of this antibody offer more accurate data.

Relationship between ICA and Type 1 Diabetes Mellitus

Before the clinical onset of the disease

Since the past decade, a great attention has been devoted to ICA as possible predictive markers for β cells dysfunction or the imminence of type 1 diabetes, as its presence in the serum can be verified several years before the clinical onset of the disease [22,59,69,75,90,125,165,166,171,174,188,262,316,319,325].

ICA in First-Degree Relatives of Type 1 Diabetic Patients

Approximately 0.9-12.0% of healthy first-degree relatives of type 1 diabetic patients are ICA-positive [42,69,125,171,188,315,316,325] and in the healthy subjects this frequency is 0-1.6% [42,125,188,231,325]. The general population (normal schoolchildren) frequency of ICA in different countries varies between 0.4 to 4.1% [90,166,178,316].

At the Onset of Type 1 Diabetes

ICA is detected in ~69% or more (69-90%) of Caucasoid individuals at the onset of type 1 diabetes [125,137,166,188,262,268,277,316]. ICA frequency in African Americans at the time of diagnosis is low [20,187,316]. This suggests that a considerable proportion of African Americans with new-onset insulin-requiring diabetes do not have autoimmune diabetes [20,187,316].

After the Establishment of the Disease

ICA frequency declines considerably following diagnosis, and no more than 5-10% of type 1 diabetic patients remain ICA-positive after 10 years [316]. Titers decline through the first year and continued to fall during subsequent years in this study population. It is thought that the persistence of ICA long after the onset of insulin-dependence is related to the presence of viable islet cells. Once the antigenic material in the pancreas is completely destroyed, the ICA disappear [42,188,231,262].

ICA and Genes (HLA and non-HLA)

The relationship of ICA with HLA has maybe created quite a disagreement among the researchers who are in search of an association of ICA as type 1 diabetes markers and the genetic factors of the disease

In most of the investigations developed in the decade of the 90´s concerning the study of HLA-DR3 or DR4 haplotypes, no association has been found between these haplotypes and ICA [188,231]. HLA-DR3 and -DR4 genotypes are the most frequent among type 1 diabetic patients. In general, the relation of the high-risk HLA antigens (DR3 and/or DR4) to islet cell antibody positivity is at best inconsistent, except perhaps in the small group of patients whose antibodies are present for an extended period after diagnosis [188].

When the study of HLA-DQ genotypes was incorporated, it has been found that the combination of ICA with the presence of HLA-DQ heterodimers (arg52 and no-asp57) can be used to identify at-risk individuals with a relative risk of ~200 times [137].

In subjects from the general population, to which ICA-persistent positivity has been detected, there is a high frequency of HLA-DR3, HLA-DR4, DQB1*0302 y DQB1*0201 [137]. Kulmala and coworkers [174] found a combination of the genetic markers (HLADR3/4 and DQB*02/0302) and the presence of ICA increases the positive predictive value (66.7% to 75%, respectively) in the detection of high-risk individuals to overt diabetes. However, because such combinations also resulted in reduced sensitivity, autoantibodies alone rather than in combination with genetic markers are recommended as the first-line screening in siblings. In conclusion, not all siblings with a broad humoral autoimmune response and/or high-risk HLA markers progress to clinical type 1 diabetes even within a long follow-up period, while some siblings with a low genetic risk and weak initial sings of humoral autoimmunity may progress to disease [174]. Another study carried out in Finland; show that there is geographical variation both in the frequency of the HLA-DQB1 genotype, which is associated with the greatest susceptibility to type 1 diabetes, and in the risk of seroconversion to ICA positivity or positivity for multiple autoantibodies. The difference in seroconversion rate could not be explained by the difference in HLA-DQB1-defined disease susceptibility, implying that the impact of environmental (possibly caused by differences in the climate and in the pattern of certain infections) triggers of diabetes-associated autoantibodies may differ between the regions studied [173].

Recently, it has been informed that the presence type 1 diabetes associated autoantibodies (ICA, IAA, GADA, IA-2A) alone were more sensitive in the prediction of future diabetes in siblings than when combined with genetic susceptibility [214]. Thus, the genetic susceptibility played an important role in whether the initial prediabetic stage progressed (progression in 29.6% of the high risk siblings compared with 6.6% of the siblings with HLA-DQB1 genotypes conferring decreased risk) and whether overt type 1 diabetes became manifest or not. Therefore, the genetic susceptibility has an important independent impact, in the initiation as well as in the progression of the autoimmune process leading to clinical diabetes in siblings of type 1 diabetics [214].

None of the type 1 diabetes associated autoantibodies (ICA, IAA, GADA, IA-2A) showed any association with CTLA-4 gene [132]. Isolated ICA positivity was independent from the HLA and INS genotypes [132]. The low ICA titers (below 20 JDFU) show no association with HLA genotypes, whereas children with multiple autoantibodies or high titers of ICA show a HLA genotype distribution resembling that seen in patients with type 1 diabetes [28,132,186,273]. However, INS - 23 Hphl AA genotype and DRB1*0401 allele show a strong association with the appearance of insulin autoantibodies (IAA). The INS and DRB1 loci seem to contribute on the pathogenesis of type 1 diabetes by initiating /modifying the insulin-specific autoimmunity. The emergence of IAA represents a crucial step in the development of β cell- autoimmunity in young children in whom the appearance of ICA, GADA and IA-2A is linked to IAA [132,322]. In conclusion, the insulin locus plays a central role in the initiation of the autoimmune process in IAA-positive individuals, while the appearance of ICA, GADA and IA-2A is a secondary phenomenon [132,322]. In addition, the HLA-DRB1*0401 variant also seems to have a role in the regulation of insulin autoimmunity. In IAA-negative individuals the development of ICA, GADA and IA-2A and progression to clinical disease is likely controlled by factors other than the INS locus [132].

ICA Frequency in Other Types of Diabetes and Disease

Type 2 Diabetes Mellitus

Some authors have described the presence of ICA in 2.2–22% of diabetic patients with an initial diagnosed clinically with type 2 diabetes, which are denominated patients with Latent Autoimmune Diabetes in Adults (LADA) or slowly progressive form of type 1 diabetes [42,47,48,49,75,117,118,122,125,137,188,202,212,237,252,288,297-299,316,326]. On the other hand, it has been proved that ICA presence is associated with a gradual decline in β-cell function in individuals with LADA [47,49,117,118,122,212,237,252,288,297-299,326].

Gestational Diabetes

In the diabetes with onset or first recognition during pregnancy, ICA frequency varies between 1.6–38% [42,86,204,205]. Presumably, the presence of ICA in gestational diabetes indicate a degree of pancreatic damage predicting, rather than due to, the pregnancy, although pregnancy in itself may accelerate the development of type I diabetes in susceptible women [188].

Viral Infections

ICA has been detected in non-diabetic patients, infected by different types of viruses [9,27,42,77,125,167,188]. In the last years, enough amount of evidence has been accumulated to show that the destruction of pancreatic β-cells is a process [59,69,125,171,174,188,316,319,325] which can take many years before their quantitative effect leads to a low production of insulin in sera, unable to maintain the glucose metabolic control. For this reason, there is relatively strong, albeit circumstantial, evidence that viral infection plays a role in the etiology of type 1 diabetes. However, the possibility that a viral infection (coxsackie, echo and others) initiate the β-cell damage and trigger type 1 diabetes in genetically susceptible patients in not excluded [9,77,125,142,167,174,180,239,255,316, 319]. ICA and other type 1 diabetes associated autoantibodies have been found in subjects infected by viruses such as rubella, mumps, rotavirus, cytomegalovirus, adenovirus and enterovirus [23,42,50,55,125,130,133,135,142,189].

Other Autoimmune Diseases

The presence of ICA has also been found in patients with organ-specific autoimmune disease. The frequency of ICA in 2049 patients was 2.4% according to the results reported by Betterle and coworkers [24]. In other studies performed in 88 persons with thyroid diseases (age 5-20 years), only two patients were ICA-positive [188]. In eight young men with

Addison´s disease one was ICA-positive too [188]. There are evidences that the rest of autoimmune endocrine diseases and the ICA are not related "per se" [188].

Islet Cell Surface Autoantibodies (ICSA)

The presence of ICSA was detected in type 1 diabetic patients by Lernmark and co-workers using freshly isolated rat islets [184]. The determination of these antibodies in much more difficult and less reproducible than those from ICA and there is a high presence of false positive among the first-degree relatives of patients with type 1 diabetes, for this reason they are not usefulness in the prediction of type 1 diabetes. Using a monoclonal technique, ICSA have been identified as belonging to the IgG and IgM class [262,296]. Similar like ICA, the ICSA have a highest prevalence at onset of type 1 diabetes patients and can precede it [262]. Some studies relate to ICA presence and the ICSA presence in the same patient [184,262], while others don't do it [296]. The difficulty in obtaining islets and the high positive rate in the control population has limited the usefulness of ICSA in the prediction of type 1 diabetes in man [262].

Insulin Autoantibodies (IAA)

The first islet autoantigen and β-cell–specific autoantigen reported was insulin [236,319]. Autoantibodies to insulin should be sought before the administration of exogenous insulin (either animal or human) because after 5–7 days of exogenous insulin treatment, insulin antibodies will arise. The immunoprecipitation assay for insulin autoantibodies does not distinguish spontaneous autoantibodies from antibodies arising from insulin immunization, which occurs as a consequence of exogenous insulin therapy [125,316].

IAAs were initially described in children at onset of type 1 diabetes [236]. They are useful as additional markers in the identification of high-risk individuals of progression to diabetes. These autoantibodies are detected with high specificity by fluid-phase radioimmunoassay [59,275,303,304,316,322,323]. Other situations, such as "Insulin autoimmune syndrome", the use of drugs and some autoimmune diseases, perhaps could be responsible for the production of IAA [303,319]. Most of the studies suggest that the presence of IAA have an inversely proportional relation with the age, besides being rarely detected in adults, as well as they are habitually the first antibody to appear in the first year of infancy [275,303,316,322]. There are also several reports which associate the presence of IAA and ICA. Ziegler and coworkers [322,325] have suggested that the combination of IAA with other markers increase the possibility to predict type 1 diabetes and show that, when IAA titers higher than 150 μU/ml are observed, and ICA which are higher to 40 JDF units, 100 % of the patients develop type 1 diabetes in a period of 5 years. The IAAs may occur more commonly in individuals who carry HLA-DR4 [316,319,324]. Techniques that detect insulin autoantibodies by an ELISA assay should not be used because IAAs so detected do not correlate with autoimmune diabetes [307,316,319].

At onset of type 1 diabetes, IAAs occur in 35–60% of children but are particularly less common in newly diagnosed adults [25,59,100,166,231,316] and latent autoimmune diabetes in adults as well [59,109,229,316]. A new IAA microassay has been developed that requires less serum than the traditional IAA assay [304,314,316]. In newly diagnosed type 1 diabetes in Australians children, IAA were present in 90% of children < 5 years old, 71% of children 5-10 years old, and 50% of children 10-15 years old [59,100,316]. Other study reported IAAs in 83% of children <10 years old and 56% of children 10 years old or older [25,316].

IAAs occur in many other autoimmune diseases incluiding autoimmune thyroid disease. IAAs were found in 13-44 % of Graves`disease patients and in 16-23 % of Hashimoto`s thyroiditis patients. IAAs have also been detected in Addison`s disease (40%), chronic hepatitis (36%), pernicious anemia (40%), systemic lupus erythematosus (29%), and rheumatoid arthritis (25%) [316]. Their meaning is unknown in the latter condition [316].

IAAs are detected in 1.3-3.7% of the first-degree relatives of type 1 diabetic patients [69,166,171,174,213], however, the general population frequency of ICA is 0.36-2.0% [25,166,178,273].

Glutamic Acid Decarboxylase Autoantibodies (GADA)

GAD is neither β-cell nor islet specific, which is expressed in all human islet cells [316,319]. GAD is expressed predominantly in the nervous system. Other tissues that express GAD include the testes, ovary, adrenal, pituitary, thyroid, and kidney [316]. For rat islets GAD is β-cell specific and levels of GAD are extremely low in mouse islet [319]. The discovery that anti-GAD autoantibodies accounted for an important component of anti-64kd autoantibodies [21] and a subset of ICA began with the discovery that patients with stiff-man syndrome expressed autoantibodies that gave rise to ICA staining and had high titers of anti-GAD autoantibodies [319]. Therefore, ICA of patient with stiff-man syndrome were termed restricted ICA or selective ICA in that the antibodies failed to react with islets of mouse pancreas and on rat islets stained only β-cell [112,114,319]. Although 64kd molecule is apparently associated with the membrane, 64kd protein does not have the typical properties of an integral protein from membrane and cannot be identified by staining in the surface of the islet cells. Islet 64kd antigen has been identified as the glutamic acid decarboxylase (GAD) is the enzyme responsible for GABA (γ-amino butyric acid-converting enzyme) synthesis within the nervous system and islet cells [2,59,319]. Currently, there are no doubt that anti-GAD autoantibodies or T cell proliferative response to GAD is present in type 1 diabetes [137,275]. It is remarkable that there is an inverse correlation between levels of GAD autoantibodies and a T cell proliferative to GAD [127,319]. Thus it is hypothesized that high levels of GAD autoantibodies may be associated with a diminished anti-islet T cell response (Th1 rather Th2) [319].

There evidences which suggest that a major component of the 64kd antigens is GAD [137,275]. Anti-64kd antibodies have been detected in 80% of new-onset cases of type 1 diabetes [137,275] and 91% of prediabetic subjects (first-degree relatives of patients with type 1 diabetes) who presented a low first-phase insulin response during intravenous glucose tolerance test (IVTT) [61,137,275].

Anti - 64 kd recognize an isoform of GAD [137,275]. Although, GAD 65 is the major immunogenic isoform [137,275,319], both form of GAD (GAD65 and GAD67) can be recognized by type 1 diabetes associated autoantibodies [137,275,319]. GAD 65 is a protein of 585 amino acids with a molecular weight of 65k encoded by a gene located on chromosome 10 (10p11) [229].

Several different radioassays for anti-GAD autoantibodies have been developed and the first Immunology of Diabetes Workshop (IDW) for measuring such antibodies was held. Four formats for determining anti-GAD autoantibodies include: 1) determination of antibody precipitation of GAD enzymatic activity, 2) radioassays utilizing affinity purified porcine brain GAD that has been labelled with I^{125}, 3) radiobinding assay using endogenously ^{35}S – labelled human recombinant GAD65 produced by in vitro transcription and translation of GAD cDNA, and 4) ELISA assays formats [59,307,319]. In particular, the immunoenzymatic assay appears to be less sensitive than either radioassay [307,319]. Radioassays using in vitro transcribed and translated GAD65 or I^{125} labelled recombinant human GAD65 can give equivalent results with high sensitivity and specificity. The Combinatorial Autoantibody International workshop of the Immunology Diabetes Society indicated that most laboratories concordantly measured anti-GAD65 and anti-IA2 autoantibodies [307,319].

Recently, sensitive and specific non-isotopic assay for measurement of autoantibodies to IA-2 and to combination of IA-2 and GAD65 have been developed [64]. This ELISA showed good agreement correlation with the abovementioned radioassays for anti-GAD autoantibodies.

GAD65 autoantibodies in type 1 diabetes seem to be mainly directed toward disease-specific epitopes, which are localized within the middle region and the COOH-terminus of the molecule [59,319]. GAD65 autoantibodies are detected in ~ 52-80% of cases of new-onset type 1 diabetes [125,136,137,229,231,275,277,316,319]. GAD67 autoantibodies are only detected in a small portion (11-18%) of type 1 diabetic patients [59,319]. The autoantibodies binding to GAD67 in type 1 diabetes seem to represent antibodies to shared epitopes with GAD65 [319], although there was report that Grave´s disease patients have been found carrying specific GAD67 antibodies in the absence of GAD65 antibodies [319].

A frequency of GAD65 autoantibodies in first-degree relatives of type 1 diabetic patients ranges between 3.0-7.0%. The general population frequency of GADA is 0.5-2.2% [25,166,178,273,316].

GADA are present between 2-31% of patient with latent autoimmune diabetes in adulthood. These are subjects with initial diagnosis of type 2 diabetes with a relatively rapid decline in insulin secretion in the first few years after diagnosis. In addition showing a number of typical characteristics similar to those with type 1 diabetes such as: Presence of type 1 diabetes associated autoantibodies (ICA and/or GADA), low body mass index, although overweight does not exclude the LADA diagnosis, low C peptide level, demand for insulin treatment in the early phase of the disease course, high prevalence of thyroid and gastric antibodies, and increased frequency of type 1 diabetes-related HLA class II haplotypes due to the presence of HLA-DR3/DR4 and DQ genes, as well as class I VNTR alleles, besides other genes [16,47,48,49,104,109,117,118,122,136,137,188,212,237,238, 252,277,288,297-299].

In LADA, the presence of GADA is much more frequent than ICA [47,49,252,298,299,316,326], although the presence of both antibodies (GADA and ICA) predicts better the insulin requirement than each of those individual antibodies [47,49,95,104,109,136,299].

GADA frequency during gestational diabetes, as well as after the delivery varies between 1.4 -9.5% [107,169,181].

Tyrosine Phosphatase Autoantibodies (ICA512/IA2 and IA2β)

In the 1990s, antigenic tryptic fragments were generated after mild trypsinization of 64 kd molecule from neonatal rat islets. Of note, mild trypsinization of 64kd molecule yields a 50, 40 and 37 kd fragments [65]. Most 64 kd –positive diabetic- sera also react with the 50kd fragment, and some sera from these patients who were negative for 64 kd reacted with 37-40kd fragments [137,275,319]. More than 90% of the diabetic sera immunoprecipitated at least with one of these three fragments [137,275]. By using this methodology in healthy identical twins of siblings with type 1 diabetes, it was reported that anti 37-40 kd autoantibodies, perhaps have a higher predictive value for type 1 diabetes than the antibodies against conventional 64kd protein and the 50 kd fragment [137,275,319]. Antibodies against 37-40 kd fragments have been detected in 50-76% of the type 1 diabetic patients at the time of diagnosis [32,137,275].

Most of type 1 diabetic patients present antibodies against triptic fragments of 37/40 kd derived from a non-identified membrane protein (different of GADA) in the islet cell. Several groups of researchers have reported autoantibodies against ICA512, which have been identified as protein tyrosine phosphatase (IA-2 protein) [32,137,180,258,275,319]. It has been proved that 40 kd fragment is related to the protein tyrosine phosphatase IA-2 (ICA512) and the 37 kd fragment to the molecule IA-2β or also known as phogrin (phosphatase of granules of rat insulinoma) [32,197,221,230,319].

The second major autoantigen, IA-2 (also known as ICA512) is a member of the transmembrane protein tyrosine phosphatase (PTP) family which is found in nervous tissue and other endocrine tissues including the pituitary [180,229,316,319]. The function of this molecule has remained a mystery, but recently it is suggested that it plays a role perhaps in the insulin secretion [126,172,229]. IA-2 (ICA512) is 929 amino acids (aa) in length, is located on chromosome 2 (2q35), and consists of an extracellular domain (aa 1-576), a transmembrane region (aa 577-600) and an intracellular domain (aa 601-979) [137,138,229]. However, molecule IA-2β is encoded by a gene on the chromosome 7 (7q36) [229] and contained 1015 amino acids [157].

The main antigenic determinants of IA2 are located in the C-terminal region from the intracellular domain [59,97,137,157,229]. The nucleotide sequence from IA-2 is virtually identical with the ones of ICA512 [137,157,229,319]. Almost all antibodies which react with IA-2β also react with ICA512, while approximately 10% of the patients developing autoimmune type 1 diabetes have autoantibodies reacting with ICA512 but not with IA-2β. Therefore it is for this reason that routinely assay for IA-2β antibodies is not done [157,319].

Several fragments located in the intracellular domain of ICA512/IA2 have been recognized by diabetic sera, among them are those placed in the IA-2 intracellular residues of molecule (IA-2ic aa 601-979), ICA512bdc (aa 256-556, 630-979), immunodominant IA-2 epitopes, termed "Fragment 1" (aa 761-964), IA-2 "Fragment 2A" (aa 256-760), IA-2 "Fragment 2B" (aa 761-928) [59,97,137,138,157,229,275,319]. The IA-2β intracellular domain is composed by amino acids 640-1015, which is 73.6% identical with IA-2/512 [157]. The IA-2 have been detected by using radioassays with a high sensitivity and specificity which include the whole molecule (aa 1-979), as well as the intracellular portions from these previously mentioned molecules [59,97,137,157,229,275,293,319]. Recently, it has been proved that the detection of IA-2 autoantibodies against the IA-2ic construct showed the highest sensitivity and specificity both in type 1 diabetes and prediabetic subjects; however, all of other IA-2 constructs aforementioned detected additional immunoreactivities with respect it. Therefore, it has been suggested the combined use into the same assay of IA-2ic, IA-2 (whole molecule) and IA-2 (aa 256-760) construct as a new strategy highly sensitive approach to the study of IA-2 autoimmunity in type 1 diabetes [293].

IA-2 (ICA512) or IA-2β (Phogrin) autoantibodies, similar to those of GADA are detected with fluid phase radioassays using ^{35}S – labelled human recombinant IA-2 produced by in vitro transcription and translation of IA-2 cDNA or I^{125} -labelled recombinant human IA-2 can give a equivalent results with high sensitivity and specificity, and also utilizing ELISA assays format have been developed [64,59,97,157,293,319]. Recently, sensitive and specific ELISA assay for measurement of autoantibodies to IA-2 have been developed [64].

The anti IA-2 (ICA512) autoantibodies have been detected in 54-86% of cases of new-onset type 1 diabetes and it ranges from 42 to 65 % in first-degree relatives who later develop diabetes [32,69,100,136,137,138,157,180,229,231,275,277,293,316]. The anti-IA-2β autoantibodies are also found in 65–70% of newly diagnosed type 1 diabetic patients and with the same frequency as IA-2A in the first-degree relatives who later develop diabetes [316, 157]. IA-2A frequencies in first-degree relatives of patients with type 1 diabetes range between 1.6-5.3%. The general population frequencies for these autoantibodies are similar to those of GADAs at 0.6-2.6% [25,166,170,178].

IA-2 autoantibodies occur in 0.1–4% of the type 2 diabetic patients [34,229,277] and in 18-23.8% of LADA patients [47,136]. In women during gestational diabetes, as well as after delivery, IA2 frequency varies between 0-6.2% [107,181].

Proinsulin Autoantibodies (PAA)

Bohmer et al [29], found a higher prevalence of PAA versus IAA in childhoods with newly diagnosed type 1 diabetes before the insulin treatment (34% vs 22.7%, respectively). Proinsulin autoantibodies were also detected in 43.8% of ICA-positive first-degree relatives of type 1 diabetes subjects and 31.3% of them were IAA- positive. However, 0.9% of ICA-negative first degree relatives were positive either for PAA or for IAA. None of normal sera contained PAA or IAA [29].

Another study reveals in newly diagnosed type 1 diabetic patients at the age of 16-40 years, 22 % of diabetic subjects but no in control subjects expressed PAA. Thus, immunity to proinsulin was lower that the reported for childhood-onset type 1 diabetes and the authors propose that, like insulin, proinsulin may be targeted less frequently in adulthood [223]. A strong correlation existed between antibody levels to proinsulin and insulin within diabetic subjects [29,140,223]. Furthermore, IAA or PAA could be completely displaced with either insulin or proinsulin in the majority of patients, suggesting that the main epitopes recognized by these antibodies at diabetes onset are on the insulin molecule. Elevated proinsulin autoantibodies in diabetic subjects confirm proinsulin is an important autoantigen in type 1 diabetes [29,140,223]. Hummel et al. suggested that proinsulin-specific humoral autoimmunity is relatively uncommon in the initial stages of type 1-associated autoimmunity [140]. The relative absence of proinsulin-specific autoantibodies during the disease process does not suggest that the screening for PAA rather than IAA would be more effective in early identification of young children at risk [140].

Glycolipid Autoantibodies

The initial studies suggesting that antibodies directed against islet glycolipids may be a component of islet cell antibodies came from evaluation of monoclononal antibodies that reacted with neuronal gangliosides and that also react with islets [43,70,84,225]. Monoclonal antibodies A2B5, 3G5, R2D6 and tetanus toxin all react with complex gangliosides and all give an ICA pattern of staining that involves all cells of the islets [12,175,224,319].

The glycolipids are components of the plasma membrane and of cytoplasm, and are involved in cell-cell interaction and in the binding to plasma membranes of hormones, toxins, viruses and autoantibodies [81,194]. Glycolipids are composed by a hydrophobic portion (the oligosaccharide chain) and a hydrophobic portion (the ceramide). The latter contains sphingosine and a fatty acid while the oligosaccharide can be of variable length with a least one sialic acid or sulfatide residue [194]. Although the antigenic properties of the glycolipids are associated with their carbohydratic part, the lipidic part is essential to ensure such properties, as well as the selective glycolization, orientation and organization of carbohydratic chains. The gangliosides as well as the sulfatides differ as to their polysacharide portions, from other glycolipids and their different characteristics consist of the presence of one or more sialic acid residues or sulfatide groups respectively. Thus, organic solvents such as methanol and chloroform remove gangliosides or sulfatides from tissue sections, while gangliosides are stable to nonpolar solvents such as acetone. Stability to acetone but removal by methanol was a quality found for most ICA [70,84,225,319]. Polar glycolipids (gangliosides and sulfatides) can readily be extracted from tissues with organic solvents and then separated from nonpolar lipids, by phase partition with chloroform, methanol and water. Extraction of human pancreas followed by the above Folch partition, followed by chromatography that separates gangliosides based on their hydrophobicity (thin-layer chromatography, TLC) or number of sialic acid residues (DEAE chromatography) allowed the isolation of ganglioside preparations that, when incubated with ICA-positive sera, removed all reactivity [41,43,70,84,225,319].

Which glycolipids are autoantigens and which are the target autoantigens for ICA?

Several candidates from glycolipid molecules have been considered as antigens. Three candidate molecules are GT3, sulfatides, and GM2-1 gangliosides (on thin-layer chromatography it has a mobility between GM2 and GM1 standards). Antibodies against these molecules have been detected, among which are the antibodies to GT3 [116], ganglioside GM2-1 [41,43,70,81,82,83,84,209,225,319] and sulfatides [38,40,43]. Antibodies to GT3 (ganglioside from rat insulinoma) have been found in 32.2% of the patients with new-onset type 1 diabetes [116].

Nayak et al. [225] have shown that the ICA autoantigen of pancreatic sections has properties of a sialic acid containing glycolipid (ganglioside), as the ICA reactivity to the pancreatic sections is lost after the digestion with neuraminidase and the incubation with a mixture of chloroform-methanol, being resistant to pronase. Other studies have proved that the sera of most ICA-positive diabetic patients reacted with a single ganglioside migrating between GM2 and GM1 standards by TLC plates, what has been termed a GM2-1 [41,43,82,83,209,253,319].

The incubation of ICA-positive sera with the upper phase of lipid extracts from human pancreas produces a marked reduction in ICA reaction to the frozen pancreas sections. The blocking effect is dose-dependent [41,43,70]. Several studies have demonstrated that the fraction of monosialogangliosides extracted from human or rat pancreas are able to block the binding of ICA to frozen sections of human pancreas (this fraction contained the ganglioside GM2-1) [41,70,81,83,84,209,253,319]. Portoukalian et al. [251] demonstrated that the majority of ICA-positive sera from patients with new-onset type 1 diabetes react to human pancreatic fucogangliosides.

Dotta et al. [84] have characterized the ganglioside GM2-1, finding a novel islet specific ganglioside molecule with unusual characteristics, such as the terminal sialic acid and two galactosamine residues (N-acetyl neuraminic acid-galactose-galactosamine-galactosamine-glucose-ceramide), which may facilitate both its antigenicity and its involvement in bet-cell autoimmunity. Like other antigens (insulin, carboxipeptidase, 38 Kd protein), it has been found that this antigen is expressed in secretory granules and is not β cell specific [85].

The anti GM2-1 antibodies have been found in 68.8% and 65% of patients with new-onset type 1 diabetes and in ICA-positive first-degree relatives of type 1 diabetes, respectively [81,82]. In 1995, Cabrera-Rode et al found after the incubation of ICA-positive sera with the upper phase of glycolipid extract from human pancreas a total inhibition of ICA positive sera to pancreatic sections in 82.3% (14/17) and 76.1% (16/21) of type 1 diabetic patients and first-degree relatives of patients with type 1 diabetes, respectively [41].

The isolation and/or synthesis of GM2-1 should allow the development of sensitive and standardized assay for autoantibodies and ELISA assays format or other biochemical methods are necessary to detect the anti GM2-1 antibodies with the aim of knowing the frequency of these antibodies in diabetic patients and for the studies to predict type 1 diabetes in the different populations.

Cabrera-Rode et al., previously shown evidences about the ability of ICA-positive sera to react with three sulfatides: SO_4-3GlcUβ1-3Galβ1-4GlcNAcβ1-3Galβ1-4Glcβ1-1Cer, SO_4-3Galβ1-1Cer y SO_4-3Galβ1-4Glcβ1-1Cer using the TLC-ELISA method [43]. These results indicate that not only gangliosides, but also sulfatides, could be targets to type 1 diabetes associated autoantibodies. In 1992, Cabrera-Rode et al reported the first international evidence about the presence of sulfatide antibodies in type 1 diabetes [43]; afterwards, Buschard et al., carried out several studies which confirm sulfatide as antigen associated with type 1 diabetes [14,38,81].

Buschard and colleagues [38], using TLC-ELISA method, the frequency of sulfatide antibodies in newly diagnosed type 1 diabetic patients have been studied, in which they found that 88% of the sera of these patients were anti-sulfatide positive and all of healthy control were negative. Electron microscopy immunogold-staining with Sulph I (anti-sulfatide monoclonal antibody) showed reactivity to α and β cells in the rat pancreas, and similar to this antibody, highly predictive value ICA stains the whole islet [38].

All this data, support the inclusion of sulfatides in the list of specific antigens that react against different ICA subsets, such as insulin, GAD, IA-2, and the GM2-1 ganglioside [19,32,43,70,81,84,123,137,197,209,221,225,277].

Cabrera-Rode et al showed that none of the ICA-positive sera of type 1 diabetic patients and first-degree relatives of type 1 diabetic patients used in the inhibitions with glycolipid extract [40,41] and acidic pancreatic fractions reduced its reactivity to pancreatic sections after preincuabation with sulfatide (SO_4-3Galβ1-1Cer), suggesting the lack of affinity to ICAs to this sulfatide [40]. These results reinforce those obtained by Buschard et al. in which anti-sulfatide antibody titer was independent of the presence of conventional ICA [38]. These data suggest that sulfatides are apparently type 1-related antigens but perhaps not ICA-specific autoantigens. As well as ICA, sulfatide antibodies could represent highly predictive value markers in type 1 diabetes, but for this to be proved; the presence of these antibodies in the sera of high risk individuals must be established. A combined detection of ICA and sulfatide antibodies may be advantageous in predicting type 1 diabetes.

Considering that sulfatides are not ICA-specific antigens, another possible interpretation could be that anti-sulfatide antibodies are present jointly with ICA in individuals with new-onset diabetes and by TLC-ELISA method, the sulfatides antibodies as well as those against GM2-1 ganglioside are detected at the same time.

Sulfatide is the major acidic glycosphingolipid in both central and peripheral myelin [14]. Buschard et al. have shown that sulfatide is a major glycophingolipid component of the islets of Langerhans and is expressed both on surface and in the secretory granules of β-cells Sulfatide is thus a potential target in the autoimmune process involved in the development of type 1 diabetes. This molecule also appears in tissues such as kidney and gallbladder, and in the choroids layer in the eyes, some of which organs are the target of late complications in type 1 diabetes [37].

In conclusion, what has been said before seems to indicate that sulfatides are antigens apparently associated with type 1 diabetes. The anti-sulfatide antibodies could represent markers with a high predictive value in the developing of type 1 diabetes. In order to verify this hypothesis it is necessary to carry out prospective studies that valuate the presence of these antibodies in the serum of high-risk individuals to overt type 1 diabetes.

Recently, Andersson and colleagues [14] found the presence of sulfatides antibodies by a new reproducible ELISA procedure in 85% (17/20) of type 1 diabetic patients and 100% (6/6) of pre-diabetic individuals (ICA-positive first-degree relatives of patients with type 1 diabetes) while none of the type 2 diabetic patients were sulfatide antibodies positive. The authors suggest that the presence and titers of sulfatide antibodies may increase the reliability of prediction when combined with other antibodies.

The answer to the previously mentioned question about Which glycolipids are autoantigens and which are the target autoantigens for ICA?. Taking into account the glycolipids previously described from the ones present in the human pancreas, the GM2-1 ganglioside and sulfatides are autoantigens associated with type 1 diabetes. However, the GM2-1 ganglioside is one of the target autoantigens of ICA.

Other Antibodies

The sensitivity and standardization of the rest of the determinations from the known antibodies are not recommendable, as well as their frequency is not so high, therefore, it is suggested that they are no used in the search for pancreatic autoimmunity or in the studies for the prediction of type 1 diabetes.

By Western blot assay, ICA69 antigen (this protein, which on SDS gel migrates at 69 Kd) has been recently determined in the surface of the islet [9,246,275]. The 69 Kd antigen is induced by interferon and show a cross-reaction with albumin. It has been reported that ICA69 have regions of identity with some regions of ABBOS peptide [9,81,275], while other studies do not show the crossed reaction existence of anti BSA antibodies and ICA69 antigens [265].

By Western blotting using recombinant ICA69 about 70% of newly diagnosed type 1 diabetes, as well as in 9% of their first degree relatives express autoantibodies to this islet protein [81,246]. However, other studies show frequency from these antibodies between 4 to 21% in type 1 diabetic patients [31,161,201]. Besides, the 38 Kd autoantigen, named Glima 38, is an amphiphilic membrane glycoprotein, specifically expressed in islet and neuronal cell lines, and thus shares the neuroendocrine expression patterns of GAD and IA-2. Glima 38 autoantibodies were detected in 19% (16/86) of newly diagnosed patients and in 14% (6/44) of prediabetic first-degree relatives up to several years before the clinical onset [3,275].

Carboxipeptidase H is a 52 Kd glycoprotein expressed by pancreatic islet cells and by other neuroendocrine cells. Within pancreatic islet β cells, carboxypeptidase H is located in insulin secretory granules where it is abundantly expressed and facilitates the conversion of proinsulin to insulin. Anti-carboxypeptidase H antibodies have been observed in 11% of new-onset cases of type 1 diabetes [31] and in 25% of ICA-positive first degree relatives of type 1 diabetic patients [81,275]. DNA topoisomerase II autoantibodies were detected in 49.2 and 47.2% of type 1 diabetic patients using purified TopII fragments and full-length TopII as antigens, respectively [63]. The presence of HSP60 Kd autoantibodies is observed between 15.5-45.0% of patients with new-onset diabetes [5,234] and finally, the SOX13 autoantibodies are present in 18-29,3% of type 1 diabetic patients [156,240].

Cellular Autoimmunity

T Cell Reactivity

Some of the target molecules of autoantibodies described in this section are also able to drive proliferation of T cells from animal models and type 1 diabetic patient or from ICA-positive individuals

To date, T cell responses in human to islet autoantigens have been particularly difficult with relatively low levels of stimulation, when stimulation is observed. This may relate to a very low frequency of autoreactive T cells outside of the islet [319]. In an international workshop with multiples laboratories studying a series of "blinded" islet antigens and peptides none of the laboratories could distinguish a small panel of patients with diabetes from control individuals [264,319]. Thus, it is likely that the assay formats will have to be greatly improved to be able to reliably detect T cell response.

Different group of researchers have reported a higher reactivity of peripheral blood mononuclear cells to GAD among the newly diagnosed type 1 patients and nondiabetic ICA-positive relatives than among the controls and NOD mice [17,18,127,196,226,294,295]. Harrinson and coworkers [127] described an inverse relationship between humoral and cellular immunity to GAD, suggesting that ICA-positive relatives who have increased T cell reactivity to GAD (and lower titer of anti-GAD antibody) represent a group with higher diabetes risk. Tisch and coworkers reported that T cell proliferative responses to GAD precede responses to other antigens [295,319].

A number of groups have found T cell responses to ICA512 (IA-2) and IA-2β [139,158,159,319], and T cells recognizing IA-2β are able to transfer diabetes in a transplant model [158].

T cell proliferative response to insulin can be detected utilizing peripheral blood of prediabetics or splenocytes of NOD mice, but again stimulation indices are low [4,13,74,87,160]. Several groups have found that a large percentage of T cells infiltrating islet of NOD mice strongly proliferate to insulin and B-chain peptide of insulin (B:9-23) [4,13,74,87,319]. In contrast, a minimal response of splenocytes to insulin is found. Subsets of these T cell clones are able to transfer diabetes into immunodeficient NOD mice and thus are sufficient for disease pathogenesis [215,319].

Recently, it has been demonstrated that CD8 T cell autoreactivity that specifically recognize target cells expressing the insulin B chain peptide is associated with β-cell destruction in type 1 diabetes in humans [249]. Nakayama and coworkers suggest that the proinsulin/insulin molecules have a sequence that is a primary target of the autoimmunity (cellular and humoral) that causes diabetes of the non-obese diabetic (NOD) mouse [222]. The author also indicate that proinsulin is a primary autoantigen of the NOD mouse, and speculate that organ-restricted autoimmune disorders with marked major histocompatibility complex (MHC) restriction of disease are likely to have specific primary autoantigens [222].

However, it has been observed that most of newly diagnosed diabetic patients or individuals at risk for type 1 diabetes, T cell reactivity to several autoantigens occurs simultaneously. In contrast, cellular reactivity to a single autoantigen is found with the same frequency in prediabetic individuals as well as in control subjects. Therefore, the autoimmune response in the inductive phase of type 1 diabetes probably targeted to pancreatic islets by the cellular and humoral reactivity to one β cell specific autoantigen, but spreading to a set of different antigens (insulin, GAD and IA-2) may be as a prerequisite for progression to destructive insulitis and clinical diseases [87].

As soon as new assays (ELISPOT or tetramer assays) with a good sensitivity, specificity and reproducibility for the quantitation of autoreactive T cells to different islet autoantigens are developed, the cell autoimmunity will offer important data for the prediction of type 1 diabetes in patients with a risk to develop the disease.

Prediction of Type 1 Diabetes: New Strategies

The long prodromal phase preceding the onset of type 1 diabetes suggests a potential to predict the disease and design trials for its prevention. The development of type 1 diabetes in relatives of type 1 diabetic patients can now be predicted with reasonable accuracy by the detection of islet associated autoantibodies. Detection of two or more autoantibodies (ICA, GADA, IA-2A, or IAA) in relatives of type 1 diabetic patients has an accumulative risk to develop type 1 diabetes of 69–90%, exceeding 90% during the 5-10 years of prospective follow-up study in the first-degree relatives of type 1 diabetic patients [6,8,22,59,69,75,90,125,166,170,213,247,316]. The combination of high-risk genes (HLA and INS genotypes), the autoantibodies previously mentioned and the use of metabolic tests (first phase of insulin responses during intravenous glucose tolerance test) contribute to the prediction of the disease and also help us to know the possible pre-clinical stage of it (either early or late), in which the patient is found [6,22,59,69,90,132,166,174,213,214,239,316].

Currently, it is possible to classify prediabetes into four preclinical stages of type 1 diabetes (no prediabetes, early, advance, late prediabetes) according to two sets of criteria. The first set based on the number of type 1 associated- autoantibodies detectable in each sample available [166,213,214]:

No Prediabetes: Negative subjects for the four type 1 diabetes- associated autoantibodies (ICA, GADA, IA-2A, or IAA)

Early Prediabetes: Subjects who show only one type 1 diabetes- associated autoantibodies

Advanced Prediabetes: Subjects with two type 1 diabetes- associated autoantibodies

Late Prediabetes: Subjects who present at least three of the four type 1 diabetes-associated autoantibodies

The second set criterion was based on a combination of type 1 diabetes associated autoantibodies and the first phase of insulin responses during intravenous glucose tolerance test [166,213,214]:

No Prediabetes: Negative subjects for the four type 1 diabetes- associated autoantibodies (ICA, IAA, GADA, IA-2A)

Early Prediabetes: Subjects who present one type 1 diabetes- associated autoantibodies but a normal first phase of insulin responses during intravenous glucose tolerance test

Advanced Prediabetes: Those subjects with two or more type 1 diabetes- associated autoantibodies but still a normal first phase of insulin responses during intravenous glucose tolerance test.

Late Prediabetes: Individuals who present an abnormal first phase of insulin responses during intravenous glucose tolerance test and at least one type 1 diabetes associated autoantibodies

ICAs: Prediction of Type 1 Diabetes

The results of perspective studies about prediction in first-degree relatives of type 1 diabetic patients suggest that high ICA titers (≥ 20 JDF units) confer a much greater risk than the low titers (< 20 JDF units) [23,30,69,90,137,261,263,316]. It has been verified that the persistence of ICA positivity is much more predictive in the clinical development of type 1 diabetes than its intermittent positivity [188,261,272]. The first-degree relatives of type 1 diabetic patients with high ICA titers were associated with an increase in the percentage of multiple autoantibodies (two or more) [170,320].

In 1990, Bonifacio et al. [30] studied subjects with different ICA levels in serum during nine years and came to the conclusion that the high ICA titers show a high predictive value in the development of type 1 diabetes; the ICA titers ≥ 80 JDF units show a predictive value of 100% to develop type 1 diabetes. The risk for type 1 diabetes after 10 years of follow-up in patients with ICA of 80 or more JDF units, was a 100%. In comparison, ICAs of 20 or more JDF units were associated with a 73% risk, and ICAs ≥ 4 JDF units with a 40% risk [90].

In a prospective study of first-degree relatives of type 1 diabetic patients from the University of Florida [263], ICA titers >40 JDF units predicted a 70% 7-year risk for type 1 diabetes, ICAs of 20–40 JDF units predicted a 20% risk, and ICAs of 10 JDF units predicted a 10% risk. The 7-year risk for type 1 diabetes in these otherwise normal ICA-positive children was 45% compared to 43% in a group of age-matched relatives of type 1 diabetic patients. Thus, ICAs appear to be as valuable for the prediction of type 1 diabetes in the general population as they are in relatives of type 1 diabetic patients [316].

The results from the last follow-up studies in first-degree relatives of type 1 diabetic patients suggest that the low ICA titers should not be used as an efficient marker for type 1 diabetes, however, the ICA titers higher or similar to 20 JDF units, remain being a good antibody to predict the risk of developing type 1 diabetes, particularly when it is associated with other antibodies (IAA, GADA, IA-2A) [30,69,90,165,170,171,174,247,320,325]. In addition, ICAs have been related to the decrease of insulin secretion after the glucose intravenous overload [69,90,137,316,325], which constitutes a destruction index from insulin secreting- cells. The presence of decreased first phase insulin responses during intravenous glucose tolerance test in ICA-positive children predicts a 5- year risk for type 1 diabetes of 50–65% [316].

Age at the time of detection of ICAs influences the risk for type 1 diabetes. In the prospective first-degree family studies, the 7-year risk for type 1 diabetes in ICA-positive individuals <10 years was ~80% versus 20% in those ICA-positive individuals >10 years of age [263,316]. The risk in children <2 years was ~90%. In the Bart's-Windsor, Bart's-Oxford prospective family studies [26], the risk for type 1 diabetes in the youngest ICA-positive quartile (<13.2 years old) was 62% versus 4% in the oldest quartile (>40.7 years old).

In first-degree relatives of type 1 diabetic patients who has ICAs in addition to GAD65 and IA-2 autoantibodies, the cumulative risk of developing type 1 diabetes was 80% at 6.7 years of follow-up, while this risk in those with GADA and IA-2A without ICA was only 14% at 10 years of follow-up. The analysis of results showed that diabetes risk was considerably associated with the ICA presence in both subjects with low titer or high titer of GADA and IA-2A. The addition, of IAAs in GAD65A positive/IA-2A-positive relatives did not increased the cumulative risk for convention to insulin-treated diabetes [247,320]. These results provide evidence that a subgroup of ICAs predicts a more rapid progression to type 1 diabetes in GAD65 and IA-2 autoantibodies positive relatives and should remain part of the assessment of type 1 diabetes risk for intervention trials. In addition, these findings provide impetus for efforts to identify a novel islet autoantigen(s) reactive with this ICA subset [247,320].

Cabrera-Rode et al. have found that 21.4% (6/28) of patients with ICA ≥ 20 JDF units developed type 1 diabetes during the 5 years of follow-up [44]. Similarly, to the one observed by ENDIT in which 29% (159/549) of the first-degree relatives of type 1 diabetic patients with ICA ≥ 20 JDF units developed type 1 diabetes in the same period of time [94]. In this study, it was observed that from the eight patients who developing type 1 diabetes during the follow-up [44], two of them presented ICA of 10 JDF units with two or more additional antibodies, as well as HLA-DR3/DR4 genes. The rest of the six patients showed ICA titers ≥ 40 JDF units and the presence of other additional type 1 diabetes associated autoantibodies. In addition, almost all of them showed an alteration of the first phase insulin response and one or more HLA-DR susceptibility allele (DR3 and/or DR4). Therefore, the authors also support the assertion that the progression to type 1 diabetes is increased in proportion with the number of antibodies and the presence of high or low risk HLA alleles who also prone to develop the disease [72,131,132,174,273,284,291]. These data also confirm that only the subjects with ICA titers < 20 JDF units who show other additional type 1 diabetes associated autoantibodies should be chosen for prevention assays because they similarly progress to type 1 diabetes [90,247,320].

Strategies for the Prediction of Type 1 Diabetes

Most of the studies involve the presence of multiple autoantibodies for the prediction of type 1 diabetes, but this strategy should not be generalized for all type of diabetes. Therefore, it is necessary to find the combination of autoantibodies which is able to predict with more sensitivity, efficiency and accuracy the individuals with a high risk of progression to type 1 diabetes and should be eligible for the prevention of the disease.

Screening programs for prediction of type 1 diabetes should be undertaken in children and adolescent on at least two occasions: between age 2-5 and before puberty [166,315,316,322]. This is because diabetes appears first near age 5 and then peaks with puberty [261,316].

The strategies for the prediction of type 1 diabetes in children and adolescent with relation to the presence of type 1 diabetes associated autoantibodies varies among the different group of researchers. Some of them prefer to star the screening with the combination of only the GADA and IA-2 antibodies [25,26,69,316]. Others consider to carry out the previous ones first and later the ICA determination [25,136,316], others suggest to test three autoantibodies (IAA, GADA and IA-2A) [8,22,59,75,90,170,306,316]. This last strategy mainly includes the IAA for the screening in children <10 years [59,90,316,322] and the ICA should be included as a secondary screening [59,170]. Another strategy is the use of the combination of the four type 1 diabetes- related autoantibodies (ICA, IAA, GADA, IA-2A) during the first years of life, particularly when there are high titers [6,111,171,191,247,263,271,307], the presence of the high risk HLA genes, as well as the loss of the first phase insulin response can be used as additional markers in the prediction [6,22,171,191,263,271]. Barker and coworkers [22], suggest that the use of the level of autoantibody can provide additional predictive information for the persistence of autoantibodies and development of type 1 diabetes and may be used to further stratify individuals for epidemiological and preventive studies.

In my opinion, generally the presence of two or more autoantibodies from the four (ICA, IAA, GADA, IA-2A) along with the persistence and high titers of these, should be the strategy for the prediction before the 20 years of age in first-degree relatives of type 1 diabetic patients or in schoolchildren. In subjects <10 years may be it necessary to verify initially the presence of ICA and IAA. Just in case of being positive for some of these antibodies, we recommend to carry out the determinations of GADA and IA-2 antibodies. However, in subjects >10 years, we suggest to determine initially the presence of ICA, in case it is positive, to carry out the determinations of GADA and IA-2A or vice versa [22,136,316]. This suggestion is based on the fact that the risk for diabetes increases when the ICA are associated with GADA and/or IA-2A [26,111,191,247].

The strategy for the prediction of LADA in type 2 diabetic patients, type 1 diabetes in women after having diagnosed gestational diabetes or type 1 diabetes in adults it is suggested that should be the detection GADA and/or ICA antibodies [90,104,107,109,136,229,238,299], because anti-IA-2 autoantibodies and anti-insulin autoantibodies are found in a low frequency [34,107,109,136,229,238]. IA-2A in LADA patients or type 1 diabetes in adults when they are present, are generally associated with GADA and/or ICA. For this reason, the strategy to be followed in these entities initially is the combination of the determinations of GADA and ICA. It is suggested that the presence of high GADA titers and directed against C-terminal epitopes of GAD or the presence of both GADA and ICA, discriminates patients with clinical characteristics very similar to those of a slowly progressive form of type 1 diabetes [95,96,136,212,288]. On the other hand, the presence of low levels GADA, in the absence of ICA or other immune markers, such IA-2 autoantibodies, characterizes a subgroup of patients with clinical characteristics almost indistinguishable from those of typical type 2 diabetes [95,96,136].

A Japanese study found that GAD autoantibodies in LADA patients recognize unique N-terminal linear epitopes that are located on the anchoring domain of GAD65 molecules and GADA titers was inversely correlated with the time in which insulin was not required [168]. However, an Italian study proved the autoantibody binding specific epitopes from the middle and C-terminal portion of GAD65 in subjects with type 2 diabetes. Sardinian type 2 diabetic patients with middle and C-terminal predominant GAD65 antibodies reactivity have clinical features more similar to those of type 1 diabetic patients. Thus GAD65 antibodies epitope analysis may help to define type 1 diabetes phenotypes among newly diagnosed GADA-positive patients classified with type 2 diabetes [193].

Achenbach and colleagues [8], suggest a strong association between risk of type 1 diabetes and high titer, bread antibody responses to IA-2 and insulin. The highest risks were associated with high-titer IA-2A and IAA, IgG2, IgG3, and/or IgG4 subclass of IA-2A and IAA, and antibodies to the IA-2-related molecule IA-2β. Using models based on these antibody characteristics, autoantibody-positive relatives can be classified into groups with risks of diabetes ranging from 7 to 80% within 5 years. For all this previously mentioned, the authors consider that the combination of autoantibody titer, subclass, and/or epitope reactivity may improve type 1 diabetes risk stratification, which could be effectively stratified on the basis of these characteristics in a single sample.

Other option with special reference to the IAA, in which it is suggested that the presence of high affinity IAA predict much better the risk for type 1 diabetes than low affinity IAA [7, 106]. Therefore, the detection of these antibodies in the prediction of type 1 diabetes should be included in the previously stated strategies. High-affinity IAA responses were more frequent when IAAs developed at very young age and in relatives who had HLA-DRB1*04 allele. IAA were of high affinity already in the first IAA-positive sample in almost all IAA-positive relatives who developed multiple islet autoantibodies and all who developed type 1 diabetes. In contrast, relatives who remained positive only for IAAs or became islet autoantibody-negative usually had lower affinity IAAs that did not increase in affinity on follow-up. All high-affinity IAAs required conservation of human insulin A chain residues 8-13 and were reactive with proinsulin. In contrast, most lower-affinity IAAs were dependent on C-terminal B chain residues and did not bind proinsulin [7,106]. These data are consistent with the concept that type 1 diabetes is associated with sustained early exposure to (pro)insulin in the context of HLA-DR4 and show that the high-affinity proinsulin-reactive IAAs identify those children with the highest diabetes risk [7,106,147,222].

In conclusion, scientists should establish the screening strategy according to the characteristics of each country, region or ethnic group. The identification of subjects with high risk for progression of type 1 diabetes should be efficient, simple, sensitive and accurate. This would be of great value for the selection of individuals for future prevention trials aiming at delaying or preventing the development of the disease.

Acknowledgements

I appreciate the cooperation offered by Professor Oscar Diaz Diaz in the critical review of this manuscript. I also whish to express my gratitude to Claudia Olivero and Teresa Rode Boschmonar for the support offered in the preparation of this manuscript.

References

[1] American Diabetes Association. Report of the expert committee on the diagnosis and classification of diabetes mellitus. *Diabetes Care* 1997;20:1183-97.

[2] American Diabetes Association. Diagnosis and classification of diabetes mellitus. *Diabetes Care* 2006;29:S43-S48.

[3] Aanstoot HJ, Kang SM, Kim J, Lindsay LA, Roll U, Knip M, et al. Identification and characterization of glima 38, a glycosylated islet cell membrane antigen, which together with GAD65 and IA2 marks the early phases of autoimmune response in type 1 diabetes. *J Clin Invest* 1996;97:2772–83.

[4] Abiru N, Wegmann D, Kawasaki E, Gottlieb P, Simone E, Eisenbarth GS. Dual overlapping peptides recognized by insulin peptide B:9-23 reactive T cell receptor AV13S3 T cell clones of the NOD mouse. *J Autoimmun* 2000;14:231-7.

[5] Abulafia-Lapid R, Gillis D, Yosef O, Atlan H, Cohen IR. T cells and autoantibodies to human HSP70 in type 1 diabetes in children. *J Autoimmun* 2003;20:313-21.

[6] Achenbach P, Bonifacio E, Ziegler AG. Predicting type 1 diabetes. *Curr Diab Rep* 2005;5:98-103.

[7] Achenbach P, Koczwara K, Knopff A, Naserke H, Ziegler AG, Bonifacio E. Mature high-affinity immune responses to (pro) insulin anticipate the autoimmune cascade that leads to type 1 diabetes. *J Clin Invest* 2004;114:589-97.

[8] Achenbach P, Warncke K, Reiter J, Naserke HE, Williams AJK, Bingley P, et al. Stratification of type 1 diabetes risk on the basis of islet autoantibody characteristics. *Diabetes* 2004;53:384-92.

[9] Akerblom HK, Knip M. Putative environmental factors in type 1 diabetes. *Diabetes Metab Rev* 1998;14:31-67.

[10] Akerblom HK, Virtanen SM, Ilonen J, Savilahti E, Vaarala O, Reunanen A, et al. Dietary manipulation of beta cell autoimmunity in infants at increased risk of type 1 diabetes: a pilot study. *Diabetologia* 2005;48:829-37.

[11] Alberti KGMM, Zimmet PZ, WHO. Definition, diagnosis and classification of diabetes mellitus and its complications. Part 1: diagnosis and classification of diabetes mellitus. Provisional report of a WHO Consultation. *Diabetic Med* 1998;5:539-53.

[12] Alejandro R, Shienvold FL, Hajek SAV, Pierce M, Paul R, Mintz DH. A ganglioside antigen on the rat pancreatic B cell surface identified by monoclonal antibody R2D6. *J Clin Invest* 1984;74:25-38.

[13] Alleva DG, Crowe PD, Jin L, Kwok WW, Ling N, Gottschalk M et al. A disease-associated cellular immune response in type 1 diabetics to an immunodominant epitope of insulin. *J Clin Invest* 2001;107:173-80.

[14] Andersson K, Buschard K, Fredman P, Kaas A, Lidstrom AM, Masbad S, et al. Patients with insulin-dependent diabetes but not those with non-insulin-dependent diabetes have anti-sulfatide antibodies as determined with new ELISA assay. *Autoimmunity* 2002;35:463-8.

[15] Aparicio JM, Wakisaka A, Takada A, Matsuura N, Aizawa M. HLA-DQ system and insulin-dependent diabetes mellitus in Japanese: does it contribute to the development of IDDM as it does in Caucasians? *Immunogenetics* 1988;28:240-6.

[16] Arikan E, Sabuncu T, Ozer EM, Hatemi H. The clinical characteristics of latent autoimmune diabetes in adults and its relation with chronic complications in metabolically poor controlled Turkish patients with Type 2 diabetes mellitus. *J Diabetes Complications* 2005;19:254-8.

[17] Atkinson MA, Bowman MA, Campbell L, Darrow BL, Kaufman DL, Maclaren NK. Cellular immunity to a determinant common to glutamate decarboxylase and coxsackie virus in insulin-dependent diabetes. *J Clin Invest* 1994;94:2125-9.

[18] Atkinson MA, Kaufman D, Campbell L, Gibbs KA, Shah SC, Bu DF et al. Response of peripheral-blood mononuclear cells to glutamate decarboxylase in insulin-dependent diabetes. *Lancet* 1992;339:458-9.

[19] Atkinson MA, Kaufman D, Newman D, Tobin A, Maclaren N. Islet cell cytoplasmic autoantibody reactivity to glutamate decarboxylase in insulin-dependent diabetes. *J Clin Invest* 1993;91:350-56.

[20] Aviles-Santa L, Maclaren N, Raskin P. The relationship between immune-mediated Type 1 diabetes mellitus and ethnicity. *J Diabetes Complications* 2004;18:1-9.

[21] Baekkeskov S, Aanstoot HJ, Christgau S, Reetz A, Solimena M, Cascalho M, et al. Identification of the 64K autoantigen in insulin-dependent diabetes as the GABA-synthesizing enzyme glutamic acid decarboxylase. *Nature* 1990;34:151–6.

[22] Barker JM, Barriga KJ, Yu L, Miao D, Erlich HA, Norris JM, et al. Prediction of autoantibody positivity and progression to type 1 diabetes: diabetes autoimmunity study in the young (DAYSY). *J Clin Endocrinol Metab* 2004;89:3896-3902.

[23] Barker JM, Yu J, Yu L, Wang J, Miao D, Bao F, et al. Autoantibody "subspecificity" in type 1 diabetes. Risk for organ-specific autoimmunity clusters in distinct groups. *Diabetes* Care 2005;28:850-5.

[24] Betterle C, Presotto F, Pedini B, Moro L, Slack RS, Zanette F, et al. Islet cell and insulin autoantibodies in organ-specific autoimmune patients. Their behavior and predictive value for the development of type 1 (insulin-dependent) diabetes mellitus a 10 years follow-up study. *Diabetologia* 1987;30:292-7.

[25] Bingley PJ, Bonifacio E, Williams AJ, Genovese S, Bottazzo GF, Gale EA. Prediction of IDDM in the general population: strategies based on combination of autoantibody markers. *Diabetes* 1997;46:1701-10.

[26] Bingley PJ, Christie MR, Bonifacio E, Bonfanti R, Shattock M, Fonte MT, et al. Combined analysis of autoantibodies improves prediction of IDDM in islet cell antibody-positive relatives. *Diabetes* 1994;43:304-1310.

[27] Bodansky HJ, Grant PJ, Dean BM, McNally J, Bottazzo GF, Hambling MH, et al. Islet-cell antibodies and insulin autoantibodies in association with common viral infections. *Lancet* 1986;2:1351-3.

[28] Boehm BO, Manfras B, Seissler J, Schoffling K, Gluck M, Holzberger G, et al. Epidemiology and immunogenetic background if islet cell antibody positive nondiabetic schoolchildren-Ulm-Frankfurt population study. *Diabetes* 1991;40:1435-9.

[29] Bohmer K, Keilacker H, Kuglin B, Hubinger A, Bertrams J, Gries FA, et al. Proinsulin autoantibodies are more closely associated with type 1 (insulin-dependent) diabetes mellitus than insulin autoantibodies. *Diabetologia* 1991;34:830–4.

[30] Bonifacio E, Bingley PJ, Shattok M. Quantification of islet cell antibodies and prediction of insulin-dependent diabetes. *Lancet* 1990;335: 47-149.

[31] Bonifacio E, Genovese S, Braghi S, Bazzigaluppi E, Lampasona V, Bingley PJ, Rogge L, Pastore MR, Bognetti E, Bottazzo GF, et al. Islet autoantibody markers in IDDM: risk assessment strategies yielding high sensitivity. *Diabetologia* 1995;38:816-22.

[32] Bonifacio E, Lampasone V, Genovese S, Ferrari M, Bosi E. Identification of protein tyrosine phosphatase-like IA2 (islet cell antigen 512) as the insulin-dependent diabetes-related 37/40 K autoantigen and a target of islet-cell antibodies. *J Immunol* 1995;155:5419-26.

[33] Bosi E, Braghi G, Maffi P, Scirpoli M, Bertuzzi F, Pozza G, et al. Autoantibodies response to islet transplantation in type 1 diabetes. *Diabetes* 2001;50:2464-71.

[34] Bottazzo GF, Bosi E, Cull CA, Bonifacio E, Locatelli M, Zimmet P, et al. IA-2 antibody prevalence and risk assessment of early insulin requirement in subjects presenting with type 2 diabetes (UKPDS 71). *Diabetologia* 2005;48:703-8.

[35] Bottazzo GF, Dean BM, Gorsuch AN, Cudworth AG, Doniach D. Complement-fixing islet-cell antibodies in Type-I diabetes: Possible monitors of active beta-cell damage. *Lancet* 1980;1:668-72.

[36] Bottazzo GF, Florin-Christensen A, Doniach D. Islet-cell antibodies in diabetes mellitus with autoimmune polyendocrine deficiencies. *Lancet* 1974;2:1279-83.

[37] Buschard K, Josefsen K, Hansen SV, Horn T, Marshall MO, Persson H, et al. Sulphatide in islets of Langerhans and in organs affected in diabetic late complications: a study in human and animal tissue. *Diabetologia* 1994;37:1000-6.

[38] Buschard K, Josefsen K, Horn T, Fredman P. Sulphatide and sulphatide antibodies in insulin-dependent diabetes mellitus. *Lancet* 1993;342:840.

[39] Buzzetti R, Quattroocchi CC, Nistico L. Dissecting the genetics of type 1 diabetes: relevance for familial clustering and differences in incidence. *Diabetes Metab Rev* 1998;14:111-28.

[40] Cabrera-Rode E, Diaz-Horta O. Are sulfatides ICA-specific antigens? *Autoimmunity* 1995;21:149.

[41] Cabrera-Rode E, Diaz-Horta O, Fernández LE, Carr A, Marquina G, Valiente O, Gonzalez-Suarez RM, Uriarte A. Glycolipids as the major autoantigens of cytoplasmatic islet cell antibodies. *Autoimmunity* 1995;20:145–51.

[42] Cabrera-Rode E, Díaz-Horta O, Rendón A, Molina G, Vera M, Licea M, et al. Prevalence of islet cell antibodies (ICA) in diabetes mellitus and other diseases in Cubans. *Autoimmunity* 1997;26:7-9.

[43] Cabrera-Rode E, Fernandez LE, Carr A, Marquina G, Valiente O, Uriarte A, et al. Which glycolipids are the autoantigens of cytoplasmatic islet cell antibodies?. *Acta Diabetol* 1992;29:70-4.

[44] Cabrera-Rode E, Molina G, Arranz C, Vera M, González P, Suárez R,et al. Effect of standard nicotinamide in the prevention of type 1 diabetes in first degree relatives of persons with type 1 diabetes. *Autoimmunity* 2006;39:333-40.

[45] Cabrera-Rode E, Molina G, Díaz-Horta O, Rendón A, Perich P, Suárez L, et al. ICA characteristics in latent autoimmune diabetes of adults, new onset type 1 diabetic, first degree relatives of type 1 diabetics and gestational diabetes. *Rev. Cubana Endocrinol* 1999;10:85-97.

[46] Cabrera-Rode E, Morales J, Díaz-Horta O, Piquer S, Rendon A, Puig-Domingo M, et al. Glycolipid immunoreactivity of non-restricted islet cell antibodies and their relationship with other islet autoantibodies in IDDM. *Avances en Diabetologia* 1998;14:73-9.

[47] Cabrera-Rode E, Perich P, Díaz-Horta O, Molina G, Suárez LR, Tiberti C, et al. Latent autoimmune diabetes in adult´s (LADA) in type 2 diabetes: Frequency and characteristics. *Rev Cubana Endocrinol* 2001;12:22-34.

[48] Cabrera-Rode E, Perich P, Díaz-Horta O, Tiberti C, Molina G, Arranz C, et al. Slowly progressing type 1 diabetes: Persistence of islet cell autoantibodies is related to glibenclamide treatment. *Autoimmunity* 2002;35:469-74.

[49] Cabrera-Rode E, Perich P, Licea M. Latent autoimmune diabetes in adults (LADA) or slowly progressing type 1 diabetes: Type 1 or type 1.5 diabetes?. *Revista de la Asociación Latinoamericana de Diabetes* 2002; X:76- 84.

[50] Cabrera-Rode E, Sarmiento L, Molina G, Pérez C, Arranz C, Galvan JA, et al. Islet cell related antibodies and type 1 diabetes associated with echovirus 30 epidemic: a case report. *J Med Virol* 2005;76:373-7.

[51] Cabrera-Rode E, Sarmiento L, Tiberti C, Molina G, Barrios J, Hernández D, et al. Type 1 diabetes islet associated antibodies in subjects infected by echovirus 16. *Diabetologia* 2003;461348-53.

[52] Cabrera-Rode E, Suárez Fonseca L, Díaz-Horta O, Díaz O. New criteria for the classification of the diabetes mellitus. *Rev Cubana Endocrinol* 2000;11:51-5.

[53] Cabrera Rode E, Suárez Fonseca L, Díaz Horta O, Díaz Díaz O. Physiopathologic classification of diabetes mellitus. *Rev Cubana Endocrinol* 1998;9:91-4.

[54] Cabrera-Rode E, Suárez L, Díaz-Horta O, Rendón A. Can mithocondrial diabetes mellitus and myopathies be prevented?. *Neurología* 1999;14:319-20.

[55] Cabrera-Rode E, Uriarte A, Ventura R, Vargas J, Napoleon O, Acosta B. Immunological study in children at risk of developing type 1 diabetes as sequel of mumps infection. *Rev Cubana Epidemiol* 1988;26:64-70.

[56] Caillat-Zucman S, Garchon HJ, Timsit J, Assan R, Boitard C, Djilali-Saiah I, et al. Age-dependent HLA genetic heterogeneity of type 1 insulin-dependent diabetes mellitus. *J Clin Invest* 1992;90:2242-50.

[57] Cardwell CR, Carson DJ, Patterson CC. Parental age at delivery, birth order, birth weight and gestational age are associated with the risk of childhood type 1 diabetes: a UK regional retrospective cohort study. *Diabetes Med* 2005;22:200-6.

[58] Castaño L, Russo E, Zhou L, Lipes MA, Eisenbarth GS: Identification and cloning of a granule autoantigen (carboxypeptidase-H) associated with type I diabetes. *J Clin Endocrinol Metab* 1991;73:1197–1201.

[59] Casu A, Trucco M, Pietropaolo M. A look to the future: Prediction, prevention, and cure including islet transplantation and stem cell therapy. *Pediatr Clin N Am* 2005;52:1779-1804.

[60] Cepedano A, Barreiro J, Pombo M, y grupo de diabetes infantil de Galicia. Incidence and clinical manifestations at onset of type 1 diabetes mellitus in Galicia (Spain, 2001-2002). *Ann Pediatr* 2005;62:123-7.

[61] Chaillous L, Delamaire M, Elmansour A, Maugendre D, Rohmer V, Joseph MG, et al. Combined analysis of islet cell antibodies which cross-react with mouse pancreas, antibodies to the Mr 64,000 islet protein, and antibodies to glutamate decarboxylase in subjects at risk for IDDM. *Diabetologia* 1994;37:491-9.

[62] Chaillous L, Delamaire M, Martignat L, Maugendre D, Marre M, Mathieu E, et al. Combined analysis of islet cell antibodies that cross-react with mouse pancreas, antibodies to the Mr 64,000 islet protein, and antibodies to glutamate decarboxylase in type I diabetic patients. *Diabetes Care* 1994;17:1115-23.

[63] Chang YH, Hwang J, Shang HF, Tsai ST. Characterization of human DNA topoisomerase II as an autoantigen recognized by patients with IDDM. *Diabetes* 1996;45:408–14.

[64] Chen S, Willis J, Maclean C, Ananieva-Jordanova R, Amoroso MA, Brooking H, et al. Sensitive non-isotopic assays for autoantibodies to IA2 and to a combination of both IA2 and GAD65. *Clin Chem Acta* 2005;357:74-83.

[65] Christie MR, Tun RY, Lo SS, Cassidy D, Brown TJ, Hollands J, et al. Antibodies to GAD and tryptic fragments of islet 64K antigen as distinct markers for development of IDDM: studies with identical twins. *Diabetes* 1992;41:782–7.

[66] Clark CM, Qiu C, Amerman B, Porter B, Fineberg N, Aldasouqi S, et al. Gestational diabetes: should it be added to the syndrome of insulin resistance?. *Diabetes Care* 1997;20:867-71.

[67] Collado-Mesa F, Barcelo A, Arheart KL, Messiah SE. An ecological analysis of childhood-onset type 1 diabetes incidence and prevalence in Latin America. *Rev. Panam Salud Pública* 2004;15:388-94.

[68] Collado Mesa F, Díaz Díaz O, Hernández Cuesta I. Comportamiento epidemiológico de la diabetes mellitus insulino dependiente en menores de 15 años de edad. Cuba, 1990-1993. *Rev Cub Endocrinol* 1997;8:119-25.

[69] Colman PG, Mc Nair P, Margetts H, Schmidli RS, Werther GA, Alford FP, et al. The Melbourne Pre-Diabetes Study prediction of type 1 diabetes mellitus using antibody and metabolic testing. *Med J. Aust* 1998;69:81-4.

[70] Colman PG, Nayak RC, Campbell IL, Eisenbarth GS. Binding of cytoplasmic islet cell antibodies is blocked by human pancreatis glycolipid extracts. *Diabetes* 1988;37:645-52.

[71] Corcoy R, Morales J. Puig-Domingo M. Mauricio D, Adelantado JM, de Leiva A. Increased frecuency and lack of protection effect of restrictive islet cell autoantibodies in gestational diabetes. *Autoimmunity* 1995;21:73.

[72] Craig ME, Howard NJ, Silink M, Rawlinson WD. Reduced frequency of HLA DRB1*03-DQB1*02 in children with type 1 diabetes associated with enterovirus RNA. *J Infect Dis* 2003;187:1562-70.

[73] Cruz TD, Valdes AM, Santiago A, Frazer deLlado T, Raffel LJ, Zeidler A, et al. DPB1 alleles are associated with type 1 diabetes susceptibility in multiple ethnic groups. *Diabetes* 2004;53:2158-63.

[74] Daniel D, Gill RG, Schloot N, Wegmann D. Epitope specificity, cytokine production profile and diabetogenic activity of insulin-specific T cell clones isolated from NOD mice. *Eur J Immunol* 1995;25:1056-62.

[75] Devendra D, Liu E, Eisenbarth GS. Type 1 diabetes: recent developments. *BMJ* 2004;328:750-4.

[76] Diabetes Prevention Trial-Type 1 Diabetes Study Group. Effects of insulin in relatives of patients with type 1 diabetes. *N Engl J Med* 2002;346:1658-91.

[77] Díaz-Horta O, Bello M, Cabrera-Rode E, Suarez J, Mas P, Garcia I, et al. Echovirus 4 and type 1 diabetes mellitus. *Autoimmunity* 2001;34:275-81.

[78] Díaz-Díaz O, Carvajal F, Fernández L, Rodríguez J. Epidemiología de la diabetes mellitus tipo 1 en menores de 15 años. Evidencias de variaciones estacionales. *Rev Cub Invest Biom* 1983;2:316-25.

[79] Donner G, Thoelke H, Mohnike A, Schneider H. High food supply in perinatal life appears to favour the development of insulin-treated diabetes mellitus (ITDM) in later life. *Exp Clin Endocrinol* 1985;85:1-6.

[80] Dorman JS, LaPorte RE, Stone RA, Trucco M. Worldwide differences in the incidence of type 1 diabetes are associated with amino acid variation at position 57 of the HLA-DQ ß chain. Proc. *Natl. Acad. Sci.* 1990;87:7370-4.

[81] Dotta F, Anastasi E, Tiberti C, Di Mario U. Autoantigens in type 1 diabetes mellitus. *J Endocrinol Invest* 1994;17:497-508.

[82] Dotta F, Falorni A, Tiberti C, Dionisi S, Anastasi E, Torresi P, et al. Autoantibodies to the GM2-1 islet ganglioside and to GAD-65 at type 1 diabetes onset. *J Autoimmun* 1997;10:585–8.

[83] Dotta F, Gianani R, Previti M, Lenti L, Dionisi S, D´Erme M, et al. Autoimmunity to the GM2-1 islet ganglioside before and at the onset of type I diabetes. *Diabetes.* 1996;45:1193-6

[84] Dotta F, Previti M, Lenti L, Dionisi S, Casetta B, D'Erme M, et al. GM2-1 pancreatic islet ganglioside: identification and characterization of a novel islet-specific molecule. *Diabetologia* 1995;38:1117-21.

[85] Dotta F, Previti M, Neerman-Arbez M, Dionisi S, Cucinotta D, Lenti L, et al. The GM2-1 ganglioside islet autoantigen in insulin-dependent diabetes mellitus is expressed in secretory granules and is not beta-cell specific. *Endocrinology* 1998;139:316-9.

[86] Dozio N, Beretta A, Belloni C, Castiglioni M, Rosa S, Bosi E, et al. Low prevalence of islet cell autoantibodies in patients with gestational diabetes mellitus. *Diabetes Care* 1997;20:81-3.

[87] Durinovic-Bello I. Autoimmune diabetes: the role of T cells, MHC molecules and autoantigens. *Autoimmunity* 1998;27:159-77.

[88] Eisenbarth GS. Type 1 diabetes: a chronic autoimmune disease. *N Engl J Med* 1986; 314:1360-7.

[89] Eisenbarth GS, Morris MA, Sceararce RM. Cytotoxic antibodies to cloned islet cells in serum of patients with diabetes mellitus. *J Clin Invest* 1981;67:403–8.

[90] Eisenbarth GS. Prediction of type 1 diabetes: The natural history of the prediabetic period. In: George S Eisenbarth, ed. *Immunology of type 1 diabetes*. New York: Eurekah.com and Kluwer Academic/ Plenum Publishers; 2004.p.268-85.

[91] Emery LM, Babu S, Bugawan TL, Norris JM, Erlich HA, Eisenbarth GS, et al. Newborn HLA-DR, DQ genotype screening: age- and ethnicity-specific type 1 diabetes risk estimates. *Pediatr Diabetes* 2005;6:36-144.

[92] Erlich HA, Bomer JL, Chang JD, Shaw SD, Raffel LJ, Klitz W, et al. Association of HLA-DPB1*0301 with insulin-dependent diabetes mellitus in Mexicans-Americans. *Diabetes* 1996;45:610-4.

[93] Erlich HA, Griffith RL, Bugawan TL, Ziegler R, Alper C, Eisenbarth GS. Implication of specific DQB1 alleles in genetic susceptibility and resistance by identification of IDDM siblings with novel HLA-DQB1 allele and unusual DR2 and DR1 haplotypes. *Diabetes* 1991;40:478-81.

[94] European Nicotinamide Diabetes Intevention trial (ENDIT) Group. European Nicotinamide Diabetes Intervention Trial (ENDIT): a randomized controlled trial of intervention before the onset of type 1 diabetes. *Lancet* 2004;363:925-31.

[95] Falorni A. Immunologic and genetic aspects of latent autoimmune diabetes in the adult. *Minerva Endocrinol* 2003;28:297-312.

[96] Falorni A, Brozzetti A. Diabetes-related antibodies in adult diabetic patients. *Best Pract Res Clin Endocrinol Metab* 2005;19:119-3.

[97] Farilla L, Tibert C, Luzzago A, Yu L, Eisenbarth GS, Cortese R, et al. Application of phage display peptide library to autoimmune diabetes: identification of IA-2/ICA512bdc dominant autoantigenic epitopes. *Eur J Immu*nol 2002;32:1420-7.

[98] Fava D, Garner S, Pyke D, Leslie RDG. Evidence that the age at diagnosis of IDDM is genetically determined. *Diabetes Care* 1998;21:925-9.

[99] Federlin K, Otten A, Hemke K. Islet cell antibodies and viral infections. *Exp Clin Endocrinol* 1987;89:368-74.

[100] Feeney SJ, Myers MA, Mackay IR, Zimmet PZ, Howard N, Verge CF, et al. Evaluation of ICA512As in combination with other islet cell autoantibodies at the onset of IDDM. *Diabetes Care* 1997;20:1403-7.

[101] Feillet H, Bach JF. On the mechanism of the protective effect of infections of type 1 diabetes. *Clin Dev Immunol* 2004;11:191-4.

[102] Feltbower RG, Bodansky HJ, McKinney PA, Houghton J, Stephenson CR, Haigh D. Trends in the incidence of childhood diabetes in south Asians and other children in Bradford, UK. *Diabet Med* 2002;19:162-6.

[103] Forbes LV, Brown LJ, Scott RS. HLA-DQ beta typing and non-Asp57 alleles in IDDM and non-diabetic subjects in New Zealand. *Diabetes Care* 1993;16:1179-83.

[104] Fourlanos S, Dotta F, Greenbaum CJ, Palmer JP, Rolandsson O, Colman PG, et al. Latent autoimmune diabetes in adults (LADA) should be less latent. *Diabetologia* 2005;48:2206-12.

[105] Fourlanos S, Narendran P, Byrnes GB, Colman PG, Harrison LC. Insulin resistance is a risk factor for progression to type 1 diabetes. *Diabetologia* 2004;47:1661-7.

[106] Franke B, Galloway TS, Wilkin TJ. Developments in the prediction of type 1 diabetes mellitus, with special reference to insulin autoantibodies. *Diabetes Metab Res Rev* 2005;21:395-415.

[107] Fuchtenbush M, Ferber K, Standl E, Ziegler AG. Prediction of type 1 diabetes postpartum in patients with gestational diabetes mellitus by combined islet cell autoantibody screening: a prospective multicenter study. *Diabetes* 1997;46:1459-67.

[108] Gale EAM. The rise of childhood type 1 diabetes in the 20th century. *Diabetes* 2002; 51:3353-61.

[109] Gale EAM. Latent autoimmune diabetes in adults: a guide for the perplexed. *Diabetologia* 2005;48:2195-99.

[110] Gambelunghe G, Ghaderi M, Cosentino A, Falorni A, Brunetti P, Falorni A, et al. Association of MHC Class I chain-related A (MIC-A) gene polymorphism with Type I diabetes. *Diabetologia* 2000;43:507-514.

[111] Gardner SG, Gale EAM, Williams AJK, Gillespie KM, Lawrence KE, Bottazzo GF, et al. Progression to diabetes in relatives with islet autoantibodies. *Diabetes Care* 1999;22:2049-54.

[112] Genovese S, Bonifacio E, McNally JM, Dean BM, Wagner R, Bosi E, et al. Distinct cytoplasmic islet cell antibodies with different risk for type 1 (insulin-dependent) diabetes mellitus. *Diabetologia* 1992;35:385-8.

[113] Gerling I, Baekkeskov S, Lernmark A. Islet cell and 64K autoantibodies are associated with plasma IgG in newly diagnosed insulin-dependent diabetic children. *J Immunol* 1986;137:3782–5.

[114] Gianani R, Pugliese A, Bonner-Weir S, Shiffrin AJ, Soeldner JS, Erlich H, et al. Prognostically significant heterogeneity of cytoplasmic islet cell antibodies in relatives of patients with type 1 diabetes. *Diabetes* 1992;41:347-53.

[115] Gibbon C, Smith T, Egger P, Betts P. Phillips D. Early infection and subsequent insulin dependent diabetes. *Arch Dis Child* 1997;77:384-5.

[116] Gillard BK, Thomas JW, Nell LJ, Marcus DM. Antibodies against ganglioside GT3 in the sera of patients with type I diabetes mellitus. *J Immunol Methods* 1989;142:3826-32.

[117] Gottsater A, Landin-Olsson M, Fernlund P, Lernmark A, Sundkvist G. β-Cell function in relation to islet cell antibodies during the first 3 yr after clinical diagnosis of diabetes in type II diabetic patients. *Diabetes Care* 1993;16:902-10.

[118] Gottsater A, Samuelsson U, Nilsson S, Lernmark A, Sundkvist G. Islet cell antibodies and fasting plasma C-peptide during the first 10 yr after diagnosis in patients with diabetes mellitus diagnosed in adult age. *Diabetes Nutricion & Metabolism* 1992;5:243-8.

[119] Green A, Patterson CC, on behalf of the EURODIAB TIGER Study Group. Trends in the incidence of childhood-onset diabetes in Europe 1989-1998. *Diabetologia* 2001;44:B3-B8.

[120] Greenbaum CJ, Cuthbertson D, Eisenbarth GS, Shatz DA, Zeidler A, Krisher JP. Islet cell antibody-positive relatives with human leukocyte antigen DQA1*0102, DQB1*0602: identification by the Diabetes Prevention Trial-type 1. *J Clin Endocrinol Metab* 2000;85:1255-60.

[121] Greenbaum CJ, Palmer JP, Yamaguchi NY, Molenaar JL, Van Beers WAM, Maclaren NK, et al. Improved specificity of ICA assays in the fourth international immunology of diabetes serum exchange workshop. *Diabetes* 1992;41:1570-4.

[122] Groop LC, Miettinen A, Groop PH, Meri S, Koskimies S, Bottazzo GF. Organ-specific autoimmunity and HLA-DR antigens as markers for β-cell destruction in patients with type II diabetes. *Diabetes* 1988;37:99-103.

[123] Guazzarotti L, Thivolet C, Tardivel I, Chevalier A, European prediabetes study group and Carel JC. Reactivity of islet cell antibodies (ICA) to recombinant glutamic acid decarboxylase (GAD). *J Autoimmunity* 1995;8:901-14.

[124] Haider MZ, Shaltout A, Alsaeid K, Al-Khawari M, Dorman JS. High frequency of HLA-DQB1 non-Asp(57) alleles in Kuwaiti children with insulin-dependent diabetes mellitus. *Hum Hered* 2000;50:242-6.

[125] Haller MJ, Atkinson MA, Schatz D. Type 1 diabetes mellitus: Etiology, presentation, and management. *Pediatr Clin N Am* 2005;52:1553-78.

[126] Harashima S, Clark A, Christie MR, Notkins AL. The dense core transmembrane vesicle protein IA-2 is a regulator of vesicle number and insulin secretion. *Proc Natl Acad Sci USA* 2005;102:8704-9.

[127] Harrison LC, Chu SX, DeAizpurua HJ, Graham M, Honeyman MC, Colman PG. Islet-reactive T cells are a marker of preclinical insulin-dependent diabetes. *J Clin Invest* 1992;89:1161-5.

[128] Haverkos HW, Battula N, Drotman DP, Rennert OM. Enterovirus and type 1 diabetes mellitus. *Biomed Pharm* 2003;57:379-85.

[129] Haverkos HW. Could the aetiology of IDDM be multifactorial?. *Diabetologia* 1997;40:1235-40.

[130] Helmke K, Otten A, Willenis W. Islet cell antibodies in children with mumps infection. *Lancet* 1980; II: 211-2.

[131] Hermann R, Knip M, Veijola R, Simell O, Laine AP, Akerblom HK, et al. Temporal changes in the frequency of HLA genotypes in patients with type 1 diabetes – indication of an increased environmental pressure?. *Diabetologia* 2003;46:420-5.

[132] Hermann R, Laine AP, Veijola R, Vahlberg T, Simell S, Lahde J, et al. The effect of HLA Class II, insulin and *CTLA4* gene regions on the development of humoral beta cell autoimmunity. *Diabetologia* 2005;48:1766-75.

[133] Hiltunen M, Hyoty H, Knip M, Ilonen J, Reijonen H, Vahasalo P, et al. Islet cell antibodies seroconversion in children is temporally associated with enterovirus infections. *J Infect Dis* 1997;175:554-60.

[134] Holick MF. Vitamin D: importance in the prevention of cancers, type 1 diabetes, heart disease, and osteoporosis. *Am J Clin Nutr* 2004;79:362-71.

[135] Honeyman MC, Coulson BS, Stone NL, Gellert SA, Goldwater PN, Steele CE, et al. Association between rotavirus infection and pancreatic islet autoimmunity in children at risk of developing type 1 diabetes. *Diabetes* 2000;49:1319-24.

[136] Hosszufalust N, Vatay A, Rajcy K, Prohaszka Z, Pozsonyi E, Horvath L, et al. Similar genetic features and different islet cell autoantibody pattern of latent autoimmune diabetes in adults (LADA) compared with adult-onset type 1 diabetes with rapid progression. *Diabetes Care* 2003;26:452-7.

[137] House DV, Winter WE. Autoimmune diabetes. The role of autoantibody markers in the prediction and prevention of insulin-dependent diabetes mellitus. *Clin Lab Med* 1997;3:499-545.

[138] Hu YE, Zhang HL, Cai T, Harashima S, Notkins AI. The IA-2 interactome. *Diabetologia* 2005;48:2576-81.

[139] Hummel M, Durinovic-Bello I, Ziegler A-G. Relation between cellular and humoral immunity to islet cell antigens in type I diabetes. *J Autoimmun* 1996;9:427-30.

[140] Hummel M, Williams AJ, Norcross A, Standl E, Bonifacio E, Ziegler AG, et al. Proinsulin-specific autoantibodies are relatively infrequent in young offspring with pre-type 1 diabetes. *Diabetes Care* 2001;24:1843-4.

[141] Hviid A, Stellfeld M, Wohlfahrt J, Melbye M. Childhood vaccination and type 1 diabetes. *N Engl J Med* 2004;14:1398-1404.

[142] Hyoty H, Taylor KW. The role of viruses in human diabetes. *Diabetologia* 2002;45: 1353-61.

[143] Hypponen E, Laara E, Jarvelin MR, Virtanen SM. Intake of vitamin D and risk of type 1 diabetes: a birth-cohort study. *Lancet* 2001;358:1500-3.

[144] Hyttinen V, Kaprio J, Kinnunen L, Koskenvuo M, Tuomilehto J. Genetic liability of type 1 diabetes and the onset age among 22,650 young Finnish twin pairs. *Diabetes* 2003;52:1052-5.

[145] IDF Diabetes atlas-Incidence. www.eatlas.idf.org. 2005

[146] Int Veld PA, Bruining J. Genetic syndrome and diabetes mellitus. In: Pickup J, Williams G, eds. *Textbook of diabetes*. London: The Blackwell Science, 1998.p.1-28.

[147] Jasinski JM, Eisenbarth GS. Insulin as a primary autoantigen for type 1A diabetes. *Clin Dev Immunol* 2005;12:181-6.

[148] Johansson C, Samuelsson U, Ludvigsson J. A high weigh gain early in life is associated with increased risk of type 1 (insulin-dependent) diabetes mellitus. *Diabetologia* 1994;37:91-4.

[149] Johansson S, Lie BA, Pociot F, Nerup J, Cambon-Thomsen A, Kockun I, et al. HLA associations in type 1 diabetes DPB1 alelles may act as markers of other HLA-complex susceptibility genes. *Tissue Antigens* 2000;61:344-51.

[150] Johnson JH, Crider BP, McCorkle K, Alford M, Unger RH. Inhibition of glucose transport into rat islet cells by immunoglobulins from patients with new-onset insulin-dependent diabetes mellitus. *N Engl J Med* 1990;332:653–9.

[151] Johnston C, Pyke DA, Cudworth AG, Wolf E. HLA-DR typing in identical twins with insulin-dependent diabetes: a difference between concordant and discordant pairs. *BMJ* 1983;286:253-85.

[152] Jones DB, Hunter NR, Duff GW. Heat-shock protein 65 as a beta cell antigen of insulin-dependent diabetes. *Lancet* 1990;336:583–5.

[153] Karounos DG. Convergence of genetic and environmental factors in the immunopathogenesis of type 1 diabetes mellitus. *J Clin Ligand Assay* 1998;21:262-71.

[154] Karounos DG, Thomas JW. Recognition of common islet antigen by autoantibodies from NOD mice and humans with IDDM. *Diabetes* 1990;39:1085–90.

[155] Karvonen M, Viik-Kajander M, Moltchanova E. Libman I, LaPorte R, Tuomilehto J. Incidence of childhood type 1 diabetes worldwide. *Diabetes Care* 2000;23:1516-26.

[156] Kasimiotis H, Myers MA, Argentaro A, Mertin S, Fida S, Ferraro T, et al. Sex-determining region Y-related protein SOX13 is a diabetes autoantigen expressed in pancreatic islets. *Diabetes* 2000;49:555–61.

[157] Kawasaki E, Yu L, Rewers MJ, Hutton JC, Eisenbarth GS. Definition of multiple ICA512/Phogrin autoantibody epitopes and detection of intramolecular epitope spreading in relatives of patients with type 1 diabetes. *Diabetes* 1998;47:733-42.

[158] Kelemen K, Crawford ML, Gill RG, Hutton JC, Wegmann D. Cellular immune response to phogrin in the NOD mouse: cloned T-cells cause destruction of islet transplants. *Diabetes* 1999;48:1529-34.

[159] Kelemen K, Gottlieb PA, Putnam AL, Davidson HW, Wegmann DR, Hutton JC. HLA-DQ8-associated T cell responses to the diabetes autoantigen phogrin (IA-2beta) in human prediabetes. *J Immunol* 2004;172:955-62.

[160] Keller RJ. Cellular immunity to human insulin in individuals at high risk for the development of type 1 diabetes mellitus. *J Autoimmun* 1990;3:321-7.

[161] Kerokoski P, Ilonen J, Gaedigk R, Dosch HM, Knip M, Hakala M, et al. Production of the islet cell antigen ICA69 (p69) with caculovirus expression system: analysis with solid-phase time-resolved fluorescence method of sera from patients with IDDM and rheumatoid arthritis. *Autoimmunity* 1999;29:281-9.

[162] Kida K, Kaino Y, Ito T, Hirai H, Nakamura K. Immunogenetics of insulin-dependent diabetes mellitus. *Acta Paediatr* 1999;Suppl 427:3-7.

[163] Kim YJ, Zhou Z, Hurtado J, Wood DL, Choi AS, Pescovitz MD, et al. IDDM patient's sera recognize a novel 30-kD pancreatic autoantigen related to chymotrypsinogen. *Immunol Invest* 1993;22:219–27.

[164] Kimpimaki T, Kupila A, Hamalainen AM, Kukko M, Kulmala P, Savola K, et al. The first signs of beta-cell autoimmunity appear in infancy in genetically susceptible children from the general population: the Finnish Type 1 Diabetes Prediction and Prevention Study. *J Clin Endocrinol Metab* 2001;86:4782-8.

[165] Knip M. Prediction and Prevention of type 1 diabetes. *Acta Paediatr* 1998;425:54-62.

[166] Knip K. Natural course of preclinical type 1 diabetes. *Horm Res* 2002;57:6-11.

[167] Knip M, Akerblom HK. Environmental factors in the pathogenesis of type 1 diabetes mellitus. Exp Clin Endocrinol Diabetes 1999;107:S93-100.

[168] Kobayashi T, Tanaka S, Okubo M, Nkanishi K, Murase T, Lernmark A. Unique epitopes of glutamic acid decarboxylase autoantibodies in slowly progressive type 1 diabetes. *J Clin Endocrinol Metab* 2003;88:4768-75.

[169] Kousta E, Lawrence NJ, Anyaoku V, Johnston DG, McCarthy MI. Prevalence and features of pancreatic islet cell autoimmunity in women with gestational diabetes from different ethnic groups. *BJOG* 2001;108:716-20.

[170] Krischer J, Cuthbertson DD, Yu L, Orban T, Maclare N, Jackson R, et al. Screening strategies for the identification of multiple antibody-positive relatives of individuals with type 1 diabetes. *J Clin Endocrinol Metab* 2003;88:103-8.

[171] Krischer J, Schatz D, Riley W, Spillar R, Silverstein J, Schwartz S, et al. Insulin and islet cell autoantibodies as time-dependent covariates in the development of insulin-dependent diabetes: A prospective study in relatives. *J Clin Endocrinol Metab* 1993;77:743-9.

[172] Kubosaki A, Nakamura S, Notkins AL. Dense Core Vesicle Proteins IA-2 and IA-2{beta}: Metabolic Alterations in Double Knockout Mice. *Diabetes* 2005;54:S46-S51.

[173] Kukko M, Virtanen SM, Tovoinen A, Simell S, Korhonen S, Ilonen J, et al. Geographical variation in risk HLA-DQB1 genotypes for type 1 diabetes and signs of β-cell autoimmunity in a high-incidence country. *Diabetes Care* 2004;27:676-81.

[174] Kulmala P, Savola K, Reijonen H, Veijola R, Vahasalo P, Karjalainen J, et al. Genetic markers, humoral autoimmunity, and prediction of type 1 diabetes in siblings of affected children. *Diabetes* 2000;49:48-58.

[175] Kundu SK, Pleatman MA, Redwine WA, Boyd AE, Marcus DM. Binding of monoclonal antibody A2B5 to gangliosides. *Biochem Biophys Res Commun* 1983;116:836-42.

[176] Kuzuya T, Matsuda A. Classification of diabetes on the basis of etiologies versus degree of insulin deficiency. *Diabetes Care* 1997;20:219-20.

[177] Kyvik KO, Nystrom L, Gorus F, Songini M, Oestman J, Castell C et al. The epidemiology of type 1 diabetes mellitus is not the same in young adults as in children. *Diabetologia* 2004;47:377-84.

[178] LaGasse JM, Brantley MS, Leech NJ, Rowe RE, Monks S, Palmer JP, et al. Successful prospective prediction of type 1 diabetes in schoolchildren through multiple defined autoantibodies: An 8-year follow-up of the Washington state diabetes prediction study. *Diabetes Care* 2002;25:505-11.

[179] Lammi N, Karvonen M, Tuomilehto J. Do microbes have a causal role in type 1 diabetes?. *Med Sci Monit* 2005;11:RA63-69.

[180] Lan MS, Wasserfall C, Maclaren NK, Notkins A. IA-2, a transmembrane protein of the protein tyrosine phosphatase family, is a major autoantigen in insulin-dependent diabetes mellitus. *Proc Natl Acad Sci USA* 1996;93:6367–70.

[181] Lapolla A, Fedele D, Pedini B, Dal Fra MG, Sanzari M, Masin M, et al. Low frequency of autoantibodies to islet cell, glutamic acid decarboxylase, and second-islet antigen in patients with gestational diabetes mellitus: a follow-up study. *Ann NY Acad Sci* 2002;958:263-6.

[182] Larsson K, Elding-Larsson H, Cederwall E, Kockum K, Neiderud J, Sjoblad S, et al. Genetic and perinatal factors at risk for childhood type 1 diabetes. *Diabetes Metab Res Rev* 2004;20:429-37.

[183] Lernmark A. Type 1 diabetes-Does suppressing T cells increase insulin?. *N Engl J Med* 2005;352:2642-4.

[184] Lernmark A, Freedman ZR, Hofmann C, Rubenstein AH, Steiner DF, Jackson RL, et al. Islet-cell surface antibodies in juvenile diabetes mellitus. *N Engl J Med* 1978;299:375–80.

[185] Lernmark A, Kolb H, Mire-Sluis T. Toward a World Health Organization (WHO) approved standard sample for islet cell antibodies, GAD65 and IA2 autoantibodies. *Diabetologia* 1999;42:381-2.

[186] Levy-Marchal C, Ticket J, Fajardy I, Gu XF, Dubois F, Czernichow P. Islet cell antibodies in normal French schoolchildren. *Diabetologia* 1992;35:577-82.

[187] Libman IM, Pietropaolo M, Trucco M, Dorman JS, LaPorte RE, Becker D. Islet cell autoimmunity in white and black children and adolescents with IDDM. *Diabetes Care* 1998;21:1824-7.

[188] Lipton R, LaPorte RE. Epidemiology of islet cell antibodies. *Epidemiologic Reviews* 1989;11:182-203.

[189] Lonnrot M, Salminen K, Knip M, Savola K, Kulmala P, Leinikki P, et al. Enterovirus RNA in serum is a risk factor for beta-cell autoimmunity and clinical type 1 diabetes: a prospective study. Childhood Diabetes in Finland (DiMe) Study Group. *J Med Virol* 2000;61:214-20.

[190] Maclaren NK, Huang SW. Antibody to cultured human insulinoma cells in insulin-dependent diabetes. *Lancet* 1975;1:997–9.

[191] Maclaren N, Lan M, Coutant R, Schatz D, Silverstein J, Muir A, et al. Only multiple autoantibodies to islet cells (ICA), insulin, GAD65, IA-2 and IA-2 beta predict immune-mediated (Type 1) diabetes in relatives. *J Autoimmun* 1999;12:279-87.

[192] MacCuish AC, Irvine WJ, Barnes EW, Duncan LJ. Antibodies to pancreatic islet cells in insulin-dependent diabetics with coexistent autoimmune disease. *Lancet* 1974;2:1529-31.

[193] Maioli M, Alejandro E, Tonolo G, Gilliam LK, Bekris L, Hampe CS, et al. Epitope-restricted 65-kilodalton glutamic acid decarboxylase autoantibodies among new-onset Sardinian type 2 diabetes patients define phenotypes of autoimmune diabetes *J Clin Endocrinol Metab* 2004;89:5675-82.

[194] Makita A, Taniguchi N. Glycosphingolipids. In: Wiegandt, ed. *Glycolipids.* Elsevier Science Publishers B.V; 1985.p.1.

[195] Maldonado M, Hampe CS, Gaur HL, D'Amico S, Iyer D, Hammerle LP, et al. Ketosis-prone diabetes: Dissection of a heterogeneous syndrome using an immunogenetic and ß-cell functional classification, prospective analysis, and clinical outcomes. *J Clin Endocrinol Metab* 2003;88:5090-8.

[196] Mallone R, Kochik SA, Laughlin EM, Gersuk VH, Reijonen H, Kwok WW et al. Differential recognition and activation thresholds in human autoreactive GAD-specific T-cells. *Diabetes* 2004;53:971-7.

[197] Mansson L, Torn C, Landin-Olson M. Islet cell antibodies represent autoimmune response against several antigens. *Int J Exp Diabetes Res* 2001;2:85-90.

[198] Maron R, Elias D, DeJongh BM, Bruining GF, VanRood JJ, Shechter Y, et al. Autoantibodies to the insulin receptor in juvenile onset insulin-dependent diabetes. *Nature* 1983;303:81–8.

[199] Marsh SG, Albert ED, Bodmer WF, Bontrop RE, Dupont B, Erlich HA, et al. Nomenclature for factors of the HLA system. *Tissue Antigens* 2002;60:407-64.

[200] Martin N, Boomsma D, Machin G. A twins-pronged attack on complex traits. *Nat Genet* 1997;17:87-92.

[201] Martin S, Kardorf J, Schulte B, Lampeter EF, Gries FA, Melchers I, Wagner R, bertrams J, Roep BO, Pfutzner A. Autoantibodies to the islet antigen ICA69 occur in IDDM and in rheumatoid arthritis. *Diabetologia* 1995;38:351-5.

[202] Maruyama T, Shimada A, Kanasutka A, Kasuga A, Takei I, Yokoyama J, et al. Multicenter prevention trial of slowly progressive type 1 diabetes with small dose of insulin (the Tokyo study): preliminary report. *Ann N Y Acad Sci* 2003;1005:362-9.
[203] Maruyama T, Takei I, Matsuba I, Tsuruoka A, Taniyama M, Ikeda Y, et al. Cell-mediated cytotoxic islet cell surface antibodies to human pancreatic beta cells. *Diabetologia* 1984;26:30–3.
[204] Mauricio D, Balsells M, Morales J, Corcoy R, Puig-Domingo M, de Leiva A. Islet cell autoimmunity in women with gestational diabetes and risk of progression to insulin dependent diabetes mellitus. *Diabetes Metab Rev* 1996;4:275-85.
[205] Mauricio D, Leiva A. Autoimmunity and gestational diabetes. *Avances en Diabetologia* 1992;5:17-22.
[206] Mire-Sluis AR, Das RG, Lernmark A. The development of a World Health Organization international standard for islet cell antibodies: the aim and design of an international collaborative study. *Diabetes Metab Res Rev* 1999;15:72-7.
[207] Mire-Sluis AR, Gaines Das R, Lernmark A. The World Health Organization International Collaborative Study for islet cell antibodies. *Diabetologia* 2000;43:1282-92.
[208] Mire-Sluis AR, Gaines Das R, Lernmark A. Standardization of antibody preparations for use in immunogenecity studies: a case study using the World Health Organization International Collaborative Study for Islet Cell Antibodies. *Dev Biol* 2003;112:153-63.
[209] Misasi R, Dionisi S, Farilla L, Carabba B, Lenti L, Di Mario U, et al. Gangliosides and autoimmune diabetes. *Diabetes Metab Rev* 1997;13:163-79.
[210] Moghaddam PH, Zwinderman AH, de Knijff P, Roep BO, Schipper RF, Van der Auwera B, et al. TNF-a microsatellite polymorphism modulates the risk of IDDM in Caucasians with the high-risk genotype HLA DQA1*0501-DQB1*0201/DQA1*0301-DQB1*0302. Belgian Diabetes Registry. *Diabetes* 1997;46:1514-5.
[211] Moltchanova E, Rytkonen M, Kousa A, Taskinen O, Tuomilehto J, Karnoven M, et al. Zinc and nitrate in the ground water and the incidence of type 1 diabetes in Finland. *Diabet Med* 2004;21:256-61.
[212] Monge L, Bruno G, Pinach S, Grassi G, Maghenzani G, Dani F, et al. A clinically orientated approach increases the efficiency of screening for latent autoimmune diabetes in adults (LADA) in a large clinic-based cohort of patients with diabetes onset over 50 years. *Diabet Med* 2004;21: 456-9.
[213] Mrena S, Savola K, Kulmala P, Akerblom HK, Knip M, and the childhood diabetes in Finland study group. Staging of preclinical type 1 diabetes in siblings of affected children. *Pediatrics* 1999;104:925-30.
[214] Mrena S, Savola K, Kulmala P, Reijonen H, Ilonen J, Akerblom HK, et al. Genetic modification of risk assessment based on staging of preclinical type 1 diabetes in siblings of affected children. *J Clin Endocrinol Metab* 2003;88:2682-9.
[215] Mukherjee R, Chaturvedi P, Qin HY, Singh B. CD4+CD25+ regulatory T cells generated in response to insulin B:9-23 peptide prevent adoptive transfer of diabetes by diabetogenic T cells. *J Autoimmun* 2003;21:221-37.
[216] Muntoni S, Cocco P, Aru G, Cucca F, Muntoni S. Nutritional factors and worldwide incidence of childhood type 1 diabetes. *Am J Clin Nutr* 2000;71:1525-9.

[217] Muntoni S, Muntoni S. New insights into the epidemiology of type 1 diabetes in Mediterranean countries. *Diabetes Metab Res Rev* 1999;15:133-40.

[218] Murao S, Makino H, Kaino Y, Konoue E, Ohashi J, Kida K, et al. Differences in the contribution of HLA-DR and DQ haplotypes to susceptibility to adult- and childhood-onset type 1 diabetes in Japanese patients. *Diabetes* 2004;53:2684-90.

[219] Mustonen A, Knip M, Akerblom K. An association between complement-fixing cytoplasmic islet cell antibodies and endogenous insulin-dependent diabetes mellitus. *Diabetes* 1983;32:743-7.

[220] Myers MA, Mackay IR, Rowley MJ, Zimmet PZ. Dietary microbial toxins and type 1 diabetes—a new meaning for seed and soil. *Diabetologia* 2001;44:1199-1200.

[221] Myers MA, Rabin DU, Rowley MJ. Pancreatic islet cell cytoplasmic antibody in diabetes is represented by antibodies to islet cell antigen 512 and glutamic acid decarboxylase. *Diabetes* 1995;44:1290-5.

[222] Nakayama M, Abiru N, Moriyama H, Babaya N, Liu E, Miao D, et al. Prime role for an insulin epitope in the development of type 1 diabetes in NOD mice. *Nature* 2005;435:220-3.

[223] Narendran P, Williams AJ, Elsegood K, Leech NJ, Dayan CM. Humoral and cellular immune responses to proinsulin in adults with newly diagnosed type 1 diabetes. *Diabetes Metab Res Rev* 2003;19:52-9.

[224] Nayak RC, Attawia NA, Cahill CJ, King GL, Ohashi O, Moromisato R. Expression of a monoclonal antibody (3G5) defined ganglioside antigen in renal cortex. *Kidney Int* 1992;41:1638-45.

[225] Nayak RS, Omar MAK, Rabizadeh A, Srikanta S, Eisenbarth GS. "Cytoplasmic" islet cell antibodies: evidence that the target antigen is a sialoglycoconjugate. *Diabetes* 1985;34:617-9.

[226] Nepom GT, Lippolis JD, White FM, Masewicz S, Marto JA, Herman A et al. Identification and modulation of a naturally processed T cell epitope from the diabetes-associated autoantigen human glutamic acid decarboxylase 65 (hGAD65). *Proc Natl Acad Sci USA* 2001;98:1763-8.

[227] Noble JA, Valdes AM, Cook M, Klitz W, Thompson G, Erlich HA. The role of HLA class II genes in insulin-dependent diabetes mellitus: molecular analysis of 180 Caucasian, multiplex families. *Am J Hum Genet* 1996;58:1134-48.

[228] Norris JM, Barriga K, Klingensmith G, Hoffman M, Eisenbarth GS, Erlich HA, et al. Timing of initial cereal exposure in infancy and risk of islet autoimmunity. *JAMA* 2003;290:1713-20.

[229] Notkins AL. Immunologic and genetic factors in type 1 diabetes. *J Biol Chem* 2002; 277:43545-8.

[230] Notkins AL, Lu J, Li Q, VanderVegt FP, Wasserfall C, Maclaren NK, et al. IA-2 and IA-2 beta are major autoantigens in IDDM and the precursors of the 40 kDa and 37 kDa tryptic fragments. *J Autoimmun* 1996;9:677-82.

[231] Ongangna JC, Levy-Marchal C. Sensitivity at diagnosis of combined β-cell autoantibodies in insulin-dependent diabetic children. *Diabetes & Metabolism* 1997;23:155-60.

[232] Onkamo P, Väänanen S, Karvonen M, Tuomilehto J. Worldwide increase in incidence of type 1 diabetes: the analysis of the data on published incidence trends. *Diabetologia* 1999;42:1395-1403.

[233] Otonkoski T, Rovainen M, Vaarala O, Dinesen B, Leipälä JA, Hovi T, et al. Neonatal type 1 diabetes associated with maternal echovirus 6 infection: a case report. *Diabetologia* 2000;43:1235-8.

[234] Ozawa Y, Kasuga A, Nomaguchi H, Maruyama T, Kasatani T, Shimada A, et al.Detection of autoantibodies to the pancreatic islet heat shock protein 60 in insulin-dependent diabetes mellitus. *J Autoimmun* 1996;9:517-24.

[235] Pak CY, Cha CY, Rajotte RV, McArthur RG, Yoon JW. Human pancreatic islet cell specific 38 kilodalton autoantigen identified by cytomegalovirus-induced monoclonal islet cell autoantibody. *Diabetologia* 1990;33:569–72.

[236] Palmer JP, Asplin CM, Clemons P, Lyen K, Tatpati O, Raghu PK, et al. Insulin antibodies in insulin-dependent diabetics before insulin treatment. *Science* 1983;222:133–9.

[237] Palmer JP. Latent autoimmune diabetes in adults (LADA) –Overview, epidemiology, current issues. *Diabetes Metabolism Research Reviews* 2001;17:S11.

[238] Palmer JP, Hirsch IB. Latent autoimmune diabetes or adults, type 1.5, adult-onset, and type 1 diabetes. *Diabetes Care* 2003;26:536-8.

[239] Park Y. Prediction of the risk of type 1 diabetes from polymorphisms in candidate genes. *Diab Res Clin Pract* 2004;66S:S19-S25.

[240] Park Y, Park H, Yoo E, Kim D. SOX13 autoantibodies are likely to be a supplementary marker for type 1 diabetes in Korea. *Am N Y Acad Sci* 2003;1005:253-8.

[241] Paronen J, Knip M, Savilahti E, Virtanen SM, Ilonen J, Akerblom HK, et al. Effect of cow's milk exposure and maternal type 1 diabetes on cellular and humoral immunization to dietary insulin in infants at genetic risk for type 1 diabetes. Finnish trial to reduce IDDM in the genetically at risk study group. *Diabetes* 2000;49:57-1665.

[242] Parslow RC, McKinney PA, Law GR, Bodansky HJ. Population mixing and childhood diabetes. *Int J Epidemiol* 2001;30:533-8.

[243] Patterson CC, Dahlquist G, Soltéz G, Green A. Is childhood-onset type 1 diabetes a wealth-related disease?. An ecological analysis of European incidence rates. *Diabetologia* 2001;44:B9-B16.

[244] Pérez-Bravo F, Oyarzun A, Carrasco E, Albala C, Dorman JS, Santos JL. Duration of breast feeding and bovine serum albumin antibody levels in type 1 diabetes: a case-control study. *Pediatr Diabetes* 2003;4:157-61.

[245] Petersen JS, Kyvic KO, Bingley PJ, Gale EAM, Green A, Dyrberg T, et al. Population based study of prevalence of islet cell antibodies in monozygotic and dizygotic Danish twins pairs with insulin-dependent diabetes mellitus. *BMJ* 1997; 314: 1575-1579.

[246] Pietropaolo M, Castaño L, Babu S, Buelow R, Kuo Y-LS, et al. Islet cell autoantigen 69 kD (ICA69): molecular cloning and characterization of a novel diabetes-associated autoantigen. *J Clin Invest* 1993;92:359–71.

[247] Pietropaolo M, Yu S, Lipman IM, Pietroapolo SL, Riley K, LaPorte RE, et al. Cytoplasmic islet cell antibodies remain valuable in defining risk of progression to type 1 diabetes in subjects with other islet autoantibodies. *Pediatr Diabetes* 2005;6:184-92.

[248] Pilcher C, Elliott RB. Improved sensitivity of islet cell cytoplasmic antibody assay in diabetics. *Lancet* 1984;1:1352.

[249] Pinkse GG, Tysma OH, Bergen CA, Kester MG, Ossendorp F, van Veelen PA, et al. Autoreactive CD8 T cells associated with beta cell destruction in type 1 diabetes. *Proc Natl Acad Sci USA* 2005;102:18425-30.

[250] Pitkäniemi J, Onkamo P, Tuomilehto J, Arjas E. Increasing incidence of type 1 diabetes- role for genes?. *BMC Genet* 2004;5:5.

[251] Portoukalian J, Rebbaa A, Thivolet C. Detection on thin layer plates of antibodies to human pancreatic fucogangliosides in the sera of type 1 diabetes patients. *Diabetologia* 1990;33:155A.

[252] Pozzilli P, Di Mario U. Autoimmune diabetes not requiring insulin at diagnosis (Latent Autoimmune Diabetes of the Adult): Definition, characterization and potential prevention. *Diabetes Care* 2001;24:1460-7.

[253] Previti M, Tiberti C, Dotta F, Lenti L, Pontieri GM, Andreani D,et al. Ganglioside characterization of human and rat pancreas: their role in endocrine autoimmunity. *J Endocrinol Invest* 1990;13:63.

[254] Pugliese A, Bugawan T, Moromisato R, Awdeh ZL, Alper CA, Jackson RA, et al. Two subsets of HLA-DQA1 alleles mark phenotypic variation in levels of insulin autoantibodies in first degree relatives at risk for insulin-dependent diabetes. *J Clin Invest* 1994;93:2447-52.

[255] Pugliese A, Eisenbarth GS. Type 1 diabetes mellitus of man: Genetic susceptibility and resistance. In: George S Eisenbarth, ed. *Immunology of type 1 diabetes*. New York: Eurekah.com and Kluwer Academic/ Plenum Publishers; 2004.p.170-203.

[256] PuglieseA, Gianani R, Moromisato R, Awdeh ZL, Alper CA, Erlich HA, Jackson RA, Eisenbarth GS. HLA-DQB1*0602 is associated with dominant protection from diabetes even among islet cell antibody-positive first-degree relatives of patients with IDDM. *Diabetes* 1995;44:608-13.

[257] Pundziute-Lycka A, Urbonaite B, Dahlquist G. Infections and risk of type 1 (insulin-dependent) diabetes mellitus in Lithuanian children. *Diabetologia* 2000;43:1229-34.

[258] Rabin DU, Pleasic SM, Shapiro JA, Yoo-Warren H, Oles J, Hicks JM, et al. Islet cell antigen 512 is a diabetes-specific islet autoantigen related to protein tyrosine phosphatases. *J Immunol* 1994;152:3183–8.

[259] Redondo MJ, Fain PR, Eisenbarth GS. Genetics of type 1A diabetes. *Recent Prog Horm Res* 2001;56:69-89.

[260] Redondo MJ, Fain PR, Krischer JP, Yu L, Cuthbertson D, Winter WE, et al. Expression of beta-cell autoimmunity does not differ between potential dizygotic twins and siblings of patients with type 1 diabetes. *J Autoimmun* 2004;23:275-9.

[261] Rewers M, Norris J, Dabelea D. Epidemiology of type 1 diabetes. In: George S Eisenbarth, ed. *Immunology of type 1 diabetes*. New York: Eurekah.com and Kluwer Academic/ Plenum Publishers; 2004.p.219-46.

[262] Riley WJ, Maclaren NK. Islet cell antibodies. In: Samols E, ed. *The Endocrine Pancreas*. New York: Raven Press; 1991.p.409-22.

[263] Riley WJ, Maclaren NK, Kricher J, Spillar RP, Silvertein JH, Schatz DA, et al.. A prospective study of the development of diabetes in relatives of patients with insulin-dependent diabetes. *N Engl J Med* 1990;323:1167-72.

[264] Roep BO, Atkinson MA, Van Endert PM, Gottlieb PA, Wilson SB, Sachs JA. Autoreactive T cell Responses in Insulin-dependent (Type 1) Diabetes Mellitus. Report of the First International Workshop for Standardization of T cell assays. *J Autoimmun* 1999;13:267-82.

[265] Ronningen KS, Atrazhev A, Luo L, Luo C, Smith DK, Korbutt G, et al. Anti-BSA antibodies do not cross-react with the 69-kDa islet autoantigen ICA69. *J Autoimmun* 1998;11:223-31.

[266] Ronningen KS, Keiding N, Green A on behalf of Genomic Marker Contributors and the EURODIAB ACE Study Group. Correlations between the incidences of childhood-onset type 1 diabetes in Europe and HLA genotypes. *Diabetologia* 2001;44:B51-B59.

[267] Rorsman F, Husebye ES, Winqvist O, Bjork E, Karlsson FA, Kampe O. Aromatic-L-amino-acid decarboxylase, a pyridoxal phosphate-dependent enzyme, is a beta-cell autoantigen. *Proc Natl Acad Sci USA* 1995;92:8626–9.

[268] Rulli M, Kuusisto A, Salo J, Kojola H, Simell O. Time-resolved fluorescence imaging in islet cell antibody quantitation. *J Immunol Methods* 1997;208:169-79.

[269] Sai P, Boitard C, Debray-Sachs M, Pouplard A, Assan R, Hamburger J. Complement-fixing islet cell antibodies from some diabetic patients alter insulin release in vitro. *Diabetes* 1981;30:1051–7.

[270] Sai P, Elmansour A, Audrian M, Chanbonnel B, Bardet S. Quantification of human cytoplasmic islet-cell antibodies which cross-react with mouse pancreas: a follow up study in type 1 (insulin-dependent) diabetic patients and first degree relatives. *Diabetologia* 1993;36:778-84.

[271] Schatz D, Krisher J, She JX. To screen or not to screen for pre-type 1diabetes? *Horm Res* 2002;57:12-17.

[272] Schimidli RS, DeAizpurua HJ, Harrison LC, Colman PG. Antibodies to glutamic acid decarboxylase in at-risk and clinical insulin-dependent diabetic subjects: relationship to age, sex and islet cell antibody status, and temporal profile. *J Autoimmun* 1994;7:55-66.

[273] Schlosser M, Strebelow M, Wassmuth R, Arnold Ml, Breuning I, Rjasanowski I, et al. The Kalsburg type 1 diabetes risk study of a normal schoolchild population: association of beta-cell autoantibodies and human leucocyte antigen-DQB1 alleles in antibody-positive individuals. *J Clin Endocrinol Metab* 2002;87:2254-61.

[274] Schott-Ohly P, Lgssiar A, Partke HJ, Hassan M, Friesen N, Gleichmann H. Prevention of spontaneous and experimental induced diabetes in mice with zinc sulfated-enriched drinking water is associated with activation and reduction of NF-Kappa B and AP-1 in islets, respectively. *Exp Biol Med* 2004;229:1177-85.

[275] Schranz DB, Lernmark A.. Immunology in Diabetes: An Update. Diabetes *Metabolism Reviews* 1998;14:3-29.

[276] Scott-Morgan L, Keller U, Heitz P, Mirza I, Diaz Jl, Casey C, et al. Insulin autoantiboides (IAA) may cause false positive islet cell antibody (ICA) results in the indirect inmunofluorescence test. *Diabetes Res* 1988;8:45-8.

[277] Seissler J, Sonnaville JJJ, Mongenthaler NG, Steinbrenner H, Glawe D, Khoo-Morgenthaler UY, et al. Immunological heterogeneity in type 1 diabetes: presence of distinct autoantibody patterns in patients with acute onset and slowly progressive disease. *Diabetologia* 1998;41:891-7.

[278] Sepa A, Wahlberg J, Vaarala O, Frodi A, Ludvigsson J. Psychological stress may induce diabetes-related autoimmunity in infancy. *Diabetes Care* 2005;28:290-5.

[279] Serrano-Rios M, Goday A, Martinez LT. Migrant populations and the incidence of type 1 diabetes mellitus: an overview of the literature with a focus on the Spanish-heritage countries in Latin America. *Diabetes Metab Res Rev* 1999;15:113-32.

[280] Service EJ, Rizza RA, Zimmerman BR, Dyck PJ, O'Brien PC, Melton III LJ. The classification of diabetes by clinical and C-peptide criteria. *Diabetes Care* 1997;20: 198-201.

[281] Shaltout AA, Moussa MA, Qabazard M, Abdella N, Karvonen M, Al-Khawari M, et al. Further evidence for the rising incidence of childhood Type 1 diabetes in Kuwait. *Diabet Med.* 2002;19:522-5.

[282] Skyler JS, Krischer JP, Woldsdorf J, Cowie C, Palmer JP, Greenbaum C, et al. Effect of oral insulin in relatives of patients with type 1 diabetes. The Diabetes Prevention Trial-Type 1. *Diabetes Care* 2005;28:1068-76.

[283] Staples JA, Ponsonby AL, Lim LLY, McMichael AJ. Ecologic analysis of some immune-related disorders, including type 1 diabetes, in Australia: latitude, regional ultraviolet radiation, and disease prevalence. *Environ Health Perspect* 2003;111:518-3.

[284] Steck AK, Bugawan TL, Valdes AM, Emery LM, Blair A, Norris JM, et al. Association of non-HLA genes with type 1 diabetes autoimmunity. *Diabetes* 2005;54:2482-6.

[285] Stene LC, Barriga K, Norris JM, Hoffman M, Erlich HA, Eisenbarth GS, et al. Perinatal factors and development of islet autoinmunity in early childhood: the diabetes autoimmunity study in the young. *Am J Epidemiol* 2004;160:3-10.

[286] Stene LC, Barriga K, Norris JM, Hoffman M, Klingensmith G, Erlich HA, et al. Symptoms of common maternal infections in pregnancy and risk of islet autoimmunity in early childhood. *Diabetes Care* 2003;26:3136-41.

[287] Stene LC, Joner G, Norwegian Childhood Diabetes Study Group. Use of cod liver oil during the first year of life is associated with lower risk of childhood-onset type 1 diabetes: a large population-based, case-control study. *Am J Clin Nutr* 2003;78:1128-34.

[288] Stenstrom G, Gottsater A, Bakhtadze E, Berger B, Sundkvist G. Latent autoimmune diabetes in adults: Definition, prevalence, {beta}-cell function, and treatment. *Diabetes* 2005;54:S68-S72.

[289] Strachan DP. Family size, infection and atopy: the first decade of the"hygiene hypothesis". *Thorax* 2000;55:S2-S10.

[290] Taniguchi T, Okazaki K, Okamoto M, Seko S, Uchida K, Seino Y. Presence of autoantibodies to carbonic anhidrase II and lactoferrin in type 1 diabetes: proposal of the concept of autoimmune exocrinopathy and endocrinopathy of the pancreas. *Diabetes Care* 2001;24:1695–6.

[291] The European Nicotinamide Diabetes Intervention Trial (ENDIT) Group, Gale EAM. Intervening before the onset of type 1 diabetes: baseline data from the European Nicotinamide Diabetes Intervention Trial (ENDIT). *Diabetologia* 2003;46:339-46.

[292] Thorsdottir I, Ramel A. Dietary intake of 10- to 16-years-old children and adolescents in central and northern of Europe and association with the incidence of type 1 diabetes. *Ann Nutr Metab* 2003;47:267-75.

[293] Tiberti C, Verrienti A, Fiore B, Yu L, Eisenbarth GS, Dotta F,et al. IA-2 combined epitope assay: a new, highly sensitive approach to evaluate IA-2 humoral autoimmunity in type 1 diabetes. *Clin Immunol* 2005;115:260-7.

[294] Tisch R, Wang B, Serreze DV. Induction of glutamic acid decarboxylase 65-specific Th2 cells and suppression of autoimmune diabetes at late stages of disease is epitope dependent. *J Immunol* 1999;163:1178-87.

[295] Tisch R, Yang X-D, Singer SM, Liblau RS, Fugger L, McDevitt HO. Immune response to glutamic acid decarboxylase correlates with insulitis in non-obese diabetic mice. *Nature* 1993;366:72-5.

[296] Toguchi Y, Ginsberg-Fellner F, Rubinstein P. Cytotoxic islet cell surface antibodies (ICSA) in patients with type 1 diabetes and their first-degree relatives. *Diabetes* 1983;35:855-60.

[297] Tuomi T, Carlsson A, Li H, Miettinen A, Nilsson A, Nissen M, et al. Clinical and genetic characteristics of type 2 diabetes with or without GAD antibodies. *Diabetes* 1999;48:150-7.

[298] Tuomi T, Groop LC, Zimmet PZ, Rowley MJ, Knowles W, Mackay IR. Antibodies to glutamic acid decarboxylase reveal latent autoimmune diabetes mellitus in adults with a non-insulin-dependent onset of disease. *Diabetes* 1993;42:359-62.

[299] Turner R, Stratton I, Horton V, Manley S, Zimmet P, Mackay IR, et al. UKPDS 25: autoantibodies to islet-cell cytoplasm and glutamic acid decarboxylase for prediction of insulin requirement in type 2 diabetes. UK Prospective Diabetes Study Group. *Lancet* 1997;350:1288-93.

[300] Vadhein CM, Rotter JJ. Genetics of diabetes mellitus. In: Alberti KGMN, ed. *International textbook of diabetes mellitus*. London: John Willey;1992.p.32-98.

[301] Van Der Winkel M, Smets G, Gepts W: Islet cell surface antibodies from insulin-dependent diabetics bind specifically to pancreatic cells. *J Clin Invest* 1982;70:41–9.

[302] Vantyghem MC, Fajardy I, Pigny P, Noel C, Kerr-Conte J, Gmyr V, et al. Kinetics of diabetes associated-antibodies after sequential intraportal islet allograft associated with kidney transplantation in type 1 diabetes. *Diabetes Metab* 2003;29:595-601.

[303] Vardi P, Brik R, Barzilai D. Insulin autoantibodies: reflection of disturbed self-identification and their use in the prediction of type I diabetes. *Diabetes/Metabolism Reviews* 1991;7:209-22.

[304] Vardi P, Dib SA, Tuttleman M, Connelly JE, Grinbergs M, Rabizadeh A, et al. Competitive insulin autoantibody RIA: Prospective evaluation of subjects at high risk for development of type I Diabetes mellitus. *Diabetes* 1987;36:1286-9.

[305] Verbeke S, Cruchet S, Gotteland M, Rios G, Hunter B, Chavez E, et al. Risk markers for insulin-dependent diabetes mellitus and duration of exposure to gluten in celiac patients. *Rev Med Chil* 2004;132:979-84.

[306] Verge CF, Gianani R, Kawasaki E, Yu L, Pietropaolo M, Chase HP, et al. Number of autoantibodies (against insulin, GAD or ICA512/IA2) rather than particular autoantibody specificities determines risk of type I diabetes. *J Autoimmun* 1996;9:379-83.

[307] Verge CF, Stenger D, Bonifacio E, Colman PG, Pilcher C, Bingley PJ, et al. Combined use of autoantibodies (IA2 autoantibody, GAD autoantibody, insulin autoantibody, cytoplasmic islet cell autoantibodies) in type 1 diabetes. Combinatorial islet autoantibody workshop. *Diabetes* 1998;47:1857-66.

[308] Vidal J, Fernández-Balsells M, Sesmilo G, Aguilera E, Casamitjana R, Gomis R, et al. Effects of nicotinamide and intravenous insulin therapy in newly diagnosed type 1 diabetes. *Diabetes Care* 2000;23:360-4.

[309] Virtanen SM, Knip M. Nutritional risk predictors of ß cell autoimmunity and type 1 diabetes at a young age. *Am J Clin Nutr* 2003;78:1053-67.

[310] Virtanen SM, Läärä E, Hyppönen E, Reijonen H, Rasanen L, Aro A, et al. Cow´s milk consumption, HLA-DQß1 genotype and type 1 diabetes: a nested case-control study of siblings of children with diabetes. *Diabetes* 2000;49:912-7.

[311] Virtanen SM, Rasanen L, Aro A, Ylonen K, Lounamaa R, Akerblom HK, et al. Is Children´s or parents´ coffee or tea consumption associated with the risks for type 1 diabetes mellitus in children?. *Eur J Clin Nutr* 1994;48:279-85.

[312] Viskari H, Ludvigsson J, Uibo R, Salur L, Marciulionyte D, Hermann R, et al. Relationship between the incidence of type 1 diabetes and enterovirus infections in different European populations: Results from the EPIVIR project. *J Med Virol* 2004;72:610-7.

[313] Weintrop N, Sprecher E, Israel S, Pinhas-Hamiel O, Joong Kwon O, Bloch K, et al. Type 1 environmental factors and correspondence analysis of HLA class II genes in the Yemenite Jewish community in Israel. *Diabetes Care* 2001;24:650-3.

[314] Williams AJ, Bingley PJ, Bonifacio E, Palmer JP, Gale EA. A novel micro-assay for insulin autoantibodies. *J Autoimmun* 1997;10:473-8.

[315] Williams AJK, Bingley PJ, Moore WPT, Gale EAM and the ENDIT Screening group. Islet autoantibodies, nationality, and gender: a multinational screening study in first-degree relatives of patients with type 1 diabetes. *Diabetologia* 2002;45:217-23.

[316] Winter WE, Harris N, Schatz D. Immunological markers in the diagnosis and prediction of autoimmune type 1a diabetes. *Clin Diabetes* 2002;20:183-191.

[317] Yamashiro Y, Taniguchi H, Baba S, Taniguchi T, Aono S, Isshiki G, et al. Heterogeneity of human islet cell antibodies in terms of cross-species reactivity. *Diabetes Res and Clin Pract* 1990;8:13-18.

[318] Yanagisawa K, Uchigata Y, Sanaka M, Sakura H, Minei S, Kanamuro R, et al. Mutation in the mitochondrial tRNA(leu) at position 3243 and spontaneous abortions in japanese women attending a clinic for pregnancies. *Diabetologia* 1995;38:809-15.

[319] Yu L, Eisenbarth GS. Humoral autoimmunity. In: George S Eisenbarth, ed. *Immunology of type 1 diabetes*. New York: Eurekah.com and Kluwer Academic/ Plenum Publishers; 2004.p.247-267

[320] Yu L, Cuthbertson DD, Maclaren N, Jackson R, Palmer JP, Orban T, et al. Expression of GAD65 and islet cell antibody (ICA512) autoantibodies among cytoplasmic ICA+

relatives is associated with eligibility for the diabetes prevention trial-type 1. *Diabetes* 2001;50:1735-40.

[321] Zeidler A, Raffel LJ, Costin G, Shaw SJ, Buchanan TA, Noble J, et al. Autoantibodies and human leucocyte antigen class II in first-degree family members of Mexican-American type 1 diabetic patients. *J Clin Endocrinol Metab* 2001;86:4957-62.

[322] Ziegler AG, Hummel M, Shenker M, Bonifacio E. Autoantibody appearance and risk for development of childhood diabetes in offspring of parents with type 1 diabetes: the 2-year analysis of the German BABYDIAB Study. *Diabetes* 1999;48:460-8.

[323] Ziegler AG, Scmid S, Huber D, Hummel M, Bonifacio E. Early infant feeding and risk of developing-associated autoantibodies. *JAMA* 2003;290:1721-2.

[324] Ziegler R, Alper CA, Awdeh ZL, Castaño L, Brink SJ, Soeldner JS, et al. Specific association of HLA-DR4 with increased prevalence and level of insulin autoantibodies in first-degree relatives of patients with type I diabetes. *Diabetes* 1991;48:709-14.

[325] Ziegler AG, Dumont-Herskowitz R, Jackson RA, Soeldner JS, Einsenbarth GS. Predicting of type 1 diabetes. *Diabetes Care* 1990;13:762-75.

[326] Zimmet PZ, Tuomi T, Mackay IR, Rowley MJ, Knowles W, Cohen M, et al. Latent autoimmune diabetes mellitus in adults (LADA): the role of antibodies to glutamic acid decarboxylase in diagnosis and prediction of insulin dependency. *Diabetic Medicine* 1994;11:299-303.

Chapter II

HUMAN ENTEROVIRUS INFECTIONS

Luis Sarmiento-Pérez*

Department of Virology, PAHO/WHO Collaborating Center for Viral Diseases, "Pedro Kouri" Tropical Medicine Institute, Havana, Cuba.

ABSTRACT

The study of picornaviruses in all its aspects has been of major significance for the development .of virology. The enteroviruses, so called because most inhabit the alimentary (enteric) tract, comprise one of the most important members of human patogens. This chapter provides a state-of-the-art review of basic science, biology, clinical manifestation, epidemiology and diagnosis of infections with enterovirus. The use of the knowledge on enteroviruses may clarify the pathogenesis of virus-induced autoimmune diseases.

Keywords: enterovirus, biology, pathogenesis, clinical manifestation, epidemiology, diagnosis.

I. BIOLOGICAL CHARACTERISTICS

The enteroviruses form a genus within the family Picornaviridae (Pico meaning small; rna, RNA genome; viridae, viruses). Like all picornaviruses, the enteroviruses are small and icosahedral RNA viruses with a diameter of about 30 nm. The enteroviruses are nonenveloped viruses that possess a single-stranded, positive (messenger)-sense RNA genome that is approximately 7500 nucleotide in length [192,209]. The enteroviral genome is

* Correspondence concerning this article should be addressed to Luis Sarmiento Pérez, Department of Virology, PAHO/WHO Collaborating Center for Viral Diseases, "Pedro Kouri" Tropical Medicine Institute, Autopista Novia del Mediodía, km 6, PO Box, 601, Marianao 13, Havana, Cuba; fax: 53-7-2046051; email: sarmiento@ipk.sld.cu or lsarmientop@yahoo.com.

organized into the 5'nontranslated region (5'NTR) which is covalently linked to a small viral protein, VPg, a polyprotein coding region, a shorter 3´ NTR, and a terminal polyadenylic tail [74,107,125]. The viral coding region can be subdivided into P1, P2, and P3 regions. The P1 region encodes 4 structural proteins (VP1-4) that comprise the enteroviral capsid, while the P2 and P3 regions encode 7 nonstructural proteins [121,191]. The picornavirus capsid is made up of 60 identical building units, each containing one copy of the four structural proteins VP1-VP4. VP1 to VP3 are partially exposed on the virion surface, while VP4 is completely internalized in infectious virions [126,157]. The folding pattern of polypeptides VP1-VP3 is similar, resulting in an eight-stranded antiparallel B-barrel structure and two α helices interconnected by loops. The carboxy termini and many of the interconnecting loops are exposed at the capsid surface, whereas the amino termini of these proteins are located inside the capsid in association with protein VP4 [39,72,128].

Different parts of the genome have different functions and the rate of their evolution reflects this fact. The noncoding regions contain sequences that are recognized by the host cell ribosomal subunits as well as factors playing a role in the replication of the genome [4,183]. These specific motifs are highly conserved whereas, for instance, a sequence 100 nt long, preceding the initiation codon, shows extensive variation [5,197,224]. On the other hand, the external capsid proteins are subjected to the pressure caused by host antibodies and exhibit notable variation in length and sequence of the loop structures connecting the B-sheets. Several important functions have mapped to the structural proteins. The capsid proteins, which form the surface of the virion, contain the major antigen epitopes. VP1 carries major neutralization epitopes among the capsid protein, although the actual sites may cover VP2 and/or VP3 [28,89,146]. Determinants of attenuation of virulence [159,160,193], virion thermostability [157], altered host range [53], in vitro cell tropism [133], persistent infection [29,182], and plaque morphology [194,251] have also been mapped to the capsid-encoding region.

Non structural proteins are essential for the enterovirus life cycle because are involved in protein processing and genome replication. Protein 2A (chymotrypsin-like protease) catalyses the cleavage between VP1/2A and frees the P1 structural protein precursor from the rest of the polypeptide chain [236]. Protein P2B plays unknown role in RNA synthesis, induces cell membrane permeability and partly responsible for proliferation of membranous vesicles [109,227]. Protein P2C is highly conserved in the enteroviruses, which functions in the replication of viral RNA and possibly in the stabilization of virion structure [22,210]. Point mutations in the region of the genome which codes for the P2C protein have been identified in enteroviruses resistant to (able to replicate in the presence of) guanidinium chloride and with defective RNA synthesis [184]. Protein 3AB is a precursor of 3B, the small polypeptide covalently named VPg linked to the 5´NTR of picornavirus RNA molecules [73,80,81]. Protein 3C (chymotrypsin-like serine protease), sometimes in the form of its precursor 3CD, is responsible for the primary cleavage of P2 from P3 (between 2C and 3A) and secondary cleavage of P1 and P2 polyproteins [92,93] while 3D is the RNA-dependent RNA polymerase [73,239].

The infectious particles are relative heat resistant (when stabilized by magnesium cations), resistant to many common detergents and disinfectants including common soap, nonionic detergents, ether, chloroform, and other lipid solvents. The virus is stable for weeks at $4^{O}C$ and for days at room temperature. Drying, ultraviolet light, high heat, formaldehyde, and free chlorine, however, readily inactivate the virus. The lack of a lipid envelope contributes to the structural stability of the enteroviruses, permitting the virus to survive the gastric pH and environmental stresses [1,2,65].

II. CLASSIFICATION

The taxonomy for enteroviruses have changed several times since the isolation of an animal virus associated with foot-and-mouth disease in 1898 [136]. Based on their ability to replicate in cells of human and primate origin, infectivity and pathogenicity in different animal species, and antigenic differences, human enteroviruses were originally subgrouped into the Poliovirus (PV), the group A coxsackievirus (CVA), the group B coxsackievirus (CVB) and echoviruses (E) [149].

Poliovirus was first identified in 1909 by inoculation of specimens into monkeys. These were the first viruses to be propagated in cell cultures in 1949 [70]. In 1948, a new group of agents were recognized by inoculation into newborn mice from two children with paralytic disease. These agents were named coxsackieviruses, referring to the first geographical site of isolation [59]. Coxsackieviruses A and B were identified on the basis of the histopathological changes they produced in newborn mice [54,152]. In 1951, with the advent of tissue culture techniques, a third group that produced cytopathic changes in cell culture and was nonpathogenic for newborn mice and non-human primates were recovered. The name echovirus was chosen because their association with human disease was, at the time of their discovery, unknown (ECHO: Enteric, Cytopathogenic, Human, Orphan=no associated disease) [50]. The value of these distinctions has to some extent been diminished by the availability of cell lines permissive for a wider range of enteroviruses and by the intrinsic variability of biological phenotypes observed among naturally occurring enterovirus strains [163]. Since 1970, newly identified serotypes have not been assigned to the above groups but, rather, have been numerically classified as enterovirus serotypes (EV) 68 to 71. Thus, through serotype - specific antisera the genus enterovirus were further classified into 64 serotypes [158] (Table 1A).

The introduction of diagnostic procedures based on nucleic acid sequences in particular polimerase chain reaction increased the need for precise classification of viruses in accordance with their molecular characteristics [11,62,100,103,124,171,177,190,222]. Based on the later type of analysis all human enterovirus were reclassified on the basis of the nucleotide and deduced aminoacid sequence into 5 groups of human viruses [120,189]. Human enterovirus A includes 12 serotypes, predominantly coxsackievirus A- serotypes in the previous classification scheme. Human enterovirus B includes 36 serotypes, predominantly echoviruses and coxsackievirus B-serotypes. Human enterovirus C includes 11 serotypes, predominantly coxsackievirus A serotype. Human enterovirus D includes two serotypes, enterovirus 68 and enterovirus 70. The fifth subgroup, poliovirus, includes the three serotypes previously classified as such [120] (Table 1B). Moreover, the number of enterovirus serotypes is increasing as the new phylogenetic serotype identification is revealing new serotypes among the previously "non-typable" strains by classical identification methods. Molecular methods have enabled the rapid identification of new enterovirus serotypes such as EV73, EV74, EV75, EV76, EV77, EV78, EV89, EV90 and EV91. The identification of these new types suggests that there may be many other additional enterovirus serotypes awaiting identification (178).

Table 1. Human enterovirus genera.

A. Classification on the basis of serotype-specific antisera

Virus	Antigenic types	Number of serotypes
Polioviruses	1-3	3
Coxsackievirus, group A	1-24 [a]	23
Coxsackievirus, group B	1-6	6
Echoviruses	1-34 [b]	28
Enteroviruses	68-71.	4

B. Classification on the basis of molecular properties

Species	Antigenic types	Number of serotypes
Polioviruses	1-3	3
Human Enterovirus A	CVA2-A8, A10, A12, A14, A16, EV71	12
Human Enterovirus B	CVB1-B6, CVA9, E1-E33[b], EV69.	36
Human Enterovirus C	CVA1, CVA11, CVA13,CVA15, CVA17-CVA22[a], CVA24	11
Human Enterovirus D	EV68, EV 70	2

[a] Coxsackievirus A type 23 turns out to be serologically closely related to echovirus 9
[b] Echovirus 8 was determined to be the same serotype as a reovirus 1, echovirus 22 y 23 as parechovirus types 1 and 2, echovirus 28 as human rinovirus 1A, and echovirus 34 as coxsackievirus A24.
Data are from reference [181].

III. Epidemiology

Enteroviruses have a worldwide distribution. In tropical and semitropical regions, they are widely distributed throughout the year. In temperate climates, the highest rates of enteroviral infection occur during the summer and fall and they are present at low levels in winter and spring. Some outbreaks of enterovirus infections have continued from fall into winter months; winter outbreaks have been recorded, but they are rare. Climate appears to be an important factor in the circulation and prevalence of enterovirus. Warm weather favors the spread of virus by increasing human contacts, and the susceptibility of the host, or the dissemination of the virus by extrahuman sources [147,170].

Enteroviruses are generally considered to be obligate parasite of humans, and that is depending on human transmission for their persistence in nature. No enteroviruses have been isolated from non-primates in nature. Experimental poliovirus infections in non-human primates were used extensively in the early studies on poliovirus infection and have revealed that chimpanzees and some monkeys are susceptible to oral poliovirus infection, but to a lesser degree than humans. The low densities of such higher primate populations in the wild, their lower susceptibility to poliovirus infections, and the lack of evidence for a persistent carrier state, suggest that these animals are unlikely to sustain endemic transmission of poliovirus [66].

The enteroviruses are transmitted by both fecal-oral and respiratory routes and remain viable for prolonged periods in sewage, water, fomites, and on hands, thereby enhancing their transmissibility. Fecal-oral transmission may predominate in areas with poor sanitary conditions and is the classic mode of enterovirus spread and probably explain patterns of spread in developing countries, whereas respiratory transmission may be important in more developed areas. Respiratory transmission-acquisition might include either aerosol spread or spread via direct contact with respiratory secretion. Respiratory spread may result from passage of viruses from the bloodstream into the saliva or from virus replication in upper respiratory tract tissues during early phase of infection [181].

Understanding environmental factors controlling enteric virus survival and transport in nature could be a key to understanding the maintenance of infections within a population. Environmental conditions can greatly affect the survival and transport of viruses in nature, and there are numerous route by which excreted virus may find its way back to the human host. Survival is adversely affected by low relative humidity, low moisture content, high temperature, low pH, low organic content and high bacterial growth. Differential environmental survival associated with seasonal changes in temperature and humidity may explain the seasonality associated with the prevalence of natural enterovirus infections [71,167].

The largest amount and duration of virus shedding occurs on primary infection with a given enterovirus serotype. Infants and young children make up substantial portion of the enterovirus-susceptible population, because they still lack the repertoire of antibodies acquired by repeated exposures to enterovirus during early childhood [84,104]. Further, the large number of susceptible children, as well as the nonhygienic behavior common to this age group, favors transmission among young children. For these reasons, children are the prime targets of these viruses and thus serve as the chief vehicle for their spread [165,180]. In warmer lands and in families living under unsanitary and poor socioeconomic conditions in temperate zones, children are infected very early in life, and more than 90% may have already experienced infections with a number of the locally prevalent enterovirus before the age of 5 years. When the infections are delayed to older childhood and young adult life, the incidence and frequency of the more severe manifestations of the enterovirus infections rises.

More individuals may escape infection as young children, only to experience more serious clinical manifestations if they become infected in later childhood or adulthood [96].

The close correlation between low socioeconomic settings and the early acquisition of infection with the enterovirus has been repeatedly emphasized in both tropical and temperate environments and reflects the general level of hygiene of the group. The frequency of severe disease associated with enterovirus infections may increase as levels of hygiene and sanitation improve [108].

The best example to illustrate that transmission of enterovirus infections is influenced by different socio-economic factors is the poliovirus experience. Poliovirus infections used to be endemic but their frequency decreased rapidly towards the end of the 19th century, as the standard of living improved. Until then poliovirus infections were frequent but their clinical picture was usually mild and paralytic complications were rare. However, when the rate of infections decreased the incidence of paralytic disease increased paradoxically. At the same time, a drift in the age distribution of this disease to include adults occurred and an increase in the severity of the disease in older person was observed. The basis of this phenomenon are explicable today: Under poor sanitary conditions, nearly everyone became infected during childhood- the development of the paralytic form of the disease being rare – and thus usually acquired a life long immunity against infection by poliovirus. In contrast, under improved sanitary conditions, some children were not exposed to polioviruses until later in childhood when they were no more protected by maternal antibodies and thus were more severely affected by the infection. For this same reason, the risk of paralytic complication was much higher in countries where poliovirus infections were rare (e.g. U.S.) compared to countries where they were common (e.g. Egypt) [97,175,188].

Within a given geographic locality, some serotypes may be endemic, with little or only gradual change in the range of serotypes present from year to year. The local serotype (constantly circulating among the few non immunes) are most likely to affect infants or children early in life, since virtually the older children and adults already have protective antibody from previous infections. In contrast, other serotypes follow an epidemic mode of transmission, causing large outbreaks and then becoming quiescent for a period of several years. The agent goes through cycles of varying length [168]. For a period of a year or more, it circulates widely throughout a population, in a wave of spread that reaches a large proportion of the susceptibles. With a longer period between waves of such infection, more persons reach a later age before their initial exposure to the agent, a large population of susceptibles again builds up, and the new cycles of infections may reach the magnitude of an epidemic or even pandemic. Older children and adults are more likely to predominate in an outbreak of a serotype that has not been present in a community for several years, creating a reservoir of susceptibles among children born since the last appearance of that serotype. Dissemination of different serotypes may thus occur in waves, with one predominant type in an area succeeding another from one year to the next or even within the same summer-fall season [169].

Among the many enterovirus serotypes that cycle year to year, certain serotypes are more commonly associated with clinical disease than others. The factors influencing enterovirus prevalence are poorly understood but may include duration of serotype-specific immunity, efficiency of transmission, ease of isolation, serotype predilection for causing clinical disease, as well as changing in reporting laboratories and possibly strain tissue – tropism [52,75,91,176,180,228,230]. It is clear that tissue-tropism varies among the enterovirus serotypes. The determinants of tissue – tropism are now being studied in hope of finding a genomic explanation for the increased frequency of clinical diseases observed with certain serotypes and the virtual absence of that disease with others [94]. It is notable that, although certain enteroviruses have been more frequently responsible for epidemics involving a specific syndrome, the same serotypes may at other times and in other places be associated with sporadic infections having different clinical manifestations or producing no symptoms [181].

The results of investigations in Cuba on circulation of enterovirus in meningitis patients clearly indicate a marked difference in the yearly prevalence pattern of enterovirus types. Some serotypes follow an endemic mode of transmission, with little or only gradual change in the range of serotypes present from year to year. In contrast, other serotypes follow an epidemic mode of transmission, causing large outbreaks and then becoming quiescent for a period of several years. From 1972 to 2004, nine large meningitis outbreaks caused by an enterovirus occurred: echovirus 4 (1972 and 1985-86), coxsackievirus B5 (1976 and 1995), coxsackievirus A9 (1990-1991), echovirus 30 (1994 and 2001), echovirus 9 (1999), echovirus 16 (2000). Other enteroviruses (coxsackievirus and numerous echoviruses) were identified from sporadic cases of viral meningitis during nonepidemic periods. Over the 30-year period echovirus 6 and echovirus 11 were isolated in 9 and 8 years, respectively. Therefore, these serotypes were considered as endemic types in Cuba [12,142,214,215]. The epidemic types had large fluctuations in the yearly number of isolates. The above-mentioned serotypes generally continue to be commonly reported in other part of the world, although in any single year their predominance may be more marked, and distribution of different serotype appears to vary between different countries [33,34,166,230]. It is remarkable that echovirus 16 emerged as a predominant strain of enterovirus associated with aseptic meningitis in Cuba in 2000. The epidemic shifted temporarily and geographically and elevated frequency of echovirus 16 isolation was limited to Cuba. However, it should be noted echovirus 13 widespread dissemination was reported in U.S. Europe and Asia during 2000, when echovirus 13 was associated for the first time with outbreaks of aseptic meningitis in different countries [35,36,42,51,63,77,113,138,173,226,238].

Although the enteroviruses as a group are ubiquitous and not normally considered as "emerging pathogens," this data compilation suggests the many different serotypes circulate at different frequencies in any given year and the prevalence of a given serotype may fluctuate wildly from year to year. Apart from E16 and E13, several enterovirus serotypes have been associated with the emergence of specific diseases (for example, pandemic acute hemorrhagic conjunctivitis) and specific serotypes have emerged to cause outbreaks of major public health concern. Enterovirus 71 is a recognized cause of epidemic severe central nervous system disease in Southeast Asia. Acute hemorrhagic conjunctivitis was a newly described disease in the 1970s associated with emergence of enterovirus 70 and coxsackievirus A24 variant. In addition, the impending eradication of poliovirus and some of the challenges currently faced by the eradication program present the possibility that poliomyelitis could emerge in the posteradication era (179).

The emergence of viral infections in areas where they were previously unknown is a problem that is faced in almost every area on earth. The emergence of novel viral infections is becoming an increasingly prominent problem due to the rapid globalization of society. Increased commerce and travel afford fantastic opportunities for viruses to reach new areas and cause infections. A number of other possibilities have been proposed as being at the origin of such emergences: 1) changes in human demographics and behaviour, 2) breakdown of public health capacity required for infectious diseases at the local, state, national, and global levels, and 3) microbial adaptation and change (a factor that makes infectious diseases unique and particularly challenging). This last approach is remarkable in RNA viruses. Unlike other types of infectious agents, RNA viruses have proven difficult to control partly because of their great diversity and capacity for rapid evolution [215].

IV. Molecular Epidemiology

It has been postulated that all enterovirus serotypes pathogenic in man originate from a common ancestor, and have differentiated with mutations and recombination as fuel of evolution. Enteroviruses, like other RNA viruses, have a high mutation rate due to the lack of proofreading activity during genome replication [61,64,67,245]. Virus genome evolves rapidly during replication in humans; and populations of excreted enteroviruses can be highly heterogeneous. Thus, enterovirus populations exist as a quasispecies, a mixture of genetic microvariants with a vast potential to adapt to new environments [115]. It has been estimated that approximately one mutation is generated per newly synthesized genome [67]. In addition to mutations, recombination is involved in enterovirus evolution. Homologous recombination, which is considered to take place copy choice, has been demonstrated between vaccine poliovirus-and wild-type origin. Natural recombination among variants derived from single infecting strains is presumably even more frequent. Other phylogenetic analysis of complete enterovirus genome provided evidence suggesting that recombination also occurs between other enteroviruses and that intraspecies recombination is a relatively frequent event in the evolution of enterovirus genomes [31,78,119,195,252]. Indeed, the recent appearance of outbreaks associated with circulating vaccine-derived poliovirus (cVDPV) in countries using oral poliovirus vaccine at low rates of coverage have been vaccine/nonvaccine recombinants having some or all of their noncapsid sequences derived from species C human enteroviruses.

The high mutation rate of enterovirus enables detailed molecular epidemiological studies based on comparison of relatively short regions of the genome. A short nucleotide sequence at the junction of the capsid and nonstructural proteins has been extensively used in molecular epidemiological studies of poliovirus, resulting in a large sequence database [213].

Sequence comparisons of poliovirus isolates have revealed the existence of numerous genotypes endemic to different regions of the world. The term " genotype", which is defined as a cluster of genetically related viruses with less than 15% nucleotide divergence across the 150 nucleotide sequence, has been used for discrimination of genetic lineages of poliovirus, whereas less than 2% nucleotide divergence between strains has been considered to indicate direct epidemiological linkage [115,195]. The definitions make epidemiological sense, but there is no theoretical justification for the choice of 85 % sequence identity. The concept of a genotype is certainly similar for other enterovirus serotypes. However, the genetic diversity of different serotypes is considerable (i.e. much less diversity for enterovirus 70 and enterovirus 71 [26] compared to echovirus 30 [176]). Each serotype may contain several distinct genotypes. Within each serotype, the independent genotypes usually show a distinct geographical distribution and some genotypes are more widely distributed than others [115,134,195].

A lineage is very linked to the period of time over which the isolates are compared. A lineage could be defined as those isolates that have less difference than the numbers of years that separate the isolates. It is well known that enterovirus strains occurring in a country may comprise diverse genetic lineages within a given serotype and that the composition may show time – dependent changes. For each serotype, several lineages may survive and circulate simultaneously in different parts of the world or even within a single country [115,117].

Molecular epidemiological investigation has been used to estimate the date of emergence of newly arising enterovirus serotypes or strains [162,232] and to study their subsequent molecular evolution and global spread [25,106,116,131,132], to confirm the common source of isolates from a single enterovirus outbreak [62,68,201] and study their genetic relationship to strains from previous outbreaks [30,105,124], and to identify cocirculating strains of a single serotype [99].

V. Pathogenesis and Immunity

The entry route of enteroviruses into the body is usually the upper respiratory or gastrointestinal mucosa. Initially, virus traverses epithelial lining cells and replicates in the initial sites of virus implantation namely, Peyer's patches and tonsils. Virus then multiplies in deep cervical and mesenteric lymph nodes, leading to a minor (primary) viremia with subsequent invasion of systemic reticuloendothelial tissues, including lymph nodes, bone marrow, liver, and spleen. The infection may remain local resulting in an asymptomatic infection and virus begins to appear in the throat and in the feces and consequently, enterovirus infected individuals excrete the virus into the faeces for several weeks leading to virus shedding into the environment. From the mucosa, the virus can enter blood circulation major (secondary) viremia via the lymphatics, and then reach the various target organ (central nervous system, liver, myocardium, skin, pancreas, joints, lungs, mucous membrane, skeletal muscle, etc), where further replication occur. Most individuals control infection prior to the major viremia. Organ-specific symptom may occur later during the course of infection [40,147,206]. If clinical disease does occur, symptoms typically begin at about day 3 and their peak coincides with the peak of viremia, although the time of onset of symptom varies from 2 days to several weeks after exposure. It is not clear if and how this incubation period varies among the various enterovirus serotypes. The reason why some individuals exhibit a higher susceptibility to the virus than others is still largely a mystery. Several factors may increase susceptibility: previous immune status, immune deficiency restricted to some strains, higher pathogenic potency of mutants, genetic HLA constitution and/ or hormonal interactions with viral multiplication [204].

The major determinant of the tissue tropism of enterovirus is presumed to be the appropriate cellular receptor. The first step in viral infection is the attachment of the virus to its receptor, a cell surface molecule which viruses have adapted to gain entry into the cell. Receptors are also considered to be key determinants in tissue tropism of viruses. To date several cell surface receptors are know for enteroviruses, among them members of the integrin and immunoglobulin superfamilies normally involved in cell adhesion [159]. Three serotypes of poliovirus use poliovirus receptor (PVR), a member of the immunoglobulin superfamily and members of the human enterovirus C use intercellular adhesion molecule-1 [220]. Integrin $\alpha v\beta 3$, also known as the vitronectin receptor, works as a receptor for coxsackievirus A9 [199] and other arginine-glycine-aspartic acid motifs (RGD) containing enteroviruses [229], whereas another integrin, $\alpha 2\beta 1$ works as a receptor for echovirus 1 [18]. In addition, a complement regulatory protein, i.e. decay-accelerating factor (DAF), and a protein called human coxsackievirus and adenovirus receptor (HCAR) are used for cellular entry by coxsackieviruses and several enteroviruses [15,16,17,219,233].

Expression of a cellular receptor is a prerequisite for infection, but this is not the only factor determining tissue susceptibility. The function of these receptors in viral entry is not understood in detail and it is possible that additional host factors are needed for complete entry [186].

Binding of the virus to its receptor initiates the viral replicative cycle. The binding to the receptor triggers conformational changes in the capsid structure that are necessary for the release of the genoma into the cellular cytoplasm, where the replication occurs. The viral genome acts as messenger RNA for the synthesis of a large poliprotein which is cleaved to generate the structural and non structural protein of the virion. The viral RNA is copied into negative sense RNA, which acts as template for the synthesis of viral genomic RNA. The newly synthesized viral RNA is covalently linked to the VPg protein at the 5′end of the RNA and then only the positive sense strand of RNA is encapsided in the viral structural protein to form infectious viral particles. Enterovirus replication induces various morphological changes in the host cell, broadly termed the cytopathic effect: shrinkage of the nucleus and accumulation of membranous vesicles in the cytoplasm. The metabolic alterations mediating this cytophatic effect include inhibition of the host cell protein synthesis and redistribution of lysosomal enzymes, and changes in plasma membrane permeability. Aproximately $10^4 - 10^5$ infectious virus particles are produced in one infected cell which is finally destroyed allowing the virus to be released to infect new target cell. Lytic infection is the usual form of enterovirus infection, but also non-lytic and chronic infections in specific cell line are known [192]. The genetic heterogeneity of enteroviral quasispecies population enable new variants to be tested after each round of replication, and selective pressure can lead to the evolution of variants with altered pathogenic properties such as virulence, tissue specificity, and host range [64].

Experimental evidences indicate that enteroviral infections is generally characterized by cell destruction and tissue injury, which is frequently associated with the local presence of immune cell infiltrates. It has been assumed that virus-induced disease is a consequence of this tissue damage, which has been recognized as the "classic" hallmarks of virus infection. However, it is now clear that many RNA and DNA viruses can establish persistent infections in the absence of lymphoid cell infiltrate and/or lysis of virally infected cells. Enterovirus that are usually lytic overcome this drawback by either regulating their gene expression, generating variants with nonlytic phenotypes or, generating deletion mutants termed defective interfering particles that posses the ability to modulate the virulence and the pathogenesis of the wild type virus [49,82,98,196,208,234].

Enterovirus infections induce both cell-mediated and humoral response. Normal humoral immune responses to enterovirus infections result in the rapid production of antiviral immunoglobulin (IgM) and then IgG and IgA [13]. Antienteroviral IgM normally persists for less than 6 months, but IgA and IgG to enteroviruses can persist for years. IgM titers have been used to predict recent or ongoing infection with enterovirus. The frequency of the antienteroviral IgA and IgG seems to increase with age, suggesting an influence of anammestic enterovirus infections [83,172,237]. It is widely accepted that neutralizing-antibody titers against enteroviruses in the mucosa and circulation, provide life-long protection against enterovirus- induced diseases and restriction of the spread of infection. Transplacentally transported maternal IgG as well as maternal IgA in breast milk can provide passive humoral immunity [250].

The exact importance of T cell mediated immunity to enterovirus and its role in viral clearance and protection from re-infection is not known. The main role of the cellular immune response resides in the elimination of primary infection and regulation of the immune response. T cells may have a role in providing help for the B-cell humoral immune response, which plays a critical role in the clearance of enteroviruses. In addition, cytolytic T cells may clear the virus directly by causing lysis of virus-infected cells or by means of cytokine release [237].

VI. Clinical Manifestations

Large proportions of the enterovirus infections are subclinical and do not reach the attention of a physician. For all members of the group, however, subclinical infection is far more common than clinical manifest disease [181]. Symptomatic infection is usually a non-specific febrile illness lasting several days, often accompanied by upper respiratory symptoms [58]. Rarely, other syndromes occur, such as 1) respiratory disease (e.g. common cold, pharyngitis, herpangina, stomatitis, pneumonia, and pleurodynia) [45,88,243], 2) gastrointestinal disease (e.g. vomiting, diarrhea, abdominal pain) [41], 3) eye disease (e.g. acute hemorrhagic conjunctivitis) [8,14,21,79,95,123,130,161], 4) heart disease (e.g. miocarditis and pericarditis) [87,118], 5) skin disease (e.g. a wide array of rashes and hand, foot, and mouth disease) [198,243], 6) neurological disease (e.g. aseptic meningitis, encephalitis and paralysis) [20,55,145,204,205] (Table 2).

Thus, a multiplicity of factors has to be taken into account when the frequency and type of symptomatic enteroviral infections are being considered. These factors are divided into three main categories: (i) factors associated with the virus, i.e., serotype, strain, virulence; (ii) extrinsic factors such as portal of entry and inoculum size, and (iii) intrinsic host factors such as genetic background, age, sex, immune competence, and previous experience with specific serotypes (expressed as status immune) [58].

No disease is uniquely associated with any specific enterovirus serotype, and no serotype is uniquely associated wit any one disease. Although clinical entities associated with particular enterovirus serotypes are otherwise rare and the disease spectra of the different serotypes overlap considerably, there are defined diseases which are usually caused by a limited number of different enterovirus serotypes. Another example is hand-foot-and-mouth disease, a febrile mucocutaneous eruption that is most frequently associated with a coxsackievirus A16 infection [198,243]. However, other coxsackievirus A serotypes and enterovirus 71 [32,90] have been reported to cause hand-foot-and-mouth disease and coxsackievirus A16 has also been associated with other types of disease. On occasion, however, particular syndromes are associated with specific enteroviruses. For example, acute hemorrhagic conjunctivitis is usually caused by coxsackievirus A24 variant or enterovirus 70 [79,130,161].

Table 2. Clinical syndrome associated with enterovirus infections.

Group Virus	Major disease associations
Poliovirus 3 types (1 - 3)	Paralytic poliomyelitis, aseptic meningitis, febrile illness.
Coxsackie group A 23 types (A1-22, A24)	Aseptic meningitis, herpangina, febrile illness, conjunctivitis, hand, foot and mouth disease
Coxsackie group B 6 types (B1-6)	Aseptic meningitis, severe neonatal disease, myopericarditis, Bornholm disease, encephalitis, febrile illness
Echovirus 31 types (1-9, 11-27)	Aseptic meningitis, rash, febrile illness, conjunctivitis, severe generalized neonatal disease.
Enterovirus 4 types (68-71)	Polio-like illness, aseptic meningitis, hand, foot and mouth (E71), epidemic conjunctivitis (E70)

Data are from references [45,58,164,181,207].

One of the most distinctive diseases produced by an enterovirus is poliomyelitis. This is almost invariably caused by one of the three poliovirus serotypes [148,164], although it is important to note that other enteroviruses are occasionally associated with a polio-like illness, in particular coxsackievirus A7 [88,241] and enterovirus 71 [47].

Until the introduction of poliovaccine, an estimated 600,000 new cases of paralytic polio occurred worldwide each year. As consequence of widespread use of poliovirus vaccine of polio's cases are being restricted to fewer areas of the world [181]. The introduction of the inactivated poliovirus vaccine (IPV) and the oral poliovirus vaccine (OPV) has resulted in the elimination of poliomyelitis from most parts of the world and represents one of the greatest achievements of medical science. IPV was licensed in the United States in 1955. Though IPV was effective in providing individual protection as well as reducing poliovirus transmission in populations, it was replaced by OPV in 1961 because of the ability of OPV, through superior intestinally-induced immunity, to rapidly reduce poliovirus transmission [185,231].

In Cuba after the introduction of the OPV in 1962, drastically poliomyelitis patients decreased. Between 1957 and 1961 there were 1162 reported cases of paralysis or death due to poliomyelitis in Cuba [85,140]. However, no poliomyelitis patient by wild type virus has been reported since 1962 [139,141,143]. The last case of poliomyelitis in the Americas associated with circulating indigenous wild poliovirus was reported in Peru in 1991 [246].

The polio eradication initiative, created after the World Health Assembly resolved, in 1988, to eradicate poliomyelitis globally by 2000, has made remarkable progress. From 1988 through September 2004, the number of countries where polio was endemic decreased from > 125 to 6, and the estimated number of polio cases decreased by more than 99%. Wild-type 2 poliovirus has not been detected worldwide since October 1999, despite improving surveillance [246,247,248].

In addition to recognized associations with acute diseases, enteroviruses are suspected to be etiologic agents in some human chronic diseases linked to persistent infections. Viral infections are also suspected to be able to trigger autoimmune processes such as Cardiomyopathy [7,10,225], Chronic Fatigue Syndrome [9,48], Post-polio Syndrome [111,127,221], Amyotrophic Lateral Sclerosis [19,24] and Type 1 Diabetes Mellitus [101]. While the association of enterovirus infections with these chronic diseases are certainly not proven, in some cases considerable evidences is accumulating which gives a strong implication of some involvement.

VII. DIAGNOSIS

Enteroviral infections can not be diagnosed on clinical grounds alone due to the wide variety of clinical manifestation (i.e. fever, headache, nausea/vomiting, anorexia, rash, diarrhea, myalgias, nuchal rigity, photophobia), few of which are unique to enterovirus infections and are often indistinguishable from those of other infections [223,244].

No specific treatment is available for enteroviral diseases, and therefore for optimal patient management (avoidance of unnecessary hospitalization and presumptive treatment of the patient), the importance of enteroviral diagnosis lies mainly in distinguishing between enterovirus-induced disease and other treatable causes of clinically similar disease, to identify enterovirus outbreaks, and to assess the prognosis [43].

In outbreaks, it is often possible to determine an etiological association with confidence because the clinical case descriptions are associated with large number of people with similar symptoms who show evidence of infection with the same serotype of enterovirus-however determining the etiology of single clinical cases is difficult [207].

Because there is no pathognomonic clinical syndrome for enterovirus, final diagnosis must be confirmed in the laboratory. Conventional methods for the diagnosis of enterovirus infections include virus isolation with subsequent serotyping and measurement of enterovirus antibodies in the serum [153]. Enteroviruses are most often isolated from stool samples, but this provides only circumstantial evidence for the disease etiology since enteroviruses can be isolated from the alimentary tract of asymptomatic individuals [122]. Therefore, the significance of enterovirus isolation from stool specimens in association with illness must be critically evaluated, for enterovirus circulates abundantly, and coincidental associations are inevitable in some instances. Isolation of an enterovirus from an affected organ or associated body fluids, (e.g. cerebrospinal fluid, myocardium, pericardial fluid) provides the strongest evidence of enteroviral diseases [46,56,88] - however, attempts to isolate enteroviruses from associated body fluids are frequently unsuccessful because of the low viral titer in clinical specimens [6,44]. Although virus isolation is often considered the "golden standard" for enterovirus detection, it has several weaknesses. The most prominent drawback is poor diagnostic sensitivity, which can be due to low viral titer, inadequate collection, handling and processing of the samples, or insusceptibility of the cell line used. No single cell line currently in use supports the growth of all known enterovirus serotypes. Therefore, to ensure maximal isolation efficiency, combinations of cell lines are generally used [86,169].

Most of the enterovirus serotypes grow well in standard cell cultures [44,57,110], except that some coxsackievirus A can be isolated only in suckling mice, but because of practical difficulties this technique is rarely used. As a consequence, coxsackievirus A infections are probably underdiagnosed and underrepresented in epidemiological surveys [135,217,242].

Because changes in cell morphology (e.g., cell rounding followed by the shrinkage and degeneration of the cell sheet) are not specific for any virus group, a confirmatory assay is needed for further typing of an isolated virus strain. Isolated enteroviruses are classically identified by neutralization of infectivity with serotype-specific antisera [129,150]. Typing by neutralization with reference antisera for all serotypes individually is clearly impractical. Type-specific antisera are therefore combined in intersecting pools in such a way that antibody to any one type is present in only a limited number of pools. Neutralization typing is carried out by incubating the isolate with a panel of antiserum pools and by subsequent evaluation of the inhibition of virus growth. Finally, the suspected enterovirus type can be confirmed by neutralization with the type-specific single antiserum. The Lim Benyesh-Melnick (LBM) pool scheme consists of eight pools (designated A to H) containing antisera to 42 different enterovirus types [129,150]. Antibodies against 19 additional CVA serotypes in seven additional pools (designated J to P) can be used if identification with pools A to H cannot be achieved [151]. Alternative other intersecting pools have been developed which also allow identification of enterovirus types 68 to 71 [112].

There are several drawbacks to the use of intersecting pools for typing of enteroviruses. First, the method is time-consuming, labor-intensive, and costly. Second, the supply of antisera is limited, and WHO has advocated a conservative approach to the use of pools, which should not be used to type every clinical isolate [154]. Third, the problem of "untypeable" enteroviruses is frequently encountered [169].

Serological diagnosis of enterovirus infections is complicated by the large number of serotypes; antibody responses are often heterotypic, the occurrence of anamnestic and on the other hand no uniformly cross-reactive enterovirus group antigen has been found [207].

The demonstration of enterovirus-specific IgM antibody in a single serum, indicative of a current antigenic stimulus, provides evidence of recent infection [23,37,60,69,76,137, 144,212,235], but results must be interpreted with caution, since the IgM response may be non-specific and background levels of IgM in the general population may be high [156], particularly during epidemic seasons. The IgM assays that are generally used in epidemiologic studies have very good sensitivity and appear to be very specific for enterovirus infection; however, these assays detect heterotypic antibodies resulting from other enterovirus infections, and therefore cannot be considered strictly serotype specific [181].

A four-fold or greater of the virus-neutralizing antibody titers between the acute-and convalescent-phase serum specimens is a classical diagnostic criterion for a serological test. The neutralization assay is considered accurate and serotype-specific, but due to the large number of enterovirus serotypes the test is laborious as long as the virus type is not known [153]. This requires the use of more than 60 virus strains and therefore is not in routine diagnostic use, although occasionally utilized in epidemiological studies. If the specific serotype of an infecting enterovirus is known or suspected, e.g., in community outbreaks, confirmatory immunoglobulin G serology can be performed on individual patients to document a rise in antibody titer from the acute to the convalescent phase infection [3].

Methods for detecting an enteroviral nucleic acid in clinical specimens have been introduced over recent years. The development of polimerase chain reaction (PCR) technology [174,211] and its subsequent adaptation for the detection of the enterovirus RNA genome via reverse-transcription polimerase chain reaction (RT-PCR) [38,102] have proved useful diagnostic tools, and have therefore become extremely popular in recent years [200].

The existence of conserved regions of nucleotide identity within the enterovirus 5'NTR has been exploited for the design of oligonucleotide primers capable of near-universal amplification of the enterovirus [202,249,253]. Multiple studies using both assays developed in house and commercially developed (Amplicor Enterovirus PCR) kits have documented that RT-PCR is an extremely rapid, sensitive and specific diagnostic modality for the detection of an enterovirus in clinical specimens, as compared to the traditional "gold standard" of tissue culture [114,187,218,240].

As noted previously, the enteroviruses are responsible for a wide array of clinical diseases affecting many organ systems. From the perspective of laboratory diagnosis, in most circumstances it is sufficient to speak of disease that is of "enterovirus cause" and to diagnose "an enterovirus" in the laboratory without necessarily specifying or identifying the particular serotype. RT-PCR, will therefore assume a major role in the laboratory diagnosis of enterovirus infections. This test impacted patient management as measured by shortened patient stays, which should translate into significant health care savings [27,216,203].

Molecular typing systems of enterovirus based on nucleotide sequences have provided a valuable alternative to the existing serological methods for identifying enterovirus types and for epidemiological monitoring. As a number of major neutralization sites reside in the VP1 proteins, serotype identification of an isolate can be achieved by comparing the sequence of the isolate with known sequences in VP1 for all serotypes and looking for identities of greater than 75% in nucleotide sequence or greater than 88% in amino acid sequence. In fact, the use of molecular typing system considerably shortened the time required for reporting the results. Molecular typing have been also used for studying other properties of enteroviruses which cannot be addressed by traditional typing methods, detect antigenic variant strains, for identifying "untypeable" enteroviruses not identified by neutralization test [177].

Acknowledgements

I whish to thank the people who work at the department of Virology, "Pedro Kouri′" Tropical Medicine Institute for creating a pleasant atmosphere. Miss. Lister Nomagugu Lekhuleni is thanked for careful revision of the English language of the manuscript.

References

[1] Abad FX, Pinto RM, Bosch A. Disinfection of human enteric viruses on fomites. *FEMS Microbiol Lett* 1997;156:107-11.

[2] Ackermann W, Fujioka S, Kurtz B. Cationic modulation of the inactivation of poliovirus by heat. *Arch Environ Health* 1970;21:377-81.

[3] Alexander P, Chapman L, Pallansch M, Stephenson W, Torok T, Anderson L. Coxsackievirus B2 infection and aseptic meningitis: a focal outbreak among members of a high school football team. *J Infect Dis* 1993;167:1201-05.

[4] Andino R, Rieckhof G, Achacoso P, Baltimore D. Poliovirus RNA synthesis utilizes an RNA complex formed around the 5′-end of viral RNA. *EMBO J* 1993;12:3587–98.

[5] Andino R, Rieckhof G, Baltimore D. A functional ribonucleoprotein complex forms around the 5′ end of poliovirus RNA. *Cell* 1990;63:369-80.

[6] Andreoletti L, Damman N, Dewilde A, Vallee L, Cremer R, Hober D, et al. Comparison of use of cerebrospinal fluid, serum, and throat swab specimens in diagnosis of enteroviral acute neurological infection by a rapid RNA detection PCR assay. *J Clin Microbiol* 1998;36:589-91.

[7] Andreoletti L, Hober D, Decoene C, Copin MC, Lobert PE, Dewilde A, et al. Detection of enteroviral RNA by polymerase chain reaction in endomyocardial tissue of patients with chronic cardiac diseases. *J Med Virol* 1996;48:53-9.

[8] Aoki K, Sawada H, Ishikawa H, Shimoji T, Kamada R, Chen CW et al. An epidemic of hemorrhagic conjuctivitis due to coxsackievirus A24 in Okinawa, Japan ad Kaohsiong, Taiwan. *Jpn J Ophthalmol* 1987;41:755-58.

[9] Archard L, Bowles N, Behan P, Bell E, Doyle D. Post viral fatigue syndrome: persistence of enterovirus RNA in muscle and elevated creatine kinase. *J Roy Soc Med* 1988;81:326-29.

[10] Archard L, Freeke C, Richardson P, Meany B, Olsen E, Morgan-Capner P, et al. Persistence of enterovirus RNA in dilated cardiomyopathy: a progression from myocarditis. In Schultheiss HP, ed. *New concepts in viral heart disease.* Berlin, Germany: Springer-Verlag K;1988.p.349-62.

[11] Bailly J, Borman M, Peigue-Lafeuille H, Kean M. Natural isolates of echovirus type 25 with extensive variations in IRES sequences and different translational efficiencies. *Virology* 1996;215:83-96.

[12] Bello M, Mas P, Palomera R, Morier L, Avalos I, Acosta B, et al. Meningoencefalitis virales por enterovirus en el período 1990-1995. *Rev Arg Microbiol* 1997;29:176-83.

[13] Bendinelli M, Conaldi P, Matteucci D. Interactions with the immune system. In: Bendinelli M and Friedmas H, eds. *Coxsackievirus, a General Update.* New York: Plenum Press;1988.p.81-102.

[14] Benenson A. Enteroviral hemorrhagic conjuctivitis. In: Benenson A, ed. *Control of communicable diseases.* Washington, DC: American Public Health Association;1998.p.11-113.

[15] Bergelson J, Chan M, Solomon K, St John N, Lin H, Finberg R. Decay-accelerating factor (CD55), a glycosylphosphatidylinositol-anchored complement regulatory protein, is a receptor for several echoviruses. *Proc Natl Acad Sci USA* 1994;91:6245–9.

[16] Bergelson J, Cunningham J, Droguett G. Isolation of a common receptor for Coxsackie B viruses and adenoviruses 2 and 5. *Science*1997;275:1320-3.

[17] Bergelson J, Modlin J, Wieland-Alter W, Cunningham J, Crowell R, Finberg R. Clinical coxsackievirus B isolates differ from laboratory strains in their interaction with two cell surface receptors. *J infect Dis* 1997;175:697-700.

[18] Bergelson J, Shepley M, Chan B, Hemler M, Finberg R. Identification of the integrinVLA-2 as a receptor for echovirus 1. *Science* 1992;255:1718-20.

[19] Berger M, Kopp N, Vital C, Redl B, Aymard M, Lina B. Detection an cellular localization of enterovirus RNA sequences in spinal cord of patients with ALS. *Neurology* 2000;54:20-5.

[20] Berlin L, Rorabaugh M, Heldrich F, Roberts K, Doran T, Modlin J. Aseptic meningitis in infants <2 years of age: diagnosis and etiology. *J Infect Dis* 1993;168:888-92.

[21] Bhide V, Prasad S, Gogate S. Isolation of a variantof enterovirus 70 from a patient during an epidemic of acute haemorrhagic conjunctivitis in Pune in 1991. *Acta Virol* 1994;38:245-6.

[22] Bienz K, Egger D, Pfister T, Troxler M. Structural and functional characterization of the poliovirus replication complex. *J Virol* 1992;66:2740-47.

[23] Boman J, Nilsson B, Juto P. Serum IgA, IgG, and IgM responses to different enteroviruses as measured by a coxsackie B5-based indirect ELISA. *J Med Virol* 1992;38:32-5.

[24] Brahic M, Smith R, Gibbs C, Garruto R, Tourtellote W, Cash E. Detection of picornavirus sequences in nervous tissue of amyotrophic lateral sclerosis and control patients. *Ann Neurol* 1985;18:337-43.

[25] Brandful J, Takeda N, Yoshii T, Miyamura K, Mingle J, Addy E, et al. A study of the evolution of coxsackievirus A24 variant in Ghana by viral RNA fingerprinting analysis. *Res Virol* 1991;142:57-65.

[26] Brown B, Oberste S, Alexander J, Kennett L, Pallansch M. Molecular epidemiology and evolution of enterovirus 71 strains isolated from 1970 to 1998. *J Virol* 1999;73:9969-75.

[27] Byington C, Taggart E, Carroll K, Hillyard D. A polimerase chain reaction – based epidemiologic investigation of the incidence of nonpolioenteroviral infections in febrile and afebrile infants 90 days and younger. *Pediatrics* 1999;103:E27.

[28] Caggana M, Chan P, Ramsingh A. Identification of a single amino acid residue in the capsid protein VP1 of coxsackievirus B4 that determines the virulent phenotype. *J Virol* 1993;67:4797-4803.

[29] Calvez V, Pelletier I, Borzakian S, Colbere-Garapin F. Identification of a region of the poliovirus genome involved in persistent infection of HEp-2 cells. *J Virol* 1993;67:4432-5.

[30] Cambridge G, MacArthur C, Waterson A, Goodwin J, Oakley C. Antibodies to coxsackie B viruses in primary congestive cardiomyopathy. *Br Heart J* 1979;41:692–6.

[31] Cammack N, Phillips A, Dunn G, Patel V, Minor P. Intertypic genomic rearrangements of poliovirus strains in vaccines. *Virology* 1989;167:507-514.

[32] Cao Y, Yang X, Li J, Ren L, Lin W, Guo Y, et al. Study on the etiology of hand, foot and mouth disease (HFMD) in China. *Acta Acad Med Sin* 1985;7:333-6.

[33] Celers J, Celers P, Bertuchi A. Les enterovirus non poliomyelitiques en France de 1974 a 1985. *Pathol Biol* 1988;36:1221-66.

[34] Centers for Diseases Control and Prevention. Summary of notifiable diseases, United States, 1994. *MMWR* 1994;43:1-8.

[35] Centers for Diseases Control and Prevention. Nonpolio enterovirus surveillance-United States, 1993-1996. *MMWR* 1997;43:1-8.

[36] Centers for Diseases Control and Prevention. Enterovirus surveillance-United States, 1997-1999. *MMWR* 2000;49:913-6.

[37] Chan D, Hammond G. Comparison of serodiagnosis of group B coxsackie virus infections by an immunoglobulin M capture enzyme immunoassay versus microneutralization. *J Clin Microbiol* 1985;21:830-4.

[38] Chapman M, Tracy S, Gauntt C, Fortmueller U. Molecular detection and identification of enteroviruses using enzymatic amplification and nucleic acid hybridization. *J Clin Microbiol* 1990;28:843-50.

[39] Chen Z, Stauffacher C, Li Y, Schmidt T, Wu B, Kamer G, et al. Protein-RNA interactions in an icosahedral virus at 3.0 Å resolution. *Science* 1989;245:154-9.

[40] Cherry J. Nonpolio enteroviruses: Coxsackieviruses, echoviruses and enteroviruses. In: Feigin R, Cherry J, eds. *Textbook of Pediatric Infectious Diseases*. Philadelphia, PA:WB Saunders;1981.p.1316-65.

[41] Cherry J. Enteroviruses: coxsackieviruses, enteroviruses and polioviruses. In: Feigin R, Cherry J, eds. *Textbook of Pediatric Infectious Diseases*. 4th ed. Philadelphia, Pa: WB Saunders;1998.p.1787-1839.

[42] Chomel J, Antona D, Thouvenot D, Lina B. Three echovirus serotypes responsible for outbreak of aseptic meningitis in Rhone-Alpes region, France. *Eur J Clin Microbiol Infect Dis* 2003;22:191-3.

[43] Chonmaitree T, Baldwin C, Lucia H. Role of the virology laboratory in diagnosis and management of patients with central nervous system diseases. *Clin Microbiol Rev* 1989;2:1-14.

[44] Chonmaitree T, Ford C, Sanders C, Lucia H. Comparison of cell cultures for rapid isolation of enteroviruses. *J Clin Microbiol* 1988;26;2576-80.

[45] Chonmaitree T, Mann L. Respiratory infections. In Rotbart HA, ed. *Human enterovirus infections*. American Society for Microbiology, Washington, DC; 1995.p.255-70.

[46] Chonmaitree T, Menegus M, Powell K. The clinical relevance of CSF viral culture. A two-year experience with aseptic meningitis in Rochester. *JAMA* 1982;247:1843-7.

[47] Chumakov K, Voroshilova M, Shindarov L, Lavrova I, Gracheva L, Koroleva G, et al. Enterovirus 71 isolated from cases of epidemic poliomyelitis-like disease in Bulgaria. *Arch Virol* 1979;60:329-40.
[48] Clements G, McGarry F, Naim C, Galbraith D. Detection of enterovirus-specific RNA in serum: The relationship to chronic fatigue. *J Med Virol* 1995;45:156-61.
[49] Colbere-Garapin F, Christodolou C, Crainic R, Pelletier I. Persistent poliovirus infection of human neuroblastoma cells. *Proc Natl Acad Sci USA* 1989;86:7590-4.
[50] Committee on the ECHO viruses. Enteric cytopathogenic human orphan (ECHO) viruses. *Science* 1955;122:1187-8.
[51] Communicable Disease Surveillance Centre. Viral meningitis associated with increase in echovirus type 13. *Commun Dis Rep CDR Wkly* 2000;10:277-80.
[52] Connolly K, Hammer S. The acute aseptic meningitis syndrome. *Infect Dis Clin North Am* 1990;4:599-602.
[53] Couderc T, Hogle J, Le Blay H, Horaud F, Blondel B. Molecular characterization of mouse-virulent poliovirus type 1 Mahoney mutants:involvement of polypeptides VP1 and VP2 located on the inner surface of the capsid protein shell. *J Virol* 1993;67:3808-17.
[54] Curnen E, Shaw W, Melnick J. Disease resembling non paralytic poliomyelitis associated with a virus pathogenicin infant mice. *JAMA* 1949;141:894-901
[55] Dagan R, Jenista J, Menegus M. Association of clinical presentation, laboratory findings, and virus serotypes with the presence of meningitis in hospitalized infants with enterovirus infection. *J Pediatr* 1988;113:975-8.
[56] Dagan R, Jenista J, Prather S, Powell K, Menegus M. Viremia in hospitalized children with enterovirus infections. *J Pediatr* 1985;106:397-401.
[57] Dagan R, Menegus M. A combination of four cell types for rapid detection of enteroviruses in clinical specimens. *J Med Virol* 1986;19:219-28.
[58] Dagan R, Menegus M. Nonpolio enteroviruses and the febrile infant. In: Rotbart H, ed. *Human enterovirus Infections*. Washington, DC: American Society for Microbiology Press;1995.p.239-54.
[59] Dallford G, Sickles G. An unidentified filterable agent isolated from the feces of children with paralysis. *Science* 1948;108:61-2.
[60] Day C, Cumming H, Walker J. Enterovirus-specific IgM in the diagnosis of meningitis. *J Infect* 1989;19:219-28.
[61] de la Torre J, Giachetti C, Semler B, Holland J. High frequency of single-base transitions and extreme frequency of precise multiple-base reversion mutation in poliovirus. *Proc Natl Acad Sci USA* 1992;89:2531-5.
[62] Diedrich S, Driesel G, Schreier E. Sequence comparison of echovirus type 30 isolates to other enteroviruses in the 5' noncoding region. *J Med Virol* 1995;46:148-52.
[63] Diedrich S, Schreier E. Aseptic meningitis in Germany associated with echovirus type 13. *BMC Infect Dis* 2001;1:14.
[64] Domingo E, Holland J. Mutation rates and rapid evolution of RNA viruses. In: Morse S, ed. *The Evolutionary Biology of Viruses*. New York; Raven Press;1994.p.161-84.
[65] Dorval B, Chow M, Klibanov A. Stabilization of poliovirus against heat inactivation. *Biochem Biophys Res Commun* 1989;159:1177-83.

[66] Dowdle W, Birmingham M. The biologic principles of poliovirus eradication. *J Infect Dis* 1997;175:S286-S292.

[67] Drake J. Rate of spontaneous mutation among RNA viruses. *Proc Natl Acad Sci USA* 1993;90:4171-5.

[68] Drebot M, Nguan C, Campbell J, Lee S, Forward K. Molecular epidemiology of enterovirus outbreaks in Canada during 1991–1992: identification of echovirus 30 and coxsackievirus B1 strains by amplicon sequencing. *J Med Virol* 1994;44:340-7.

[69] El-Hagrassy O, Coltart D, Banatvala J. Coxsackie-B-virus-specific IgM responses in patients with cardiac and other diseases. *Lancet*1980; ii:1160–62.

[70] Enders J, Weller TH, Robbins F. Cultivation of the Lansing strain of poliomyelitis virus in cultures of various human embryonic tissues. *Science* 1949;109:85-7.

[71] Feachem R, Garelick H, Slade J. Enteroviruses in the environment. *Trop Dis Bull* 1981;78:185-230.

[72] Filman D, Syed R, Chow M. Structural factors that control conformational transitions and serotype specificity in type 3 poliovirus. *EMBO J*1989;8:1567-79.

[73] Flanegan J, Baltimore D. Poliovirus-specific primer-dependent RNA polymerase able to copy poly(A). *Proc Natl Acad Sci USA* 1977;74:3677-80.

[74] Flanegan J, Petterson R, Ambros V, Hewlett M, Baltimore D. Covalent linkage of a protein to a defined nucleotide sequence at the 5` terminus of virion and replicative intermediate RNAs of poliovirus. *Proc Natl Acad Sci USA* 1977;74:961-5.

[75] Fox J, Hall C, Cooney M, Luce R, Kronmal R. The Seattle Virus Watch. II. Objectives, study population and its observation, data processing and summary of illnesses. *Am J Epidemiol* 1972;96:270-85.

[76] Frisk G, Torfason E, Diderholm H. Reverse radioimmunoassay of IgM and IgG antibodies to coxsackie B viruses in patients with acute myopericarditis. *J Med Virol* 1984;14:191-200.

[77] From the Centers for Disease Control and Prevention. Echovirus type 13-United States, 2001. *JAMA* 2001;286:1831-2.

[78] Georgescu M, Balanant J, Macadam A, et al. Evolution of the Sabin type 1 poliovirus in humans: Characterization of strains isolated from patients with vaccine-associated paralytic poliomyelitis. *J Virol* 1997;71:7758-68.

[79] Gh K, Ogi P, Miyamura K, Ogino T, Yamazaki S. Acute haemorrhagic conjuctivitis: seroepidemiology of Coxsackievirus A24 variant and enterovirus 70 in Singapore. *J Med Virol 1990*;31:245-7.

[80] Giachetti C, Semler B. Molecular genetic analysis of poliovirus RNA replication bymutagenesis of a VPg precursor polypeptide. In: Brinton M, Heinz F, eds. *New aspects of positive-strand RNA viruses.* Washington, DC: American Society for Microbiology;1990.p.83-93.

[81] Giachetti C, Semler B. Role of a viral membrane polypeptide in strand-specific initiation of poliovirus RNA synthesis. *J Virol* 1991;65:2647-54.

[82] Gibson J, Righthand V. Persistence ECHOvirus type 6 in cloned human cells. *J Virol* 1985;54:219-23.

[83] Glimaker M, Samuelson A, Magnius L, Ehrnest A, Olcen P, Forsgrem M. Early diagnosis of enteroviral meningitis by detection of specific IgM antibodies with a solid-

phase reverse immunosorbent test (SPRIST) and mu-capturte EIA. *J Med Virol* 1992;36:193-201.

[84] Gondo K, Kusuhara K, Take H, Ueda K. Echovirus type 9 epidemic in Kagoshima, southern Japan: Seroepidemiology and clinical observation of aseptic meningitis. *Pediatr Infect Dis J* 1995;14:787-91.

[85] González O, Más P. Epidemiological surveillance and control of poliomyelitis in the Republic of Cuba. *J Hyg Epidemiol Microbiol Immunol* 1987;31:381-9.

[86] Grandien M, Forsgren M, Ehrnst A. Enteroviruses. In: Lennette EH, Lennette DA, and Lennette ET,eds. *Diagnostic procedures for viral, rickettsial, and chlamydial infections.* 7th ed. Washington, DC: American Public Health Association;1995.p. 279-97

[87] Grist N. Coxsackie virus infections of the heart. In: Waterson A, ed. *Recent advances in clinical virology 1.* Edinburgh, United Kingdom: Churchill Livingstone;1977.p.141-50.

[88] Grist N, Bell E, Assaad F. Enteroviruses in human disease. *Prog Med Virol* 1978;24:114-57.

[89] Haarmann C, Schwimmbeck P, Mertens T, Schultheiss T, Strauer T. Identification of serotype-specific and nonserotypespecific B-cell epitopes of coxsackie B virus using synthetic peptides. *Virology* 1994;200:381-9.

[90] Hagiwara A, Tagaya I, Yoneyama T. Epidemic of hand, foot and mouth disease associated with enterovirus type 71 infection. *Intervirology* 1978;9:60-3.

[91] Hall C, Cooney M, Fox J. The Seattle virus watch program. I. Infection and illness experience of virus watch families during a community wide epidemic of echovirus type 30 aseptic meningitis. *Am J Public Health Nations Health* 1970;60:1456–65.

[92] Hanecak R, Semler B, Anderson C, Wimmer E. Proteolytic processing of poliovirus polypeptides: antibodies to polypeptide P3-7c inhibit cleavage at glutamine-glycine pairs. *Proc Natl Acad Sci USA* 1982;79:3973-7.

[93] Hanecak R, Semler B, Ariga H, Andersson C, Wimmer E. Expression of a cloned gene segment of poliovirus in E. coli: evidence for autocatalytic production of the viral proteinase. *Cell* 1984;37:1063-73.

[94] Harvala H, Kalimo H, Dahllund L, Santti J, Hughes P, Hyypia T, et al. Mapping of tissue tropism determinants in coxsackievirus genomes. *J Gen Virol* 2002;83:1697-706.

[95] Higgins P. Enteroviral Conjuntivitis and its neurological complications, brief review. *Arh Virol* 1982;73:91-101.

[96] Honig E, Melnick J, Isacson P. An epidemiological study of enteric virus infections. Poliomyelitis, Coxsackie, and orphan (ECHO) viruses isolated in two socioeconomic groups. *J Exp Med* 1956;103:247-62.

[97] Horstmann D. Enterovirus infections of the central nervous system. The present and future of poliomyelitis. *Med Clin North Am* 1967;51:681-92.

[98] Huang A. Defective interfering viruses. *Annu Rev Microbiol* 1973;27:101-17.

[99] Hughes M, Hoey E, Coyle P. A nucleotide sequence comparison of coxsackievirus B4 isolates from aquatic samples and clinical specimens. *Epidemiol Infect* 1993;110:389-98.

[100] Huttunen P, Santii J, Pulli T, Hiyypia T. The major echovirus group is genetically coherent and related to coxsackie B viruses. *J Gen Virol* 1996;77:715-25.

[101] Hyöty H, Taylor K. The role of viruses in human diabetes. *Diabetologia* 2002;45:1353-61.

[102] Hyypia T, Auvinen P, Maaronen M. Polimerase chain reaction for human picornaviruses. *J Gen Virol* 1989;70:3261-8.

[103] Hyypia T, Hovi T, Knowles N, Stanway G. Classification of enterovirus based on molecular and biological properties. *J Gen Virol* 1997;78:1-11.

[104] Irvine D, Irvine A, Gardner S. Outbreak of E.C.H.O. virus type 30 in a general practice. *Br Med J* 1967;4:774-6.

[105] Ishiko H, Takeda N, Miyamura K, Kato N, Tanimura M, Lin K, et al. Phylogenetic analysis of a coxsackievirus A24 variant: the most recent worldwide pandemic was caused by progenies of a virus prevalent around 1981. *Virology* 1992;187:748-59.

[106] Ishiko H, Takeda N, Miyamura K, Tanimura M, Yamanaka T, Kasuga K. Phylogenetically different strains of a variant of coxsackievirus A 24 were repeatedly introduced but discontinued circulating in Japan. *Arch Virol* 1992; 126:179-93.

[107] Jacobson S, Konings D, Sarnow P. Biochemical and genetic evidence for a pseudoknot structure at the 3′ terminus of the poliovirus RNA genome and its role in viral RNA amplification. *J Virol* 1993;67:2961-71.

[108] Jenista J, Powell K, Menegus M. Epidemiology of neonatal enterovirus infection. *J Pediatr* 1984;104:685-90.

[109] Johnson L, Sarnow P. Three poliovirus 2B mutants exhibit noncomplementable defects in viral RNA amplification and display dosage-dependent dominance over wild-type poliovirus. *J Virol* 1991;65:4341-9.

[110] Johnston L, Siegel C. Presumptive identification of enteroviruses with RD, HEp-2, and RMK cell lines. *J Clin Microbiol* 1990;28:1049-50.

[111] Julen J, Leparc-Goffart I, Lina B, Fuchs F, Fory S, Janatova I, et al. Postpolio syndrome: poliovirus persistence is involved in the pathogenesis. *J Neurol* 1999;246:472-6.

[112] Kapsenberg J. Picornaviridae: the enteroviruses (polioviruses, coxsackieviruses, echoviruses). In Lennette HE, Halonen P, and Murphy FA, eds. *Laboratory diagnosis of infectious diseases. Principles and practice.* New York: Springer-Verlag;1988.p.692-722.

[113] Keino M, Kanno M, Hirasawa K, Watari T, Mikawa M, Saito K, et al. Isolation of echovirus type 13 from patients of aseptic meningitis. *Jpn J Infect Dis* 2001;54:249-50.

[114] Kessler H, Santner B, Rabenau H, Berger A, Vince A, Lewinski C et al. Rapid diagnosis of enterovirus infection by a new one-step reverse transcription-PCR assay. *J Clin Microbiol* 1997;35:976-7.

[115] Kew O, Mulders M, Lipskaya G, da Silva E, Pallansch M. Molecular epidemiology of polioviruses. In: Kew OM, Nathanson N, eds. *Molecular Epidemiology. Seminars in Virology*. New York: Academic Press;1995.p.401-14.

[116] Kew O, Nottay B, Hatch M, Hierholzer J, Obijeski J. Oligonucleotide fingerprint analysis of enterovirus 70 isolates from the 1980 to 1981 pandemic of acute

hemorrhagic conjunctivitis: evidence for a close genetic relationship among Asian and American strains. *Infect Immunol* 1983;41:631-5.

[117] Kew O, Nottay B, Rico-Hesse R, Pallansch M. Molecular epidemiology of wild Poliovirus trasmition. In: Kurstak E, Marusyk RG, Muphy FA, Van Regenmortel MHV, eds. *Applied Virology Research*.USA: Plenun Press;1990.p.199-221.

[118] Kimura H, Shibata M, Kuzushima K, Nishikawa K, Nishiyama Y, Lansdown A. Viral infections and diseases of the heart. *Prog Med Virol* 1978;24:70–113.

[119] King A. Preferred sites of recombination in poliovirus RNA: an analysis of 40 intertypic cross-over sequences. *Nucleic Acid Res* 1988;16:11705-23.

[120] King A, Brown F, Christian P, Hovi T,Hyypia T, Knowles N. Picornaviridae. In: Van Regenmortel M, Fauguet C, Bishop E, et al., eds. *Virus taxonomy: The classification and nomenclature of viruses. Seventh report of the international committee on taxonomy of viruses.* San Diego, CA: Academic Press;2000.p.657-73.

[121] Kitamura N, Semler B, Rothberg P, Larsen G, Adler C, Dorner A, et al. Primary structure, gene organization and polypeptide expression of poliovirus RNA. *Nature* 1981;291:547-53.

[122] Kogon A, Spigland I, Frothingman T, Elveback L, Williams C, Hall C, et al. The Virus Watch Program: a continuing surveillance of viral infections in metropolitan New York families. VII. Observations on viral excretion, seroimmunity, intrafamilial spread and illness association in coxsackie and echovirus infections. *Am J Epidemiol* 1969;89:51-6.

[123] Kono R. Apollo 11 disease or acute hemorrhagic conjuctivitis: a pandemic of a new enterovirus infection of the eye. *Am J Epidemiol* 1975;101:303-9.

[124] Kopecka H, Brown B, Pallansch M. Genotypic variation in coxsackie B5 isolates from three different outbreaks in the United States. *Virus Res* 1995;38:125-36.

[125] Lee Y, Nomoto A, Detjen B, Wimmer E. A protein covalently linked to poliovirus genome RNA. *Proc Natl Acad Sci USA* 1977;74:59-63.

[126] Lentz K, Smith D, Geisler C. Structure of poliovirus type 2 Lansing complexed with antiviral agent SCH48973: Comparison of the structural and biological properties of three poliovirus serotypes. *Structure* 1997;5:961-78.

[127] Leparc I, Kopecka H, Fuchs F, Janatova I, Aymard M, Julien J. Search for poliovirus in specimens from patients with the post-polio syndrome. *Ann NY Acad Sci* 1995;753:233-6.

[128] Li T, Chen Z, Johnson E, Thomas J. Conformations, interactions, and thermostabilities of RNA and proteins in bean pod mottle virus: Investigation of solution and crystal structures by laser Raman spectroscopy. *Biochemistry* 1992;31:6673-82.

[129] Lim K, Benyesh-Melnick M. Typing of virus of combination of antiserum pools: application typing of enterovirus (coxsackie and echo). *J Immunol* 1960;84:309-17.

[130] Lim K, Yin-Murphy M. An epidemic of conjunctivitis in Singapore in 1970. *Singapore Med J* 1971;12:247-9.

[131] Lin K, Takeda N, Miyamura K, Yamazaki S, Chen C. The nucleotide sequence of 3C proteinase region of the coxsackievirus A24 variant: comparison of the isolates in Taiwan in 1985–1988. *Virus Genes* 1991;5:121-31.

[132] Lin K, Wang H, Sheu M, Huang W, Chen C, Yang C. Molecular epidemiology of a variant of coxsackievirus A24 in Taiwan: two epidemics caused by phylogenetically distinct viruses from 1985 to 1989. *J Clin Microbiol* 1993;31:1160-6.

[133] Lindberg A, Crowell R, Zell R, Kandolf R, Pettersson U. Mapping of the RD phenotype of the Nancy strain of coxsackievirus B3. *Virus Res* 1992; 24:187-96.

[134] Lipskaya G, Chervonskaya E, Belova G. Geographical genotypes (geotypes) of poliovirus case isolates from the former Soviet Union: Relatedness to other known poliovirus genotypes. *J Gen Virol* 1995;76:1687-99.

[135] Lipson S, Walderman R, Costello P, Kzabo K. Sensitivity of rhabdomyosarcoma and guinea pig embryo cell cultures to field isolates of difficult-to-cultivate group A coxsackieviruses. *J Clin Microbiol* 1988;26:1298-1303.

[136] Loeffler F, Frosch P. Report of the Commission for Research on foot-and-mouth disease. In: Hahon N, ed. *Selected papers on virology*. Englewood Cliffs, NJ: *Prentice-Hall*;1964:64-8.

[137] Magnius O, Saleh L, Vikerfors T, Norder H. A solidphase reverse immunosorbent test for the detection of enterovirus IgM. *J Virol Methods* 1988; 20:73-82.

[138] Maguire H, Atkinson P, Sharland M, Bendig J. Enterovirus infections in England and Wales: laboratory surveillance data: 1975 to 1994. *Commun Dis Public Health* 1999;2:122-5.

[139] Mas P. Eradication of poliomyelitis in Cuba: a historical perspective. *Bull WHO* 1999;77:681-7.

[140] Más P, Bravo J, Andrus J, Comellas M, Galindo M, de Cuadros C, et al. Lessons from Cuba: mass campaign administration of trivalent oral polio vaccine and seroprevalence of poliovirus neutralizing antibodies. *Bull WHO* 1994;72:221-5.

[141] Más P, Caceres V, Galindo M, Gary H, Valcarcel M, Barrios J, et al. Persistence of vaccine-derived poliovirus following a mass vaccination campaign in Cuba: Implications for stopping polio vaccination after global eradication. *Int J Epidemiol* 2001;30:1029-34.

[142] Mas P, Comellas M, Marrero M, Jacobo M, Palomera R. Meningoencefalitis por enterovirus en Cuba. Estudio de 14 años. *Rev Cub Ped* 1992;64:16-21.

[143] Más P, Gary H, Sarmiento L, Caceres V, Barrios J, Palomera R, et al. Poliovirus detection in wastewater and stool following an immunization campaign in Havana, Cuba. *Int J Epidemiology* 2003;32:772-7.

[144] McCartney A, Banatvala J, Bell E. Routine use of m-antibody-capture ELISA for the serological diagnosis of coxsackie B virus infections. *J Med Virol* 1986;19:205-12.

[145] McIntyre P, Keen G. Laboratory surveillance of viral meningitis by examination of cerebrospinal fluid in Cape Town, 1981–9. *Epidemiol Infect* 1993;111:357-71.

[146] McPhee F, Zell Y, Reimann B, Hofschneider P, Kandolf R. Characterization of the N-terminal part of the neutralizing antigenic site I of coxsackievirus B4 by mutation analysis of antigen chimeras. *Virus Res* 1994;34:139-51.

[147] Melnick J. Enteroviruses. In: Evans AS, ed. *Viral Infections of Humans, Epidemiology and Control*. New York: Plenum;1989:191-263.

[148] Melnick J. Current status of poliovirus infections. *Clin Microbiol Rev* 1996;9:293-300.

[149] Melnick J. Enteroviruses: polioviruses, coxsackieviruses, echoviruses and newer enterovirus. In: Fields B, Knipe D, Howley P, et al, eds. *Fields Virology.* 3rd ed. Philadelphia, Pa: Lippincott Raven Publisher;1996.p.655-712.

[150] Melnick J, Rennick V, Hampil B. Lyophilized combination pools of enterovirus equine antisera: Preparation and test procedures for the identification of field strains of 42 enteroviruses. *Bull WHO* 1973;48:263-8.

[151] Melnick J, Schmidt N, Hampil B, Ho H. Lyophilized combination pools of enterovirus equine antisera: preparation and test procedures for the identification of field strains of 19 group A coxsackievirus serotypes. *Intervirology* 1977;8:172-81.

[152] Melnick J, Shaw W, Curnen E. A virus from patients diagnosed as non-paralytic poliomyelitis or aseptic meningitis. *Proc Soc Exp Biol Med* 1949;71:344-9.

[153] Melnick J, Wenner H, Phillips C. Enterovirus. In: Lenette E and Schmidt N, ed. *Diagnostic procedures for viral, rickettsial and chlamydial infections.* 5th ed. Washington, DC: American Public Health Association Inc; 1979.p.471-534.

[154] Melnick J, Wimberly I. Lyophilized combination pools of enterovirus equine antisera: new LBM pools prepared from reserves of antisera stored frozen for two decades. *Bull WHO* 1985;63:543-50.

[155] Mendelsohn C, Wimmer E, Racaniello V. Cellular receptor for poliovirus: Molecular cloning, nucleotide sequence, and expression of a new member of the immunoglobulin superfamily. *Cell* 1989;56:855-65.

[156] Miller A, Carmichael H, Calder B, Behan P, Bell E, McCartney R, et al. Antibody to coxsackie B virus in diagnosing postviral fatigue syndrome. *Br Med J* 1991;302:140-3.

[157] Minor P. The molecular biology of poliovaccines. *J Gen Virol* 1992;73:3065-77.

[158] Minor P, Brown F, Domingo E, Hoey E, King A, Knowles N. Picornaviridae. In: Murphy FA,. Fauquet CM, Bishop DL, et al., eds. *Virus taxonomy. Classification and nomenclature of viruses. Sixth report of the International Committee on Taxonomy of Viruses Virology Division, International Union of Microbiological Societies.* Vienna, Austria: Springer-Verlag;1995.p.329-36.

[159] Minor P, Ferguson M, Evans D. Antigenic structure of polioviruses of serotypes 1, 2 and 3. *J Gen Virol* 1986;67:1283-91.

[160] Minor P, Schild G, Bootman J. Location and primary structure of a major antigenic site for poliovirus neutralization. *Nature* 1983;301:674-9.

[161] Mirkovic N, Schmidt J, Yin-Murphy M, Melnick J. Enterovirus etiology of the 1970 Singapore epidemic of acute conjunctivitis. *Intervirology* 1974;4:119-27.

[162] Miyamura K, Takeda N, Tanimura M, Ogino T, Yamazaki S, Chen C, et al. Evolutionary study on the coxsackievirus A 24 variant causing acute hemorrhagic conjunctivitis by oligonucleotide mapping analysis of RNA genome. *Arch Virol* 1990;114:37-51.

[163] Modlin J. Introduction. In: Mandell GL, Bennett JE, Dolin R, eds. *Principles and practice of infectious diseases.* 4th ed. New York: Churchill Livingstone;1995.p.1606-13.

[164] Modlin J. Poliomyelitis and poliovirus immunization. In: Rotbart H, ed. *Human enterovirus infections.* Washington, DC: American Society for Microbiology; 1995. p.195-220.

[165] Modlin J. Update on enterovirus infection in infants and children. *Adv Pediatr Infect Dis* 1996;12:161.

[166] Moore M. Centers for Disease Control. Enteroviral disease in the United States,1970-1979. *J Infect Dis* 1982;146:103-8.

[167] Moore M, Kaplan M, McPhee J, Bregman D, Klein S. Epidemiologic, clinical, and laboratory features of Coxsackie B1-B5 infections in the United States, 1970-79. *Public Health Rep* 1984;99:515-22.

[168] Moore M, Morens D. Enterovirus, including polioviruses. In: Belshe R, ed. *Texbook of human virology*. Littleton, MA: PSG Publishing Company;1984.p.407-84.

[169] Morens D, Pallansch M, Moore M. Polioviruses and other enteroviruses. In: Belshe RB, ed. *Textbook of human virology*. St. Louis, Mo: Mosby Year Book;1991.p.427-97.

[170] Morens D, Pallansch M. .Epidemiology. In: Rotbart H, ed. *Human Enterovirus Infections*. Washington, DC: American Society for Microbiology Press;1995.p.3-23.

[171] Muir P, Ka¨mmerer U, Korn K, Mulders M, Po¨yry T, Weissbrich B, et al. Molecular Typing of Enteroviruses: Current Status and Future Requirements. *Clinical Microbiol Reviews* 1998;11:202-27.

[172] Muir P, Nicholson F, Tilzey A, Signy M, English T, Banatvala J. Chronic relapsing pericarditis and dilated cardiomyopathy: serological evidence of persistent enterovirus infection. *Lancet* 1989;i:804–807.

[173] Mullins J, Khetsuriani N, Nix W, Oberste M, LaMonte A, Kilpatrick D, et al. Emergence of echovirus type 13 as a prominent enterovirus. *Clin Infect Dis* 2004;38:70-7.

[174] Mullis K, Faloona F. Specific synthesis of DNA in vitro via a polimerase-catalyzed chain reaction. *Methods Enzymol* 1987;155:335-50.

[175] Nathanson N, Murphy F. Evolution of viral disease. In: Nathanson N, ed. *Viral pathogenesis*. 1st ed. Philadelphia, New York: Lippincott-Raven publishers;1997.p.353-69.

[176] Oberste S, Maher K, Kennett M, Campbell J, Carpenter M, Schnurr D. Molecular epidemiology and genetic diversity of echovirus type 30 (E30): genotypes correlate with temporal dynamics of E30 isolation. *J Clin Microbiol* 1999;37:3928-33.

[177] Oberste S, Maher K, Flemister R, Marchetti G, Kilpatrick D and Pallansch M. Comparison of Classic and Molecular Approaches for the Identification of untypeable Enteroviruses. *J Clin Microbiol* 2000;38:1170-4.

[178] Oberste MS, Maher K, Williams AJ, Dybdahl-Sissoko N, Brown BA, Gookin MS, et al. Species-specific RT-PCR amplification of human enteroviruses: a tool for rapid species identification of uncharacterized enteroviruses. *J Gen Virol* 2006;87:119-28.

[179] Palacios G, Oberste MS. Enteroviruses as agents of emerging infectious diseases. *J Neurovirol* 2005;11:424-33.

[180] Pallansch M. Epidemiology of coxsackie B viruses. In: Friedman H and Bendinelli M, ed. *Coxsackieviruses-a general update*. New York: Plenum Press;1988.p.399-417.

[181] Pallansch M, Raymond P. Enteroviruses: polioviruses, coxsackieviruses, echoviruses and newer enterovirus. In: Knipe D, Howley P, Griffin D, et al, eds. *Fields Virology*. 3th ed. Philadelphia, Pa: Lippincott Raven Publisher;2001.p.123-775.

[182] Pavio N, Buc-Caron H, Colbe`re-Garapin F. Persistent poliovirus infection of human fetal brain cells. *J Virol* 1996;70:6395-401.
[183] Pelletier J, Kaplan G, Racaniello V, Sonenberg N. Capindependent translation of poliovirus mRNA is conferred by sequence elements within the 5′ noncoding region. *Mol Cell Biol* 1988;8:1103-12.
[184] Pincus E, Wimmer E. Production of guanidine-resistant and –dependent poliovirus mutants from cloned cDNA: Mutations in polypeptide 2C are directly responsible for altered guanidine sensitivity. *J Virol* 1986;60:793-6.
[185] Plotkin S, Vidor E. Poliovirus vaccine inactivated. In: Plotkin SA, Orenstein WA, eds. *Vaccines.* 4th ed. Philadelphia: WB Saunders; 2004.p.625-49.
[186] Powell R, Ward T, Evans D, Almond J. Interaction between echovirus 7 and its receptor, decay-accelerating factor (CD55): Evidence for a secondary cellular factor in A-particle formation. *J Virol* 1997;71:9306-12.
[187] Pozo F, Casas I, Tenorio A, Trallero G, Echevarria J. Evaluation of a comercially available transcription-PCR assay for diagnosis of enteroviral infection in archival and prospectively collected cerebrospinal fluid specimens. *J Clin Microbiol* 1998;36:1741-5.
[188] Prevots D, Ciofi degli Atti M, Sallabanda A. Outbreak of paralytic poliomyelitis in Albania, 1996: High attack rate among adults and apparent interruption of transmission following nationwide mass vaccination. *Clin Infect Dis* 1998;26:419-25.
[189] Pringle C. Virus taxonomy at the XIth International Congress of Virology, Sydney, Australia, 1999. *Archives of Virology* 1999;144:2065-70.
[190] Pulli T, Koskimies P, Hyypia T. Molecular comparison of coxsackie A virus serotypes. *Virology* 1995;211:30-8.
[191] Racaniello V, Baltimore D. Cloned poliovirus complementary DNA is infectious in mammalian cells. *Science* 1981;214:916-9.
[192] Racaniello V. Picornaviridae: The Viruses and Their Replication. In: Knipe D, Howley P, Griffin D, et al, eds. *Fields Virology*. 3th ed. Philadelphia, Pa: Lippincott Raven Publisher;2001.p.123-775.
[193] Ramsingh A, Caggana M, Ronstrom S. Genetic mapping of the determinants of plaque morphology of coxsackievirus B4. *Arch Virol* 1995;140:2215-26.
[194] Ramsingh A, Collins D. A point mutation in the VP4 coding sequence of coxsackievirus B4 influences virulence. *J Virol* 1995;69:7278-81.
[195] Rico-Hesse R, Pallansch M, Nottay B, Kew O. Geographic distribution of wild poliovirus type 1 genotypes. *Virology* 1987;160:311-22.
[196] Righthand V, Blackbum R. Steady-state infection by ECHOvirus 6 associated with nonlytic viral RNA and an unprocessed capsid polypeptide. *J Virol* 1989;63:5268-75.
[197] Rivera V, Welsh J, Maizel J. Comparative sequence analysis of the 5′-noncoding region of the enteroviruses and rhinoviruses. *Virology* 1988;165:42-50.
[198] Robinson C, Doane W, Rhodes A. Report of an outbreak of febrile illness with pharyngeal lesions and exanthems, Toronto, summer 1957- isolation of group A Coxsackie virus. *Can Med Assoc J* 1958;79:615-21.

[199] Roivainen M, Hyypia T, Piirainen L, Kalkkinen N, Stanway G, Hovi T. RGD-dependent entry of coxsackievirus A9 into host cells and its bypass after cleavage of VP1 protein by intestinal proteases. *J Virol* 1991;65:4735-40.

[200] Romero J. Reverse-transcrption polimerase chain reaction detection of the enteroviruses. *Arch Pathol Lab Med* 1999;123:1161-9.

[201] Rossouw E, Tsilimigras C, Schoub B. Molecular epidemiology of a coxsackievirus B3 outbreak. *J Med Virol* 1991;34:165-71.

[202] Rotbart H. Diagnosis of enteroviral meningitis with the polimerase chain reaction. *J Pediatr* 1990;117:85-9

[203] Rotbart H. Enzymatic RNA amplification of the enteroviruses. *J Clin Microbiol* 1990;28:438-42.

[204] Rotbart H. Meningitis and encephalitis. In: Rotbart H, ed. *Human Enterovirus Infections*. Washington, DC: ASM Press;1995.p.271-89.

[205] Rotbart H. Enteroviral infections of the central nervous system. *Clin Infect Dis* 1995;20:971-81.

[206] Rotbart H, Kirkegaard K. Picornavirus pathogenesis: viral access, attachment and entry into susceptible cells. *Semmin Virol* 1992;3:483-99.

[207] Rotbart H, Romero J. Laboratory diagnosis of enteroviral infections. In: Rotbart H, eds. *Human enterovirus Infections*. Washington, DC: American Society for Microbiology Press;1995.p.401-18.

[208] Roux L, Simon A, Holland J. Effects of defective interfering viruses on virus replication and pathogenesis. *Adv Virus Res* 1991;40:181-211.

[209] Rueckert R. Picornaviridae: the viruses and their replication. In: Fields B, Knipe D, Howley P, et al, eds. *Virology*. 3rd ed. Philadelphia, Pa: Lippincott Raven Publisher; 1996.p.609-54.

[210] Ryan MD, Flint M. Virus encoded proteinases of the Picornavirus super-group. *J Gen Virol* 1997;78:699-723.

[211] Saiki R, Gelfand D, Stoffel S. Primer-directed enzymatic amplification of DNA with a termoestable DNA polymerase. *Science* 1988;239:487-91.

[212] Samuelson A, Skoog E, Forsgren M. Aspects on the serodiagnosis of enterovirus infections by ELISA. *Serodiagn Immunother Infect Dis* 1990;4:395-406.

[213] Santti J, Harvala H, Kinnunen L, Hyypia T. Molecular epidemiology and evolution of coxsackievirus A9. *J Gen Virol* 2000;81:1361-72.

[214] Sarmiento L, Mas P, Goyenechea A, Palomera R, Morier L, Capo V. First epidemic of echovirus 16 meningitis in Cuba. *Emerg Infect Dis* 2001;7:887-9.

[215] Sarmiento L. Enteroviral Meningitis and Emergence of Rare Enterovirus Types: Cuban Experience. In: Phyllis V Strong, ed. *Focus on Meningitis Research*. New York: Nova Science Publishers, Inc; 2004.p.1-14.

[216] Schlesinger Y, Sawyer M, Storch G. Enteroviral meningitis in infancy: potential role for polimerase chain reaction in patient management. *Pediatrics* 1994;94:157-62.

[217] Schmidt N, Ho H, Lennette E. Propagation and isolation of group A coxsackieviruses in RD cells. *J Clin Microbiol* 1975;2:183-5.

[218] Severini G, Mestroni L, Falaschi A, Camerini F, Giacca M. Nested polymerase chain reaction for high-sensitivity detection of enteroviral RNA in biological samples. *J Clin Microbiol* 1993;31:1345-9.

[219] Shafren D, Bates R, Agrez M, Herd R, Burns G, Barry L. Coxsackieviruses B1, B3, and B5 use decay accelerating factor as a receptor for cell attachment. *J Virol* 1995;69:3873-7.

[220] Shafren D, Dorahy D, Ingham R, Burns G, Barry R. Coxsackievirus A21 binds to decay-accelerating factor but requires intercellular adhesion molecule 1 for cell entry. *J Virol* 1997;71:4736-43.

[221] Sharief M, Hentges R, Ciardi M. Intrathecal immune response in patients with the post-polio syndrome. *N Engl J Med* 1991;325:749-55.

[222] Shimizu H, Utama A, Yoshii K, Yoshida H, Yoneyama T, Sinniah M, et al. Enterovirus 71 from fatal and nonfatal cases of hand, foot and mouth disease epidemics in Malaysia, Japan and Taiwan in 1997-1998. *Jpn J Infect Dis* 1999;52:12-5.

[223] Singer J, Maur P, Riley J, Smith P. Management of central nervous system infections during an epidemic of enteroviral aseptic meningitis. *J Pediatr* 1980;96:559-63.

[224] Skinner M, Racaniello V, Dunn G, Cooper J, Minor P, Almond J. A new model for the secondary structure of the 5′ noncoding RNA of poliovirus is supported by biochemical and genetic data which also show that RNA secondary structure is important to neurovirulence. *J Mol Biol* 1989;207:379-92.

[225] Sole M, Liu P. Viral myocarditis: a paradigm for understanding the pathogenesis and treatment of dilated cardiomyopathy. *J Am Coll Cardiol Suppl A* 1993;22:99A-105A.

[226] Somekh E, Cesar K, Handsher R, Hanukoglu A, Dalal I, Ballin A, et al. An outbreak of echovirus 13 meningitis in central Israel. *Epidemiol Infect* 2003;130:257-62.

[227] Sonenberg N. Poliovirus translation. Curr Top Microbiol Immunol 1990;161:23-47.

[228] Spigland I, Fox J, Elveback L, Wasserman F, Ketler A, Brandt C, et al. The Virus Watch Program: a continuing surveillance of viral infections in metropolitan New York families. II. Laboratory methods and preliminary reports on infections revealed by virus isolations. *Am J Epidemiol* 1966;83:413-35.

[229] Stanway G, Hyypia T. Parechoviruses. *J Virol* 1999;73:5249-54.

[230] Strikas R, Anderson L, Parker R. Temporal and geographic patterns of isolates of nonpolio enterovirus in the United States, 1970-1983. *J Infect Dis* 1986;153:346-51.

[231] Sutter R, Kew O, Cochi S. Live, Attenuated Poliovirus Vaccines. In: Plotkin SA, Orenstein WA, eds. *Vaccines*. 4th ed. Philadelphia: WB Saunders; 2004.

[232] Takeda N, Tanimura M, Miyamura K. Molecular evolution of the major capsid protein VP1 of enterovirus 70. *J Virol* 1994;68:854-62.

[233] Tomko R, Xu R, Philipson L. HCAR and MCAR: the human and mouse cellular receptors for subgroup C adenoviruses and group B coxsackieviruses. *Proc Natl Acad Sci USA* 1997;94:3352-6.

[234] Tonew M, Hartmann M, Schmidtke M, Stelzner A. Replication and persistence of Coxsackievirus B3 in human fibroblasts. *Int J Microbiol Parasitol and Infect Dis* 1995;282:92-101.

[235] Torfason G, Frisk G, Diderholm H. Indirect and reverse radioimmunoassay and their apparent specificities in detection of antibodies to enteroviruses in human sera. *J Med Virol* 1984;13:13-8.

[236] Toyoda H, Nicklin M, Murray M, Anderson C, Dunn J, Studier F, et al. A second virus-encoded proteinase involved in proteolytic processing of poliovirus polyprotein. *Cell* 1986;45:761-70.

[237] Tracy S, Chapman N, Rubocki R, Beck M. Host Immune Responses to Enterovirus Infections. In: Rotbart H, ed. *Human Enterovirus Infections*. Washington, DC: ASM Press;1995.p.175-91.

[238] Trallero G, Casas I, Avellon A, Perez C, Tenorio A, De La Loma A. First epidemic of aseptic meningitis due to echovirus type 13 among Spanish children. *Epidemiol Infect* 2003;130:251-6.

[239] Van Dyke A, Flanegan J. Identification of poliovirus polypeptide p63 as a soluble RNA-dependent RNA polymerase. *J Virol* 1980;35:732-40.

[240] van Vliet K, Glimaker M, Lebon P, Klapper P, Taylor C, Ciardi M. Multicenter evaluation of the amplicor enterovirus PCR test with cerebrospinal fluid from patients with aseptic meningitis. *J Clin Microbiol* 1998;36:2652-7.

[241] Voroshilova M, Chumakov K. Poliomyelitis-like properties of AB-IV-coxsackie A7 group of viruses. *Prog Med Virol* 1959;2:106-70.

[242] Wecker I, ter Meulen V. RD cells in the laboratory diagnosis of enteroviruses. *Med Microbiol Immunol* 1977;163:233-40.

[243] Wenner H. Virus diseases associated with cutaneous eruptions. *Prog Med Virol* 1973;16:269-336.

[244] Wilfert C, Lehrman S, Katz S. Enteroviruses and meningitis. *Pediatr Infect Dis* 1983;2:333-41.

[245] Wimmer E, Hellen C, Cao X. Genetics of poliovirus. *Annu Rev Genetics* 1993;27:353-436.

[246] World Health Assembly. Global eradication of poliomyelitis by the year 2000: resolution of the 41st World Health Assembly. Resolution WHA 41.28. *World Health Organization,* Geneva; 1988.

[247] World Health Organization. Report of the interim meeting of the Technical Consultation Group on the global eradication of poliomyelitis, WHO/EPI/GEN/02. *World Health Organization*, Geneva; 2002.

[248] World Health Organization. Global Polio Eradication Initiative Strategic Plan 2004-2008. *World Health Organization,* Geneva; 2004.p.22.

[249] Yang C, De L, Yang S, Gómez J, Cruz J, Halloway B, et al. Genotype-specific in vitro amplification of sequences of the wild type 3 polioviruses from México y Guatemala. *Virus Research* 1992;24:277-96.

[250] Zaman S, Carlsson B, Morikawa A, Jeansson S, Narayanan I, Thiringer K. Poliovirus antibody titres, relative affinity, and neutralising capacity in maternal milk. *Arch Dis Child* 1993;68:198-201.

[251] Zhang H, Blake W, Ouyang X, Pandolfino Y, Morgan-Capner P, Archard C. A single amino acid substitution in the capsid protein VP1 of Coxsackievirus B3 (CVB3) alters

plaque phenotype in Vero cells but not cardiovirulence in a mouse model. *Arch Virol* 1995;140:959-66.

[252] Zheng D, Zhang L, Fang Z. Distribution of wild type 1 poliovirus genotypes in China. *J Infect Dis* 1993;168:1361-7.

[253] Zoll G, Melchers W, Kopecka H, Jambroes G, van der Poel H, Galama J. General primer-mediated polymerase chain reaction for detection of enteroviruses: Application for diagnostic routine and persistent infections. *J Clin Microbiol* 1992;30:160-5.

Chapter III

Enterovirus-Induced Type 1 Diabetes

_Luis Sarmiento-Pérez_*

Department of Virology, PAHO/WHO Collaborating Center for Viral Diseases, "Pedro Kouri" Tropical Medicine Institute, Havana, Cuba.

Abstract

Enteroviruses have been examined for their possible role in the etiology of type 1 diabetes for nearly 40 years, yet the evidence remains inconclusive. This chapter provides evidences suggesting the involvement of enteroviruses in the development and/or acceleration of type 1 diabetes and discusses potential mechanisms of pathogenesis. These evidences include the isolation of coxsackievirus B4 from the pancreas of a child at diagnosis of type 1 diabetes, several epidemiological and prospective studies showing that some cases of type 1 diabetes are strongly associated with enterovirus infections, seasonal incidence studies, case-control studies that show an increased prevalence and levels of IgM antibodies to enterovirus in newly diagnosed patients. Other evidences involves several case studies in which diabetes develops after an enterovirus infections, increased T cell response to enterovirus antigens in type 1 diabetic patients, suggestions that enterovirus infections during pregnancy might initiate the events leading to childhood diabetes, and a higher frequency of enterovirus RNA in the serum/blood of type 1 diabetic patients at diagnosis. The currently available information supports the assumption that the role of enterovirus infections in the etiology of type 1 diabetes is stronger than for most other environmental agents, but the causal relationship remains to be confirmed in future studies.

Keywords: enterovirus, type 1 diabetes, autoimmunity, environmental factor, etiology, pathogenic mechanisms.

---

* Correspondence concerning this article should be addressed to Luis Sarmiento Pérez, Department of Virology, PAHO/WHO Collaborating Center for Viral Diseases, "Pedro Kouri" Tropical Medicine Institute, Autopista Novia del Mediodía, km 6, PO Box, 601, Marianao 13, Havana, Cuba; fax: 53-7-2046051; email: sarmiento@ipk.sld.cu or lsarmientop@yahoo.com.

Type 1 diabetes mellitus is an autoimmune disease of increasing incidence, associated with significant morbidity and mortality, but currently without cure or prevention. The cause of this chronic and debilitating disease is unknown. Genetic and epidemiological evidence points to an overriding environmental influence on diabetes development, and, of possible external candidates, the enterovirus has attracted the greatest attention as a putative trigger or accelerant of disease [2,24,43,70,112,124,152,171,179,189].

However, there are at least three factors that have made research into the putative enteroviral etiology of type 1 diabetes difficult to conduct and interpret: i) the widespread exposure to these and related viruses that occurs during childhood, which makes it difficult to study the natural history of these infections in target populations, ii) enterovirus infections are common whilst diabetes is relatively uncommon, and, iii) any virus effects will probably have taken place some months or years before diabetes or pre-diabetes is diagnosed, by which time host-virus interactions are hard to study.

Despite these difficulties, several lines of evidences contribute to the continued plausibility of enterovirus-induced type 1 diabetes. The main findings are listed in Table 1 and the major studies are described in detail below.

Table 1. Summary of evidence associating enteroviruses with type 1 diabetes.

Evidence	References
Virus isolation from pancreas at diabetes onset/in association with pancreas infiltration in patients with acute enterovirus infection	105, 210
Identification of enterovirus genome in islet cells of diabetic patients, but not non-diabetic controls, by in situ hybridization	209
Enterovirus-specific IgM/neutralizing antibodies more prevalent at diagnosis of type 1 diabetes vs controls	9, 56, 72
Case control and case reports showing increase in enterovirus antibodies immediately before development of islet cell antibodies, and/or type 1 diabetes.	77, 89, 120, 158
Enterovirus RNA detection in serum in relation to development of islet cell antibodies, and/or type 1 diabetes.	5, 23, 121, 122, 132

I. Serological Evidences

A possible relationship between enterovirus infection and type 1 diabetes mellitus has been under investigation for nearly 40 years. Early serological studies provided supporting serological evidence linking enteroviral infection with type 1 diabetes. The first report of higher frequency of coxsackievirus group B (CVB) antibodies in newly diagnosed diabetic patients than matched control subjects was published in 1969 [56]. Since then, there have been several studies of similar design from a great number of countries confirming this observation.

The majority of studies have found al least one positive association with specific coxsackievirus and or a greater frequency of positive serology for several enterovirus when compared to control [9,23,31,52,53,57,72,88,89,101,110,132,164]. The most consistent finding has been the elevation of IgM class CVB antibodies in newly diagnosed diabetic patients referring to quite recent infections. A Swedish group reported an extremely high prevalence of CVB IgM (67 %) among children with type 1 diabetes diagnosed during an outbreak of type 1 diabetes in Upssala in 1982 through 1984 but a complete absence of CVB IgM (0 %) in age-matched controls [50,52,72]. Nevertheless, the presence of IgM does not necessarily indicate recent primary infection. IgM may result from reactivation of a latent infection, or it may indicate lack of viral clearance.

However, not all serological studies seeking associations between enterovirus infections have reported positive results and therefore this remains a controversial area of research. Some studies have found no evidence of a correlation between the onset of type 1 diabetes and Coxsackie B viral infections, while other studies have found higher levels of anti-Coxsackie B virus-specific antibodies in non-diabetic control subjects than in recent-onset diabetic patients[65,128,134,144,148,170,188]. The inconsistent evidence for or against an association between enterovirus infection and type 1 diabetes was the finding of Green et al. [64] in a recent review of published serological controlled studies through a medline search (1966 to 2002), supplemented by references from identified papers and hand search of relevant journals (Table 2 A , B).

Table 2 A) Lack association between enteroviral infection(s) and type 1 diabetes mellitus.

Ref/ year	Study site	Number of case/ controls	Cases: Incident/ prevalent (time since diagnosis)	Cases: Age (years)	Cases and controls matched (explicit individual or frequency matching) for: Age	Sex	Place	Sample time	Enteroviral Serotypes Tested	Test used
134/1975	UK	49/49	Prevalent	7-63	Yes	Yes	Yes	Yes	CV B1–B5	NtAb
170/1978	Germany	81/80	2-4 weeks	1-54	No	No	No	Yes	CV B1–B5	HA for IgM and IgG
44/1983	USA	175/67	At diagnosis	Children	No	No	Yes	Yes	CV B1–B6	IgM IF
148/1982	USA	33/33	At diagnosis	Children	Yes	Yes	No	Yes	CV B3–B5	NtAb, CF
188/1989	Sweeden	98/94	At diagnosis	0-14	Yes	Yes	Yes	Yes	CV B1–B6	IgM RIA
65/1972	UK	34/121	At diagnosis	adult	No	No	No	No	CV B1–B6	NtAb

Reprinted from reference [64].

Various studies may demonstrate an association between virus infection and disease, but there can be numerous reasons why a study can fail to show an association, even when one exist. The discrepancies could be due to the fact that in all these studies the determination of enterovirus infection was carried out indirectly through the determination of anti - enterovirus antibodies. The serotype (or even group) specificity of many of these serological assays is poor and identification of an association between a specific viral serotype and type 1 diabetes is complicated by several factors: cross-reactivity between the more than 64 enterovirus serotypes and between enteroviruses and related picornaviruses such as hepatitis A; heterotypic antibody responses to second and subsequent infections; individual variation in antibody response; the existence of distinct viral strains (indistinguishable on standard serotype assays) within serotypes and the capricious nature of antibody response to enterovirus infection.

Another factor is the own serious limitations of the seroepidemiologic approach to studying past exposure to diabetogenic enteroviruses [42,51,60,61,73]. In addition, only a limited range of enteroviruses has been tested for in most studies; i.e. range of 3-14 serotypes in those studies employing traditional serological assays. We suggest that these studies probably should consider any enterovirus as a possible etiologic agent and should include the circulating enteroviruses in the subset to be examined.

Table 2 B) Positive association between enteroviral infection(s) and type 1 diabetes mellitus.

Ref/ year	Study site	Number of case/ controls	Cases: Incident/ prevalent (time since diagnosis)	Cases: Age (years)	Cases and controls matched (explicit individual or frequency matching) for: Age	Sex	Place	Sample time	Enteroviral Serotypes Tested	Test used
55/1969	UK	123/250	Recent onset	0-60+	No	No	No	No	CV A2, A5, A10, A16, CV B3–B5	CF, NtAb
57/1973	UK	162/319	0-16 weeks	0-20+	Yes	No	No	No	CV B1–B5	NtAb
88/1974	USA	9/36	<6 weeks	4 -13	Yes	Yes	Yes	Yes	CV B1–B6	NtAb
164/1982	Japan	103/56	Prevalent > 4 years	3-20	Yes	Yes	No	No	CV B1–B5	NtAb
110/1983	UK	28/290	2-16 weeks	3-14	No	No	No	No	CV B1–B6	NtAb
9/1985	UK	38/98	<2 weeks	<15	Yes	No	No	No	CV B1–B5	IgM Elisa
9/1985	Austria	72/82	<1month	<15	Yes	No	Yes	No	CV B1–B5	IgM Elisa
9/1985	Aus-tralia	12/24	<2weeks	2-12	Yes	Yes	No	Yes	CV B1–B5	IgM Elisa
54/1992	Swee-den	23/46	At diagnosis	<15	Yes	No	Yes	Yes	CV B1–B5	IgM RIA
72/1995	USA	128/120	New onset	<18	Yes	Yes	Yes	Yes	CV B1–B6 CVA9, E 4, 6, 9, 11, 30, 34, EV71.	Mono clonal IgM EIA

CVAs, Coxsackie A viruses; CVBs, Coxsackie B viruses; CF, complement fixation; EIA, enzyme immunoassay; NtAb, neutralizing antibodies; RT-PCR, Reverse Transcriptase-Polimerase Chain Reaction; RIA, radioimmunoassay; IF, Immunofluorescence; HA, Hemaglutination.

Reprinted from reference [64].

II. Evidences of Enteroviral RNA Detection

Though serological evidences have failed to prove or disprove the suggested diseases association and often provide conflicting conclusions from very similar study design, a link between enterovirus infections and the development of type 1 diabetes mellitus have been bolstered by recent studies using more sensitive techniques such as direct detection of the enterovirus genome by Reverse Transcriptase-Polimerase Chain Reaction (RT-PCR) in peripheral blood [116,140].

Separate research groups have described a more frequent occurrence of enterovirus RNA in the serum or blood of newly diagnosed diabetic patients than control subjects [5,20,21,25,26,27,36,48,109,132,187,206]. Some of these groups of researchers have also investigated enteroviral RNA in serum or blood from autoantibody-positive and autoantibody-negative children (132) as well as siblings of diabetic children (206). In such studies both patients, siblings and autoantibody-positive children showed a higher frequency of enterovirus RNA compared with the controls and autoantibody-negative subjects.

RT-PCR applied to blood or serum essentially indicates a viremia. During viremia, enteroviruses are transported both intracellularly by mononuclear cells (lymphocytes or monocytes) and extracellularly in serum to susceptible target organs including the pancreas. It is thus evident that the assay result is dependent on the moment of sampling, since the viremic period is believed to last only a few weeks at most. Therefore, only a fraction of enterovirus infections can be detected by RT-PCR study of serum or blood and this would explain the low frequency of enteroviral RNA detection in most studies.

As viremia is a sign of an acute infection, a significantly higher frequency of enterovirus RNA in blood or serum from type 1 diabetic children at the onset of disease, their siblings as well as in prediabetic children (defined by autoantibody analysis), than in children of a control group reveals that enterovirus infections may be aetiologically important in the development of type 1 diabetes, either by initiating the development of the disease or by operating as the final insult to β cells in individuals. This does not exclude the possibility that viremia would be a sign of chronic enterovirus infection. It is nevertheless probable that a local chronic β-cells infection could produce sufficient quantities of viruses in the circulation to be detected by RT-PCR.

It is noteworthy that other studies using this methology have also failed to detect such association. In a prospective study within a cohort of genetically high risk children no evidence was found that enterovirus infections are associated with the process leading to β-cell autoimmunity [62]. In a group of newly diagnosed type 1 diabetes children in Finland no enterovirus RNA was detectable in contrast to a group of prediabetic children with an enterovirus RNA prevalence of 22 % [122].

The detection of the enterovirus genome is usually carried out by amplification of the 5-non-translated region, which is very conserved among the enterovirus group. Accordingly, one advantage of RT-PCR method is that the assay detects RNA of all known enteroviruses as the amplified sequence is common to all. Hence, sequencing of this part of the viral genome means that comparisons of the sequence only vaguely implicate a specific serotype. Molecular typing of enteroviruses should ideally focus on regions encoding determinants for neutralization (i.e. VP1 that codes for the major antigenic sites and most type-specific neutralization determinants). Nevertheless, direct sequencing of amplicons of the 5'NTR has revealed in most studies viruses of the CVB group [5,20,21,23,132], in agreement with those serological studies that detect an increase in anti-CVB IgM at type 1 diabetes diagnosis [9,72]. The remarkable consistency of the results from these studies have provided further evidence supporting the conception that enterovirus infections are implicated in human type 1 diabetes.

III. PROSPECTIVE STUDIES

When interpreting the data and analyses described above we note that there several studies which now have detected evidence of enterovirus infection associated with type 1 diabetes. As have been noted, such a study design usually involve patients with clinical diabetes together with control subjects and therefore is not optimal for detection of infections which have occurred long before clinical manifestation of diabetes.

Large-scale prospective studies are required to firmly establish a causal relationship between enterovirus infections and development of prediabetic autoimmunity or progression from autoimmunity to clinical diabetes. Several prospective studies have been conducted to study the natural course of the β-cell damage and to test various intervention strategies for the prevention of type 1 diabetes mellitus.

The first prospective studies designed to assess the role of enterovirus infections in the induction and acceleration of type 1 diabetes mellitus were carried out under Childhood Diabetes in Finland (DiMe) scheme. This study, which was carried out during 1987-1993, initiated a new era in the investigation of the pathogenesis of type 1 diabetes mellitus. They were based in three separate series: 1) an intrauterine exposure series comprising pregnant mothers whose children subsequently manifested type 1 diabetes mellitus and control mothers whose children remained nondiabetic; 2) a cohort of initially unaffected siblings of diabetic children who were followed until they developed subclinical β–cell damage (type 1 diabetes-related autoantibodies) or clinical type 1 diabetes and control siblings who remained nondiabetic; 3) a case-control series comprising children with newly diagnosed type 1 diabetes and control subjects.

In the prospective studies was documented serologically and molecularly that initially non-diabetic siblings of diabetic patients who manifested subclinical β-cell damage or clinical type 1 diabetes acquire enterovirus infections more frequently than do their healthy siblings. Interestingly, the excess of infections was observed both closely prior to the clinical diagnosis as well as several years before overt diabetes. Furthermore, enterovirus infections appeared to coincide with increase of autoimmune markers for progression to type 1 diabetes, especially for antibodies against islet cell (ICA), and glutamic decarboxylase (GADA) or the onset of clinical disease [77,89,122,158].

These findings have been confirmed in the Finish Diabetes Prediction and Prevention trial (DIPP) which was initiated in Finland in 1994. The DIPP study is a prospective population-based birth-cohort study in which Finnish children with increased genetic risk for type 1 diabetes were studied for the appearance of diabetes-associated autoantibodies at 3- to 12-month intervals from birth over the first 2 years.

Again, enterovirus infections showed clustering at the time when autoantibodies first appeared. The frequency of enterovirus infections during the entire follow- up period was higher in the children who presented with signs of β-cell autoimmunity than in their control subjects matched for time of birth, sex, and the HLA-DQB alleles associated with type 1 diabetes mellitus. The case and control children had similar frequencies of adenovirus infections, implying that the children who developed autoantibodies are not more susceptible to viral infections in general.

The frequency of enterovirus infections verified serologically was higher in the case children during the 6-month period preceding the appearance of the first diabetes-associated autoantibodies than in the matched time interval for the control children. The difference between case subjects and control subjects was even more pronounced for enterovirus RNA detection during this interval. In addition, positive enterovirus RNA findings in case children were significantly clustered around this 6-month period. This temporal association between enterovirus infections and the onset of β-cell autoimmunity is consistent with the hypothesis that enteroviruses may be one of the factors initiating autoimmunity [114,121,163,165,166].

Other prospective study series such as the Nutritional Prevention of Type 1 Diabetes Mellitus Intervention Trial reach similar conclusions, namely, that the infants who progress to diabetes have the strongest enteroviral exposure.

IV. Type 1 Diabetes and Enterovirus Infections in Pregnancy

There are several evidences of an increased frequency of enteroviral infections during pregnancies from which children who later develop type 1 diabetes are born [32,33,34,35,36,37,38,120,121]. Clustering in time and place of birth as described in United Kingdom [162] suggest that an exposure associated with the risk of the disease would have an epidemic pattern of spread and is operating during the perinatal time of life.

Stronger indications are yielded by population-based case-control studies from researchers in Sweden looking at virus antibodies by the time of delivery in mother whose children later developed type 1 diabetes mellitus. These studies showed group-specific antibodies to enteroviruses and also type-specific CVB IgM antibody titres to be higher in mothers whose children later developed diabetes compared with control mothers. The Swedish group also demonstrated that the association was rather specific to enterovirus, since the levels of antibodies to mumps, herpesvirus, or toxoplasma did not differ between mothers of cases and control subjects [33,35,37,38].

In the intrauterine exposure series of the DiMe study previously described, maternal enterovirus infections during pregnancy were shown to entail a risk of diabetes in the offspring. The risk effect was associated with clinical diabetes manifesting before the age of 3 years [89]. The diabetes risk effect seemed to be specific for enteroviruses, as it was not associated with other virus infections documented in the same subjects. The frequency of other virus infections such as cytomegalovirus, adenovirus and Epstein Barr virus did not differ between the groups [76,89,91].

In the DIPP study the occurrence of enterovirus infections during pregnancy was also evaluated using serum samples obtained at the end of the first trimester of pregnancy from the mothers of the case-and control children as well as cord blood samples. In contrast with the DiMe study, the occurrence of enterovirus infections during pregnancy did not seem to be more common than for mothers in the control group as no differences between the groups were observed [121].

However, there are two reports from individual clinical cases which have supported the suggestion that enterovirus infections during pregnancy might initiate the events leading to childhood diabetes.

In the first report an infant was followed regularly from birth until the child progressed to clinical type 1 diabetes at the age of 14 months. He had a strong enterovirus exposure exceptionally early in life; the first enterovirus infection occurred before the age of 3 months and the second between the age of 9 and 12 months. The first infection probably occurred at birth, when the child had symptoms of a respiratory infection. This infection was followed by the appearance of β-cell autoimmunity, and clinical type 1 diabetes was diagnosed shortly after the second infection. The child had a low level of maternal enterovirus antibodies and short duration of breast-feeding, both associated with increased risk for enterovirus infections during the foetal period and infancy [120].

In a separate report a baby girl, who was born severely growth-retarded with neonatal insulin-deficient diabetes, suggested that enteroviral infections may induce β-cell autoimmunity even in utero [145]. The infant's serum contained high concentrations of circulating antibodies against islet cells and their antigens, such as insulin and GADA. The serological studies showed that the mother had contracted an enteroviral infection possibly caused by echovirus 6 or other cross-reacting agent because the serotype-specific antibody titre increased from less than 4 to 16 during pregnancy. The T cell response was clearly positive 3 months but no longer at 12 months after birth, supporting the diagnosis of an intrauterine infection. Based in this finding, the pathogenic process could have been triggered by a maternally transmitted echovirus 6 infection involving the fetal pancreas early in gestation. It is not certain whether the infection directly damaged pancreatic cells during organogenesis but it did induce an aggressive β-cell targeted autoimmune attack. This resulted in massive β-cell loss and insulin deficiency during the first half of pregnancy, subsequent severe fetal growth retardation and immediate postnatal diabetes.

In a recent study, the Swedish group revealed that intrauterine exposure to maternal enterovirus infection during pregnancy is a risk factor for development of autoimmune thyroiditis during childhood and adolescence. As type 1 diabetes mellitus and autoimmune thyroiditits are closely linked, a common pathogenetic factor like enterovirus infection was suggested [176].

It is, however, likely that exposure to other viruses during fetal life might initiate type 1 diabetes mellitus [34]. Some studies have shown an association between congenital rubella and diabetes arising later in life [44]. The most compelling evidence was the observation of a very high prevalence of diabetes occurring in children or young adults who were followed up for complications of the fetal rubella embryopathy syndrome [127]. Because the rubella embryopathy syndrome is now extremely rare due to effective population-based vaccination programmes this fetal infection would not account for a large number of cases.

To summarize, the findings of time and space clustering of birth dates for later diabetic cases suggest that enterovirus infections could also operate during the early phases of the pathogenesis.

V. Direct Evidences – Case Reports

In terms of direct evidence for the role of enterovirus infections in the etiology of type 1 diabetes mellitus, the most dramatic evidence for a role of enteroviral infection in the pathogenesis of type 1 diabetes was reported by Yoon et al., in 1979 [210]. These investigators isolated a coxsackievirus B4 from the autopsy pancreas of a 10-year-old boy who died of diabetes ketoacidosis but also developed clinical signs of meningitis. During life there was a rising serological titre to the virus cultured at autopsy, which makes it unlikely that the virus was a laboratory contaminant. Immunoflurescence did identify the virus in the brain stem of the patient. The histology of the pancreas appears to have been typical of type 1 diabetes with insulin-deficient islets and insulitis but little evidence of the dramatic β-cell necrosis which characterizes coxsackieviral pancreatitis in infants [45]. Following inoculation of the viral isolate into mice, the animals developed hyperglycemia, inflammatory cells in the islet of Langerhans, and islet endocrine cell necrosis. Virus could be demonstrated in the murine insulin containing β-cells, thereby fulfilling Koch's postulates. Although this finding has been documented only once, the isolation of an enterovirus from the pancreas of a diabetic patient at diseases diagnosis is a strong argument for suggesting the role of enteroviruses in the etiology of type 1 diabetes mellitus [98,136].

A reasonable explanation for the positive culture of a coxsackievirus B4 in the autopsy studied by Yoon et al., was done by Foulis in 1997 [47]. According to Foulis´s analysis it is possible that this child had already lost a critical number of β-cell through the typical autoimmune process and that the clinical presentation of diabetes was provoked by a severe coxsackieviral infection, accompanied by viraemia, affecting primarily the brain; i.e. the virus may not have been primarily responsible for the β-cell loss in this child.

Other study reports the isolation of another enterovirus, echovirus 9, from a 6-week-old girl with an acute onset of type 1 diabetes mellitus. The coincident onsets of type 1 diabetes mellitus during generalized severe infection with echovirus 9 strongly suggest a causal relationship between the viral infection and type 1 diabetes mellitus in the patient. At variance with previously reported case, the patient's isolate did not induced necrosis and β-cell death. In addition the patient did not had sign pointing to an autoimmune reaction [199].

There are others direct supporting evidence on the association of coxsackie B viral infection with the onset of type 1 diabetes. A girl who died of myocarditis and diabetes shortly after open heart surgery had lymphocytic infiltration of the islets and beta cell necrosis. Coxsackie B4 antigens were detected in the islets by immunofluorescence and high levels of antibody against coxsackie B4 virus were present in the child's serum. In addition, a young girl developed diabetic symptoms for a 10-day period shortly after coxsackie B5 viral infection, went into remission for 2 months, and then developed definite T1D. The virus isolated from the girl's feces caused glucose intolerance in DBA/2, SJL/J, and Swiss male mice, but not in BALB/c or C3H mice. Islet cell antibodies were found in the child a week before the onset of diabetes and immunogenetic analysis revealed that the child had markers indicating a high risk for the development of type 1 diabetes [104].

It is important to note that some studies failed to detect evidence of viral infection in diabetic pancreases [16,45] and in contrast with the apparent success of the detection of enterovirus RNA from blood, in the majority of studies no enterovirus genome could be detected when pancreas from cases of type 1 diabetes was analysed post-mortem at some stage during the first year after diagnosis [47,49].

Only one study known to us [209] provides a definite islet-cell tropism of enteroviruses in human pancreases in vivo. In this study, autopsy pancreases from 12 newborn infants who died of fulminant coxsackievirus infections, as well as pancreata from 65 deceased adolescent and adult type 1 diabetic patients were studied for presence of enteroviral RNA by in situ hybridization. In addition, 40 non diabetic control pancreases were included in the study. Enterovirus genomes could be detected in islet, but not in exocrine cells of deceased newborn infants studied (7 out of 12), as well as in type 1 diabetic patients (4 out of 65). In contrast, pancreatic control tissues from non diabetic patients were consistently negative for enteroviral RNA.

VI. Humoral and Cellular Immune Response to Enteroviruses

It is currently widely accepted that T cell mediated immunity against pancreatic β-cells plays a crucial role in the pathogenesis of type 1 diabetes. Although the important role of cell mediated immunity in the pathogenesis of type 1 diabetes is accepted, studies on the characteristics of cellular immunity against enterovirus infections and their relationship with type 1 diabetes are few.

Some studies have found an increased T-cell proliferation to enterovirus antigens among newly diagnosed type 1 diabetic patients when compared to non-diabetic donors [99,100,111]. Other studies found no differences in T-cell proliferation against coxsackievirus B4-infected lysate between diabetic patients and healthy non-diabetic donors [190]. In contrast, some groups have reported a reduced percentage of responders to purified coxsackievirus B4 amongst children with new- onset type 1 diabetes compared to control children [101].

One of the most representative studies evaluating the cellular immune responses to enterovirus antigens was reported by Juhela S and coworkers [168]. This study showed that children with diabetes for 4-72 months more often had T-cell responses to the coxsackievirus B4-infected cell lysate antigen than children with new-onset diabetes ($P < 0.01$) or control children ($P < 0.01$). Responses to recombinant nonstructural protein 2C of coxsackievirus B4 were also more frequent in children with type 1 diabetes for 4-72 months when compared with control subjects ($P = 0.03$), whereas the responses to purified coxsackievirus B4 and recombinant VP0 protein, which did not contain nonstructural proteins, did not differ. These data suggest that T-cell responses to coxsackievirus B4 proteins and particularly to the antigens containing the nonstructural proteins of the virus are increased in children with type 1 diabetes after the onset of the disease. However, in children with new-onset diabetes, responses were normal or even decreased [101]. The low proliferative response against coxsackievirus B4 antigens at disease onset is in agreement with a previous study showing reduced T-cell proliferation against selected enterovirus peptide at time of diagnosis [168].

These studies were interpreted as indicating that coxsackievirus B4-reactive T cells are absent from the circulation because of redistribution into the inflamed pancreas and therefore unavailable for detection in peripheral blood. An alternative explanation for normal or reduced proliferation of T cells to enterovirus antigens was proposed by the research group headed by Professor Peakman. These researchers also found a lower frequency of T-cell proliferation to coxsackievirus B4 antigens in patients contrasted with the marked enhanced production of the inflammatory cytokine IFN-γ in response to coxsackievirus B4 antigens. The relative lack of proliferation, but enhanced IFN-γ production by anti- coxsackievirus B4 memory T- cell in type 1 diabetic patients was attributable to a different balance of phenotypically distinct populations of memory cells, when compared with control subjects. Accordingly, it was suggested that diabetes diagnosis is characterized by a state in which anti- coxsackievirus B4 effector cells (primed memory cell subset that produce the proinflammatory cytokine IFN-γ) are mobilized from the central memory pools (primed memory T-cells with the capacity to proliferate), which may in consequence become depleted. From this study it is possible that the explanation for the predominance of coxsackievirus B4-specific effector memory cells in patients with type 1 diabetes at diagnosis lies in either a recent or persistent exposure to coxsackievirus B4 infection [190,191].

Enterovirus-induced T cell responses also generate several other proinflammatory cytokines (e.g. interferon-α and-β), which can promote the activation of autoreactive T-cell clones [100]. By 1987, special interest was focused on interferon α when it was found that β cells express interferon-α in diabetic patients at autopsy [46]. Several year later, French investigators reported an increased level of interferon-α in the blood of patients with newly diagnosed type 1 diabetes and, interestingly, the presence of enterovirus RNA was found in half of the interferon-α positive patients, compared to no virus RNA detected among the interferon-α negative patients [21].

As interferon-α is part of the innate system, which is activated early during an infection, the increased interferon concentrations would be a reliable indicator of ongoing enterovirus infections. In fact, coxsackievirus B4 seems able to induce the synthesis of interferon-α in human β cells in vitro, thus mimicking the expression of this cytokine in the pancreas of type 1 diabetic patients [20,21]. In addition, it has been demonstrated that coxsackievirus B4 can strongly induce the production of interferon-α by peripheral blood mononuclear cells from patients with type 1 diabetes [79]. Finally, it is noteworthy that several data supports the contention that the abnormal localization of interferon-α in the pancreas of type 1 diabetic patients reflects a recent and/or silent viral infection at the time of diagnosis [87,92,174,191].

With regard to humoral response, several reports have shown that enterovirus infections may induce islet cell autoantibody seroconversión or increased level of several islet autoantibodies. Furthermore, the children who converted to islet cell autoantibody positivity during an enterovirus infection more often had the high-risk HLA-DQB1 genotype than did children who were constantly islet cell autoantibody - negative [77,89]. As has been noted elsewhere, other reports on individual cases reinforce the conclusion that enterovirus infection triggers the development of islet cell autoantibodies [120,145,173,199].

However, it is proposed in one study carried out in Italy that the autoimmune reaction develops after infection is likely to be transient and not related to diabetes progression or spreading to diabetes associated islet antigens. In such study, a small number of patients with acute coxsackievirus infection were prospectively followed and both humoral and cellular responses to a GAD-65 peptide sharing homology with a peptide from the non-structural CVB protein P2C were evaluated. Sixty percent of the subjects developed anti-GAD-65 antibodies and 78 % developed a T-cell response against two peptides encompassing the GAD-65/P2C homology region 247 to 279. After one year of follow-up, none of the subjects developed clinical disease or continued to show signs of anti-GAD-65 autoantibodies or T-cell immune responses to GAD-65 peptides [18].

VII. Epidemiological Evidence Suggesting Involvement of Enterovirus

As has been shown in chapter I, the incidence of type 1 diabetes varies depending on the geographical area and is the highest in northern Europe and Sardinia (21 new cases per year for every 100.000 inhabitants), medium in the rest of Europe and U.S (4-14 cases) and low in Asia and South America (less one per 100.000 per year). The incidence varies also remarkably amongst geographically closely located countries, and for example in Finland the incidence is three to five times higher than in the neighbouring countries Estonia and the Karelian Republic of Russia [113,142,151,185]. In addition, the incidence of type 1 diabetes increases in most Western Countries [63] and show temporary variations. For example, in Finland the incidence of type 1 diabetes has registered an increment of 13/100.000 in 1953 to near 40/100.000 in the 2000s which is four times higher than in the early 1950s [151,186].

The reasons behind this epidemiological pattern are largely unknown. Part of the international variation might be explained by variable frequencies of diabetes associated genes in different populations. However, the increase in the incidence rate has been so rapid that it cannot be explained only by genetic factors but rather by an increasing impact of some environmental factors. The marked seasonal variation in the incidence of type 1 diabetes mellitus has been interpreted as evidence of an infectious agent or agents for such environmental impact. Increasing rates of type 1 diabetes in some countries and epidemic of type 1 diabetes have been attributed to several enteroviruses viruses [92]. Several studies have been proposed or are in progress to assess the epidemiological association between type 1 diabetes and enterovirus infections.

Epidemiological Association Between Type 1 Diabetes and Enterovirus Infections

The seasonal variation in the incidence of type 1 diabetes parallels that of enteroviral infections. The annual peak of enterovirus diseases (August through September) [131,147] precedes the major peak of type 1 diabetes incidence (October through January) [55]. Many studies in both the northern and southern hemispheres have confirmed these findings, which have generally been interpreted as coinciding with the time of enterovirus infections. Moreover, epidemiological studies have been showed an increased incidence of type 1 diabetes after epidemics caused by enterovirus.

Gleason and co-workers [59] related temporal changes in the number of type 1 diabetes cases seen in Massachusetts, from 1964 through 1973 to the reported incidence of several infectious diseases, including enteroviral meningitis outbreaks. In 1974, an outbreak of 12 cases of type 1 diabetes was reported from Florida, U.S. Three of 9 cases tested, compared to 2 of 36 controls, had elevated neutralizing antibodies to coxsackievirus B3 [88] A report from Sweden found that 1 of 22 Swedish soldiers who contracted symptomatic coxsackieviris B infection (most likely with coxsackievirus B4) developed type 1 diabetes 10 weeks later [137].

A circumstantial association between the occurrence of an outbreak of coxsackievirus B5 occurred in Jefferson County, Alabama, USA during June to October, 1983 and a subsequent increase in the incidence of type 1 diabetes provides the best example of a temporal association between a enterovirus outbreak and increased disease incidence in the general population [200]. In this report, staticallly significant increases in the incidence of type 1 diabetes occurred immediately following the epidemic of coxsackievirus B5. The average annual incidence of type 1 diabetes in Jefferson County for the period 1979-1988 was relatively stable with the exception of 1983-1984 in which peaks in the rates were observed, corresponding temporally to the coxsackievirus B5 - meningitis epidemic. The number of type 1 diabetes cases diagnosed in the 12-month periods beginning July, 1983, significantly exceeded the average number of cases diagnosed in the previous four 12-month periods; the annual incidence rate in the peak period was 18.4/100 000 person-years while the previous average annual rate was 11.7/100.000 person – year. Overall, an excess of 6.7/100.00 person-years over the average annual incidence for the previous 4 years was reported. It is important to note that, the peak incidence of type 1 diabetes occurred 2 months after the peak incidence of aseptic meningitis.

Other investigators have reported "epidemics" of type 1 diabetes which occurred in the same time period. The 1984 epidemic of childhood diabetes in Poland was associated with a concurrent epidemic of aseptic meningitis [154]. A case – control study conducted during this period yielded an association with only one enterovirus, coxsackievirus B5. The overall incidence of type 1 diabetes almost doubled compared with the previous 12 years, from 3.5/100.000 in 1970 through 1981 to 6.6/100.000 in 1982 through 1984. A number of consistencies between Jefferson County and Poland data were observed. First, the magnitude of the increase was similar in Poland and Jefferson County, a doubling of incidence rates was observed in the early 1980s. Second, the increased incidence in Jefferson County corresponded temporally with an epidemic of illness attributed to coxsackievirus B5, the same enterovirus which produced a significant association with diabetes in Poland. It is noteworthy that in contrast to other coxsackievirus B, coxsackievirus B5 infections occur primarily in outbreaks with comparatively few cases occurring during intervening years. According to the U.S. enterovirus surveillance data obtained during the years 1961-1995, coxsackievirus B5 has an epidemic pattern of occurrence in the United States. In fact, prior to 1983 coxsackievirus B5 was last U.S. epidemic in 1972 and during non epidemic years it was isolated infrequently [147]. Furthermore, alterations of the normal seasonal pattern were similar in both epidemic areas; an exaggerated autumn-winter peak occurred between August and April in Jefferson County (1983) and in Poland (1984) [201].

Data from the U.S. Virgin Island indicate a striking increase in type 1 diabetes incidence in 1983 and 1984, over a baseline incidence of virtually zero; the incidence rate nearly quadrupled in 1984 [183]. Numerous other reports from around the world also show an increased incidence of type 1 diabetes in the early 1980 [32,97,129,155,172].

Taken together, these findings, reported from geographically distant populations, resulted in similar changes in type 1 diabetes incidence at the same time. Such unusual circumstances suggest that similar changes in environmental factors, like enterovirus infections, were responsible for the changes in incidence.

There are instances where the diagnosis of diabetes in one member of a family has been rapidly followed by its appearance in other members of the same family [133,150]. A clinical report from United Kingdom describes classical type 1 insulin deficient diabetes mellitus arising in twins aged 14 months, both of whom had evidence of enterovirus infection. The diagnosis of type 1 diabetes was made in the second twin within 12 days of the first. Both twins were negative for enterovirus by PCR five months following diagnosis, although both were then positive for islet cell antibodies. Sequencing of the amplicons produced by PCR suggested that the viruses from each twin were not the same but that they were both variants related to echovirus 6 [173]. A recent study revealed a simultaneous type 1 diabetes onset in mother and son coincident with an enteroviral infection. The results of such study showed that the whole family had a proven enterovirus infection at the time of type 1 diabetes diagnosis of the mother and the 10-years-old boy. Such cases indicate that infection is likely to have been from a common source within the family. They add further weight to the strong epidemiological evidence for the association of enterovirus infection with the onset of type 1 diabetes.

Nevertheless, temporal relationship between the peak seasons for enteroviral infections, late summer/early fall, preceding peak onset of diabetes in fall and winter, was noted by some but not all investigations [1,22,50,55,131,135,181,184,202]. For example, Hierholzer and Harris [74] found no diabetes among 109 children 4 years after the children had contracted coxsackievirus B3 or/and coxsackievirus B4 infection. Similarly, Dippe et al., [40] did not find any-one with glucose intolerance among 136 young residents of the isolated Pribilof Islands 5 years after an outbreak of coxsackievirus B4.

As has been show the epidemiological evidence remains as inconclusive today; but continues because of intriguing clues and epidemiologic evidence supporting the hypothesis that at least some cases of type 1 diabetes are caused by enterovirus infections [10,11,54,121,165,178,206].

Correlation between the Epidemiology of Enterovirus Infections and International Variation of Diabetes Incidence

According to the "environmental" hypothesis, the putative environmental factors in countries of lower incidence should be less than or as frequent as in those countries of higher incidence. Contrary to the "environmental" hypothesis, it has been shown an inverse correlation between the incidence of type 1 diabetes and enterovirus infections [86].

Lönnrot and co-workers [119] studied the frequency of antibodies to enterovirus in two populations (Finland and Lithuania) with an important difference of type 1 diabetes incidence. As has been previously noted, Finland has the highest incidence of type 1 diabetes mellitus in the world, whereas Lithuania the incidence is substantially lower. They found significantly higher enterovirus antibody levels in Lithuanian children than in their age-and sex-matched Finnish counterparts, which implies a higher frequency of enterovirus infections in Lithuania. Accordingly, the results suggest inverse relationship between the frequency of enterovirus infections and the incidence of type 1 diabetes in Lithuania and Finland. They conclude that a high frequency of enterovirus infections does not necessarily lead to an increased incidence of type 1 diabetes.

In other study, the level of responsiveness in two neighbouring countries, Finland and Estonia, with different poliovirus immunization practices and striking differences in the incidence of type 1 diabetes was also compared. Enterovirus-specific cellular immunity was studied in Estonian and in Finnish children at the age of 9 months and the results showed that Finnish children have weaker cellular immunity against enteroviruses at the age of 9 months compared.with Estonian children at the same age. In that study was hypothesed that stronger T cell immunity which cross-reacts with other enterovirus serotypes could explain the lower incidence of type 1 diabetes in Estonia by providing effective protection against diabetogenic enterovirus strains in Estonian children [102]. The poliovirus vaccine, in theory, could modulate the protection against other enteroviruses by inducing cross-reactive T cell immune responses; however, no signs of cross-reactivity of polivirus-induced antibodies with diabetes associated epitopes of islet cell autoantigens were found in sera collected after poliovirus vaccination in a small pilot study carried out in Finland [67, 78]. Nevertheless, with regard to the influence of immunization by poliovirus vaccines in the pathogenesis of type 1 diabetes, Sadeharju K et al., [163] demonstrated that poliovirus antibodies induced by uniform vaccinations did not differ between the prediabetic and control children suggesting that the regulation of antibody responses to enteroviruses is not disturbed.

Further report evaluated the relationship between the epidemiology of enterovirus infections and type 1 diabetes at the population level. Enterovirus antibodies were examined in the background population (1-year-old and 10-14-year-old children) in seven countries with either exceptionally high (Finland and Sweden) or low/intermediate incidence of diabetes (Estonia, Germany, Hungary, Lithuania, Russia). Again, the results suggested that the countries with high incidence of type 1 diabetes have lower frequency of enterovirus infections compared to countries where type 1 diabetes is less common. Thus, an inverse relationship may exist between the frequency of type 1 diabetes and enterovirus infections in the background population [194].

A recent study analysed the maternal enterovirus antibodies from serum samples taken from pregnant women between 1983 and 2001 in Finland and Sweden using enzyme immunoassay and neutralisation assays. Comparable samples were also taken between 1999 and 2001 in countries with a lower incidence of diabetes (Estonia, Germany, Hungary, Israel, Lithuania, Russia). The results showed a clear decrease in maternal enterovirus antibody levels over the past 20 years ($p<0.0001$) and the frequency of enterovirus antibodies was higher in countries with a low or intermediate incidence of type 1 diabetes compared with high-incidence countries ($p<0.0001$) [196]. Indeed, during the foetal life, maternal antibodies are needed to compensate for the immaturity of the fetal and neonatal immune system. However, if the mother lacks an antibody repertoire against enteroviruses the infant will be poorly protected against these infections. This may be the case in Finland and Sweden: a low frequency of enterovirus infections has led to poor maternal immunity against these infections. Thus, the total frequency of enterovirus infections may have also decreased among infants, but the occurrence of severe enteroviral disease may have increased since the infants lack maternal enterovirus antibodies [186].

The inverse relationship, as observed in such studies, could be taken as evidence against the role of enterovirus infections in type 1 diabetes. However, in seroepidemiological studies we cannot exclude the possibility that certain diabetogenic virus variants, which cannot be detected by the present methods, circulate in the countries with a high diabetes incidence.

The observed correlation, although inverse, may also reflect some true biological phenomenon related to possible role of enteroviruses in the pathogenesis of type 1 diabetes. This finding is in line with the proposed polio hypothesis, as described elsewhere in this volume, according to which the complications of enterovirus infections become more common in an environment with a decreased rate of infections [92,195]. In both instances, a dramatic decrease in the frequency of enterovirus infections has led to a new epidemiological situation favourable for the frequent occurrence of complications, such as poliomyelitis or β-cell autoimmunity. Accordingly, a low frequency of these infections in the background population would increase the susceptibility of young children to the diabetogenic effect of such viruses. This may partly explain why the incidence of type 1 diabetes has rapidly increased in Finland during the past 15 years although the frequency of enterovirus infections has decreased during the same period of time [195]. This could also explain the observation indicating higher incidence of type 1 diabetes in rural than in urban areas as low population density is associated with low transmission rate of enteroviruses.

These facts suggest that the development of type 1 diabetes in humans could be reduced in the presence of high amounts of pathogens. It is well known that viruses can cause but also prevent autoimmune disease: the exposure of NOD mice to mouse hepatitis virus decrease cumulative incidence of diabetes. Virally induced cytokines and chemokines can influence the progression of autoimmunity and depending on the time, location and level of expression, can prevent the disease. Thus, the timing of the infection, the viral strain, the antigenic load, and other unknown factors are crucial in the protection or predisposition to the disease.

Epidemiological Modes of the Enteroviruses Involvement in the Pathogenesis of Type 1 Diabetes

Among the more than 60 different enterovirus serotypes, CBV serotypes have been most frequently implicated in the pathogenesis of type 1 diabetes and more recently other serotypes, such as the echoviruses, have emerged as being of potential importance [54,90,92]. However, it is not clear whether we should assume that only a few strains of enterovirus are specifically diabetogenic or whether diabetogenicity should be taken as a general property of enterovirus infections. Nor is it known whether certain genetic determinants of the virus are more important than antigenic structure with respect to diabetogenic potential [86].

It has been postulated that several different enterovirus serotype could be involved in type 1 diabetes. In that case serotype distribution of enterovirus in different countries may affect diabetes incidence as well. The results from DiMe study have suggested that several different serotypes might play a role in the pathogenesis of type 1 diabetes. The infections detected during a prospective observation included several CVB serotypes (i.e. coxsackievirus B1, B2, B3, B5) but also other coxsackievirus serotype (coxsackievirus A9). In all these cases the infection was associated temporally with increases in type 1 diabetes-associated autoantibodies or the onset of clinical disease [158]. Interestingly, a relative excess of some serotypes (coxsackievirus B5 and coxsackievirus A9) were found in Finnish children [85] if compared to those isolated in U.S. (about 24.000 strains isolated during years 1969-1981) and in WHO surveys [175].

Also the sequence analyses of enterovirus RNA detected in prospective serum samples suggest that the infections were caused by various non-polio enterovirus, although the genetic conservation of the amplified sequence between enterovirus serotypes hampered specific identification [77,121,122]. These findings support the hypothesis that several enterovirus infections bring about a progressive loss of β-cells which in certain susceptible individuals may eventually lead to the manifestation of clinical type 1 diabetes.

Taking into account the large number of serotypes and the extensive genetic variability within each serotype, it has been speculated that not necessarily all strains, but only certain endemically circulating genotypes are diabetogenic. This hypothesis would be the best one to explain the difference of type 1 diabetes incidence due to the geographical restrictions of endemic transmission of the lineages [85,51,167].

Roivainen and co-workers [160] have demonstrated that multiples enterovirus serotype including poliovirus type 1/Mahoney, coxsackievirus A13, human parechovirus 1 and several echovirus (serotypes 6, 7, 11) were capable of causing significant functional impairment and beta-cell death. Importantly, in her studies in vitro Dr. Roivainen showed that although prototypic strains of some echovirus serotypes (i.e. echovirus serotype 9 and 30) may demonstrate minimal β cell destruction, field *isolates* of the same serotype can be highly potent in this respect. In human islets, Dr Rovainen analysed infections of different echovirus 30 strains isolated from different countries at different time and she found that some of the strains were clearly more destructive than the others. For example, different strains isolates of echovirus 30 in Holland 1977, 1979, 1987 and in France 1996 were clearly more destructive than others and the corresponding prototype strain. It was concluded that a wide range of serotype could be potentially diabetogenic but the capacity of an enterovirus to destruct human β-cells or impair their function is not entirely defined by the serotype, but by as yet unidentified characteristics of the virus strains involved. A further consequence of these results is that all serotype appear to include strains capable of damaging β-cells. It is possible that striking differences in tissue tropism and virulence are based on very few or even single aminoacid differences in defined key locations in the genome [160].

The ability of different strains of a single virus type to produce different pathogenic expressions is well documented within the picornavirus group. Research on coxsackievirus B4 has demonstrated that antigenic changes at the epitope level occur at a frequency greater than 1/100. This suggests that even within the same virus pool, there may be many antigenic variants with different tissue tropism and different physiological properties, which would account for the wide spectrum of clinical diseases produced by the coxsackievirus B. The genetic variability of encephalomyocarditis virus (EMCV) strains, a murine picornavirus, appears to define their tropism to β cells and their diabetogenicity. In genetically susceptible mice, the EMCV-D variant can infect and destroy pancreatic β-cells, while the EMCV-B variant is generally nondiabetogenic [104]. Moreover, only certain strains of enterovirus, derived from human diabetic patients can evoke diabetes in animals [92].

While within-serotype variation of enterovirus genomes can be extensive, several examples exist where individual point mutations could dramatically affect the virulence of a virus both in humans and in animal models. In the case of neurovirulent poliovirus [153], neurovirulent Theiler´s encephalomyelitis virus [213], and diabetogenic EMCV [8], a single aminoacid change in the VP1 capsid protein determines the virulent or pathogenic phenotype. Replicaction of coxsackievirus B4 in the mouse acinar pancreas is shown to be dependent on only one residue, Thr-129 of VP1 [17]. It has been hypothesised that a host range restriction of virus through the substitution in the capsid protein probably determines the virus´pathogenic effect. In the ECMV model, the diabetogenic protein variant probably allows the virus to attach to the pancreatic β-cells [106,161]. In cell cultures, a single – point mutation on the EMCV polyprotein that correspond to amino acid 152 of VP1 has been observed to occur only to change a diabetogenic to a nondiabetogenic variant, i.e., from G to A (Ala to Thr) [8]. Interestingly, induction of diabetes by a diabetogenic EMCV strain has been prevented by prior inmunization with non diabetogenic EMCV variant [138].

As in the case of EMCV, not all CVB strains are diabetogenic, explaining why type 1 diabetes appears to be associated with coxsackieviral B infections in infrequent isolated cases. In addition only certain strains of mice develop diabetes after infection. Furthermore, a comparative analysis of the enterovirus RNA sequences from type 1 diabetes children, their siblings and healthy controls revealed differences that may be related to the diabetogenic properties of enteroviruses [207].

Since 1983, the existence of diabetogenic variants has been demonstrated for the coxsackievirus B4 [69]. In this report, the Edwards isolate of coxsackievirus B4 (coxsackievirus B4-Edwards, which is of human origin and induce diabetes in mice) and three of its plaque-purified virion "strains designated as Edwards isolate-1 (E1), Edwards isolate-2 (E2), and Edwards isolate-3 (E3), were compared to demonstrate existence of virion heterogeneity within the human isolate. The results showed that, coxsackievirus B4-Edwards, E1, E2, and E3 were serologically similar by infectivity neutralization tests, had identical plaque morphology, and replicated to a similar level in the mouse pancreas. However, virus isolate (strain) E2 showed the most intense accumulation in islet cells of mice during acute infection. These observations suggest that the Edwards isolate of coxsackievirus B4, like other human isolates of coxsackievirus B4, probably exists as a heterogeneous population of virion strains. The pathogenic consequences and expression of any diabetogenic potential is, therefore, dependent on virus strain selection.

Later on, the complete nucleotide sequence of E2 strain and its comparison with non diabetogenic coxsackievirus B4 JBV strain revealed a total of 111 aminoacid substitutions in the E2 strains, scattered throughout the genome. Of them, 82 aminoacid changes were located in the non-capsid region and 29 aminoacid changes among the capsid proteins. It has been suggested that some of the aminoacid changes may be involved in the determination of its diabetogenicity [105].

Another report examined another coxsackievirus B4 variant which directly affects human pancreatic islets in tissue culture. This strain can produce a persisting infection of islets with concomitant effects on insulin secretion and proinsulin synthesis. It is speculated that the ability of this coxsackievirus B4 strain to establish a persistent infection might be due to substitution of 11 amino acids located at the surface of the structural protein VP1, adjacent to the predicted receptor binding canyon of the virus [207,208].

The entire genome of a strain of echovirus 9, which was isolated from a 6-week-old child at the clinical onset of type 1 diabetes as well as from the prototype strain echovirus 9 Barty-IFN were sequenced. According to the sequencing results, the echovirus 9 strain isolated from diabetic patient had several aminoacid differences both in capsid proteins and in non-structural proteins when compared to the prototype strains. Some of these changes could be involved in the diabetogenicity, but at this stage it is impossible to say which of them are important for the pathogenic phenotype [146,199].

Recently, a laboratory strain of coxsackievirus B5 was passaged repeatedly in mouse pancreas in vivo. After 15 passages, the virus phenotype was clearly changed and infection of the variant resulted in a diabetes-like syndrome in mice characterized by chronic pancreatic inflammation together with dysregulation in glucose metabolism, loss of pancreatic acinar tissue, and mild insulitis. In order to characterize the genetic determinants involved in mouse pancreas adaptation, the passaged virus variant together with the parental virus strain was cloned for molecular characterization. The whole genome sequencing of both virus strains revealed only limited differences. Altogether, eight nucleotides were changed resulting in five amino acid substitutions, of which three were located in the capsid proteins [3].

As far, it is not known what genomic regions could regulate diabetogenicity of enteroviruses. The knowledge from polio and other enterovirus diseases clearly points out that virulence is associated with specific mutations, but the mutations regulating e.g. neurovirulence of polioviruses may be completely different than those regulating the diabetogenicity of enteroviruses. In addition, recombinations between enterovirus strains occur frequently, and they may also play a role in the diabetogenic properties. Therefore, it is important to sequence the complete genome of a large number of isolates from diabetic, prediabetic and control subjects to identify what mutations could be associated with type 1 diabetes. Comparative studies on pathogenic differences of parallel variants from relevant virus strains may reveal the aminoacids and/or nucletides of the virus genome, which are the most critical for pathogenesis of type 1 diaberes.

From these studies, it is clear that much further work needs to be carried out to decide those nucleotide structures which cause enteroviruses to be diabetogenic. However, allow one to hypothesize that some specific strains of enterovirus are most important one with regard to diabetogenic potential. As a consequence of error-prone replication of the genomic RNA, the enteroviruses exist as mixtures of microvariants or quasispecies in clinical isolates, highlighting the possibility that β-cell-tropic and potentially diabetogenic variants could circulate in nature or may emerge sporadically during systemic infection, possibly driven by the host immune response [191].

VIII. Possible Mechanism of Enterovirus – Induced Type 1 Diabetes

On the basis of data described in this volume, we can infer that considerable progress has been made in research leading to a better understanding of the natural course of type 1 diabetes and its relationship with enterovirus infection. There are numerous proposed mechanisms explaining how viral infection could induce type 1 diabetes. However, the actual mechanisms by which enterovirus may contribute to destruction of pancreatic β-cells remains to be established. Several mechanisms that are not mutually exclusive have been suggested. The virus may destruct β cells either directly by a lytic infection, or indirectly by a virus-directed immune response against infected β cells.

Direct β Cell Lysis by Enterovirus Infections

The issue of whether enterovirus infects β-cells, causing lytic destruction and precipiting the development of type 1 diabetes is controversial. It has been demonstrated that some enterovirus group has variant that can replicate in the pancreas and may cause direct β-cell lysis by the cytotoxic life cycle of the virus [13,19,69,177]. As noted before, autopsy case reports have documented insulitis in newborns and young children who died of fulminant CVB infection, and CVB antigens have been found in their β-cells, suggesting that CVB are able to infect β-cells also in vivo [98,136,210]. In vitro studies have shown that enteroviruses can replicate in insulin – producing β-cells, and that infection may result in functional impairment or death of the β-cells [159,160,191].

Recent works provides convincing evidences that enterovirus infections can be detected in situ in human islets. This finding suggests that enteroviruses play a part in the development of type 1 diabetes and that this part is based on direct action by enteroviruses on β-cells. This study showed that the cell surface molecules, PVR, HCAR and integrin αvß3, which act as enterovirus receptors in established cell lines, are expressed in primary human islets and specifically in β-cells, and that these receptors are responsible for viral infections resulting in destruction of β-cells [209].

Chronic enterovirus infections have also been described. Indeed, a persistence of coxsackievirus B4 has been demonstrated in a murine model of type 1 diabetes [12]. In addition, a study suggests the possibility that the CVB group is able to replicate at a low level in human islet cells *in vitro* with no obvious cytolytic effect [20,21]. However, this hypothesis is controversial in human. The question of enterovirus persistence in human pathology is unresolved with several studies suggesting that it does occur in idiopathic dilated cardiomyopathy [15,41] and chronic inflammatory muscle disease [14] but there have been doubters [75,117].

In DiMe prospective study, a significant association was found between the development of diabetes associated antibodies and a preceding enterovirus infection. However, in one child who had multiple enterovirus infections, phylogenetic analysis of sequences demonstrated that genetically distinct enteroviruses were detected at different time points, and no enterovirus RNA was detected in samples taken between the RNA-positive samples, which suggests that chronic infection was unlikely [122].

Although convincing evidence for persistent enteroviral infection of human β-cells is missing, it is plausible that persistent infection with a defective noncytopathic enterovirus may cause diabetes [58]. Accordingly, these hypotheses, suggesting either acute lytic β-cell destruction or a chronic infection leading to gradual impairment of insulin secretion, are both basically possible pathogenetic models.

Both hypotheses assume that no autoimmunity is required for progression to type 1 diabetes. It is worth noting, that β-cell autoimmunity is a key element in the pathogenesis of type 1 diabetes and in the vast majority of patients an autoimmune component is evident [7]. This raises provocative questions about the relevance of this mechanism in the pathogenesis of type 1 diabetes, which is associated in 70 to 90 % of cases with the presence of ICA.

Thus, the mechanism of acute cytolytic infection of β-cells, proposed by earlier studies, appears to be incompatible with the long preclinical period of autoimmunity preceding type 1 diabetes. It is therefore likely that this mechanism can explain the pathogenesis in those very few cases that progress to type 1 diabetes without autoimmunity. A case report has indeed demonstrated progression to type 1 diabetes without preceding autoimmunity [143]. Japanese researchers [96] have confirmed that some patients with type 1 diabetes have a novel form of the disease, so called fulminant type 1 diabetes, that's not caused by immune cells attacking the pancreas. Recently [95] the same researchers have demonstrated high titres of IgA antibodies to enterovirus in the fulminant diabetic patients without islet-related autoantibodies, indicating higher susceptibility to enteroviral infections among them. It is interesting that, EMCV (the best characterized model of virus-induced diabetes in mice) produce acute lytic infection of pancreatic β cells and diabetes whose severity correlates with the degree of β-cell lysis [28,71]. In this model there is no indication that the EMCV triggers humoral β cell autoimmune, as evidenced by lack of ICA.

In summary, the existence of diabetogenic variants, or variants that preferentially replicate in β-cells, in the enteroviruses could potentially trigger diabetes by replication of the virus in islets in susceptible individuals, leading to rapid onset non-autoimmune diabetes. Results from studies on pancreases from human autopsies and cultured human islets support the idea that during systemic enterovirus infections, the virus may reach pancreatic islets and cause direct β-cell damage. However, except for rare cases, the vast majority of human type 1 diabetes does not appear to result from an acute cytolitic enteroviral infection. Alternatively it has been postulated that in individuals who have already lost substantial β cell mass through ongoing autoimmunity damage by another mechanism, acute cytolytic infection could provide the final insult in the β-cell- damaging process leading to clinical manifestation of the disease [94].

Virus-Directed Immune Response Against Infected β Cells

A more common scenario could be represented by an acute/persistent infection in the pancreas of individuals that would trigger the induction of autoimmunity. Autoreactive T cells and/or autoantibodies cause autoimmune diseases by destroying or functionally impairing targeted tissues. Several mechanisms may be responsible for the activation of autoreactive T cells in autoimmune diseases. These include: molecular mimicry; release of autoantigens during inflammation; superantigens, and bystander activation. Of them, two major hypotheses have been elaborated to account for putative associations between enteroviruses and autoimmunity: Molecular Mimicry [123] and Bystander Activation [191]. In the former, an immune response directed against the virus cross-reacts with islet cell self-antigens leading to disappearance of normal tolerance to self-antigens and mis-directed immune response. In the case of bystander damage, a virus up-regulates nonspecific immune responses that lead to pathology.

i) Molecular Mimicry

The concept of molecular mimicry describes a situation in which the sequence or structural similarities between virus and autoantigens determinants can lead to functional T and B cells cross-reactivity (anti-virus with anti-self) with resultant tissue damage and perpetuation of the autoimmune response. Nevertheless, the finding of sequence homology is, by itself, insufficient evidence of biologically meaningful mimicry. Wucherpfennig K and Strominger J in 1995 [205] demonstrated that structural similarity rather than sequence identity between peptides is the key determinant for mimicry between environmental and autoantigenic epitopes, and that functional cross reactivity exists in the context of a human autoimmune disease. Interestingly, the induction of cross-reactivity would not require a replicating agent, and the immunologically mediated injury could occur after removal of the pathogen, a hit-and-run event. Clearly, the virus infection that initiates an autoimmune phenomenon need not be present at the time overt disease develops. Functional molecular mimicry has proved difficult to study, and despite impressive recent studies in autoimmune gastritis [4], it remains an attractive but elusive hypothesis in human autoimmune diseases.

Regarding to type 1 diabetes and enterovirus, it has been postulated that type 1 diabetes may result from a misdirected immunologic attack on pancreatic β-cells by lymphocytes responding to an acute or chronic viral infection.

Evidence for molecular mimicry as a potential pathogenic mechanism underlying type 1 diabetes was enhanced in 1992 by the finding of a sequence homology between the 65kDa isoform of glutamic acid decarboxylase (GAD65) and the CVB P2C protein [108,123]. From table 3, we see that the viral P2C sequence with homology with GAD 65 is highly conserved in the group B of enteroviruses. It should be noted the enterovirus belonged to this group are highly prevalent, which implies that exposure to the mimicry motif will occur frequently throughout life [197,198].

It has been observed that immunization of mice with coxsackievirus 2C protein or the coxsackievirus peptide containing the region of sequence similarity with GAD 65 can induce T-cell immune responses that cross-react with GAD 65 or GAD 65 peptides corresponding to the region of sequence similarity [83,103]. There is indeed a murine model of diabetes where coxsackieviral infection of the pancreas is followed by the appearance of anti 64 kDa antibodies and diabetes [29,30,84]. In addition, T cell cross-reactivity between coxsackievirus and glutamate decarboxylase has been associated with a murine diabetes susceptibility allele [180].

Table 3. Aminoacid sequence comparisons between human GAD 65 and protein 2C of various enteroviruses. Grey shaded areas represent a six aminoacid identity.

GAD 65	F	K	M	F	P	E	V	K	E	K	G	M	A
CVB4 -2C(Group B)	V	K	I	L	P	E	V	K	E	K	H	E	F
CVB1-2C (Group B)	V	K	I	L	P	E	V	K	E	K	H	E	F
CVB3-2C (Group B)	V	K	I	L	P	E	V	K	E	K	H	E	F
CVB5-2C (Group B)	V	K	I	L	P	E	V	K	E	K	H	E	F
E4-2C (Group B)	V	K	I	L	P	E	V	K	E	K	H	E	F
E30-2C (Group B)	V	K	I	L	P	E	V	K	E	K	H	E	F
E12-2C (Group B)	V	K	I	L	P	E	V	K	E	K	H	E	F
E16-2C (Group B)	V	K	I	L	P	E	V	K	E	K	H	E	F
CVA2-2C (Group A)	V	K	I	I	P	E	A	K	D	K	V	E	F
CVA4-2C (Group A)	E	R	I	I	P	E	A	K	D	K	V	E	F
CVA16-2C(Group A)	E	K	I	I	P	A	A	K	E	K	V	E	F
E70-2C (Group D)	T	K	I	L	P	E	A	R	E	K	H	E	F
PV1-2C (Poliovirus)	E	K	I	I	P	Q	A	R	D	K	L	E	F
PV2-2C (Poliovirus)	E	K	I	I	P	Q	A	R	D	K	L	E	F
PV3-2C (Poliovirus)	E	K	I	I	P	Q	A	R	D	K	L	E	F

Cross-reactive antibodies have also been induced during peptide immunization in rabbit. Lonrrot and her colleague [118] demonstrated that rabbit antibodies raised against coxsackievirus B4 P2C-derived peptides cross-react with GAD 65 peptides derived from the homology region and vice versa.

Antibodies against the peptides derived from the region with sequence homology have been induced during enterovirus infections in prediabetic subjects, and were also shown to present in patients with newly diagnosed type 1 diabetes. However, similar peptide antibody responses were seen during enterovirus infections in control children who did not progress to diabetes, and the diabetic patients matched non-diabetic control children had levels of peptide antibodies equal to those in the patients. This is in line with a report by Ritcher and coworkers [156] showing an equal frequency of antibodies against coxsackievirus B4 protein in GADA-positive patients with type 1 diabetes and GADA-negative non diabetic subjects, but conflict with another report showing that antibodies against peptides carting the homology sequences were not more frequent in type 1 diabetes patients than in non-diabetic controls [83].

Interestingly, the homology sequence in GAD 65 and CVB has been shown to be presented by HLA-DR3 and not HLA-DR1 or DR4, which suggest that a putative role of enteroviral infections by means of molecular mimicry will indeed be restricted by HLA-DR alleles. In support to this finding an association has been reported of diabetes with group B enterovirus infections in HLA-DR3 positive (which define the risk for type 1 diabetes), rather than in HLA-DR3 negative patients [126].

Controversy exists as to whether the PEVKEK motif itself is recognized. Much works has focused on immune responses against this region of sequence similarity between GAD 65 and P2C [118,145,157,158,169,188,193,197]. To characterize coxsackievirus B4-specific T-cell epitopes, overlapping peptides covering the 2C protein were synthesized and coxsackievirus B4-specific T-cell lines were established from healthy and diabetic subjects. In this study, the authors concluded that the coxsackievirus B4 2C protein is strongly immunogenic for T-cells and PEVKEK is included in a T-cell epitope, however, PEVKEK region seems does not represent a major T cell epitope presented by HLA-DR3 and DR4 [125]. Other studies have suggested that this epitope may be more recognized by T-cells in diabetic patients, but this is not a demonstration of cross reactivity [7].

At present, there are no definitive data to support a role for this region in initiating islet autoimmunity through molecular mimicry. However, studies performed by Varela-Calvino and associates clearly shows that the P2C protein is a major target of the T cell response to coxsackievirus B4, and therefore it remains important to focus on this part of the virus, but not necessarily on the PEVKEK homology region. This group of researcher found specific T-cell response to the CB4 lysates and the purified P2C protein in individuals with and without high-risk haplotypes, suggesting that HLA antigens is not a determining factors in responsiveness to these antigens. In contrast, HLA type is likely to have a strong influence on selection of the epitope of P2C that are targeted, and this is the major factor in determining the potential for molecular mimicry between viral and autoantigens [190,192].

It is possible that other coxsackievirus B4 antigens may also harbor cross-reactive epitopes. Moreover, in relation to molecular mimicry, it is well established that similarities between regions of antigens leading to T–cell cross-reactivity are the consequence of shared structural features rather than simply reflection of sequence identity [205]. These may not require aminoacid sequence identity and are therefore difficult to identify by database searches [77].

Several other possible cross-reactivities between CVB proteins/epitopes and autoantigens important in type 1 diabetes have been suggested. Studies with animals models indicates that one of the reactive β- cell autoantigens is the heat shock protein 60 (HSP60) [66]. The immunogenic region in HSP60 share a sequence homology with two regions in enterovirus capsid proteins, one in the VP1 protein and the other in the VP0, the precursor of VP2 and VP4 proteins. The cross-reactivity between some of these enterovirus group B proteins (i.e VP1, and/or VP2) and heat shock proteins has been demonstrated by Harkonen et al [68] by using EIA and immunoblotting assay.

The carboxy-terminal (C-terminal) part of tyrosine phosphatases (a major target autoantigen in type 1 diabetes) has a 5-amino acid sequence identity, followed by five amino acid similarity with the conservative motif in the VP1-protein of enteroviruses (PALTAVETGA/HT), which is a highly immunogenic B- and T-cell epitope in enterovirus infection-induced immune responses. The potential humoral cross-reactions between immune responses induced by tyrosine phosphatases and enteroviruses was also studied by Harkonen and coworker [66] and their results indicated that enterovirus infection in humans may also occasionally induce a humoral response that cross-reacts with IA-2/IAR. Moreover, there is indication that immunization with coxsackievirus B4 (strain E2) in the non-obese diabetic mice induce humoral immune response to tyrosine phosphatase IA-2, heat shock protein 60, and some other regions of autoantigens [39,103].

These studies suggest that apart from well-documented sequence homology between the 2C protein of coxsackieviruses and the β-cell autoantigen glutamic acid decarboxylase [6] there are other motifs in picornavirus proteins homologous to islet cell autoantigens, which might induce cross-reacting immune-responses during picornavirus infections. However, in several studies; proof of the hypothesis of molecular mimicry is hindered by the fact that healthy control groups also show reactivity to islet cell autoantigens.

From the studies in transgenic mice it appear that sequence homology alone may not be sufficient to break immunological non-responsiveness to autoantigens. According to these studies a natural infection can break T-cell non-responsiveness, whereas immunization with the homologous viral antigens did not, suggesting that non-specific factors such as local inflammation will contribute to the pathological process [141,212].

ii) Bystander Activation

This mechanism consists in the non-specific activation of autoreactive T cells-that have escaped thymic selection- in a chronic inflammatory environment induced by virus.

In this scenario, autoreactive T cell clones become activated, acquire a Th1 bias and become pathogenic as a result of cell/tissue damage associated with a strongly pro-inflammatory environment in which dendritic cell activation is a key component (Figure 1). The importance of bystander activation in the context of type 1 diabetes receives considerable support from studies on animal models. This includes (i) evidence that β cell damage accelerates diabetes in appropriate models [80,81,82] and (ii) the strong requirement for islet co-stimulation in numerous models (eg through B7.1 or cytokine expression under the rat insulin promoter) [203,204].

Two important parameters in viral – mediated diabetes induction have been identified [80,81,82]. First, prior to infection a significant population of diabetogenic lymphocytes must infiltrate the pancreas and establish a degree of insular infiltration and damage. This level of preexisting islet damage is however manageable and clinical disease is not observed. Second, viral infection and replication must occur within cells of the Islets of Langerhans. Therefore, the primary role of virus in the development of diabetes is reach the pancreas and to infect tissue [149]. During this process, individual β-cells may become damaged resulting in the presentation of sequestered islet antigen, the stimulation of preexisting autoreactive T cells, and thereby induce the development of autoimmune disease. Since no direct viral damage to the β- cells has been observed in the animal model following viral infection, infection of islet cells most likely activates an indirect anti-viral defense that is responsible for presenting β-cells to the diabetogenic T cells and, subsequently, inducing disease.

Strong evidences for bystander activation by enteroviruses leading to accelerated autoimmune diabetes in animal models has been obtained by Horwitz and coworkers [82], and in these studies there was no evidence of a role for mimicry or induction of anti-viral T cells. This study involves the use of BDC2.5 mice, which carry a transgene encoding a diabetogenic T-cell receptor specific to an islet granule antigen that is distinct from GAD65 and does not cross-react with coxsackievirus B4 [82]. Inoculation of this mouse with coxsackievirus B4 led to the rapid development of diabetes mellitus. The infected BDC2.5 mice were found to have infiltration of the islet cells with lymphocytes carrying the transgenic T-cell receptor, even though the target cell for this virus is the exocrine pancreas and not the islet cells. It is presumed that this acceleration of diabetes is caused by bystander cells that respond to the release of proinflammatory cytokines, leading to activation of T cells that destroy the islet cells.

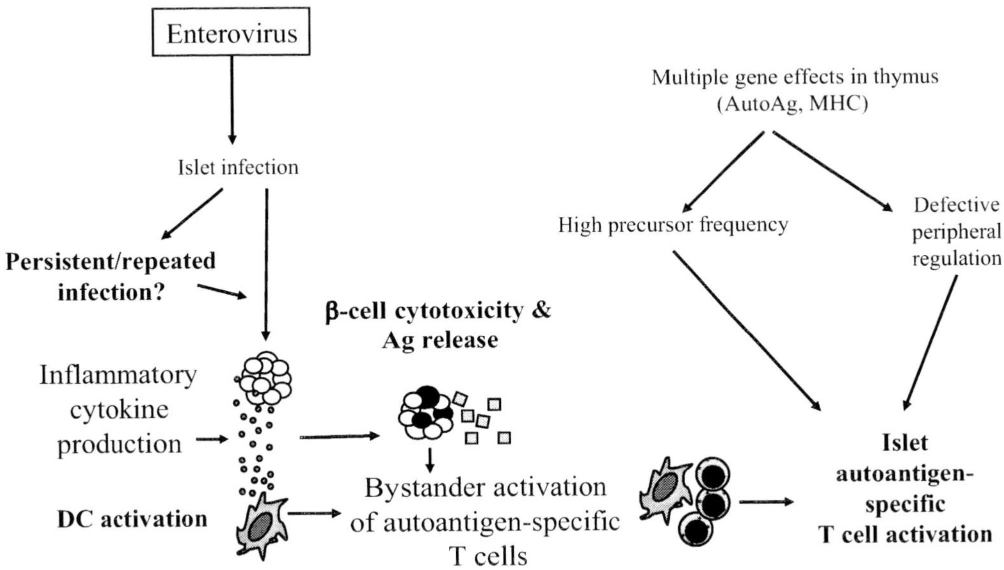

Figure 1. Model for the bystander effect of enteroviruses in inducing islet autoimmunity. Modified from Varela - Calvino et al in ref. 191, and used with permission (Dr. Mark Peakman).

Involvement of bystander mechanism is also supported by the results of Chehadeh et al. who showed that patients with newly diagnosed type 1 diabetes had increased levels of IFN-α in their blood. The enterovirus infection was most probably the trigger in the study since enterovirus RNA was found in the blood of half of the IFN-α positive patients [20]. According to a study published by Vreugdenhil and colleagues [200] the majority of the enterovirus are avid triggers of production of pro-inflammatory cytokines by human leukocytes such as IL-1β, TNF-α, and, notably, the type 1 interferons, including interferon-α and -β. In agreement with this finding, other study showed that CVB infect endothelial cells, with pro-inflammatory cytokine release and functional up-regulation of adhesion molecules [211]. Recent work suggests that coxsackievirus B4 infection can induce the production of proinflammatory cytokines through a TLR4-dependent pathway in human pancreatic cells, and these cytokines seem to be involved in the damage to the insulin-producing cells [182].

IX. Conclusion

Many of the bacteria, parasites, and viruses linked to the development of chronic diseases are common throughout the world, but only some infected people develop severe outcomes. Like most infectious and chronic diseases, clinical type 1 diabetes is just the tip of the iceberg of a broad spectrum of pathology. Enteroviruses cause a wide spectrum of both common and uncommon illnesses among infants and children. This implies that if enteroviruses are involved in the development type 1 diabetes, it is a rare consequence of a common event. It is thus evident that most enterovirus infections are not associated with progression to diabetes. Indeed, everyone has one or more enteroviral infections during childhood and adolescence, however, only a few children and young adults develop type 1diabetes.

The mechanism behind enterovirus induced type 1 diabetes is unknown, but it has been shown that the genetics of the virus as well as the genetics of the host are important. The former might also explain why not all individuals with a high risk HLA develop type 1 diabetes after an infection with an enterovirus since the diabetogenic variants probably are in minority.

The role of genetic susceptibility of the host has been demonstrated in coxsackie B-induced diabetes in animals models. Yoon and coworkers infected several different species of monkeys, including rhesus, cynomolgus, cebus and patas with monkey -cell- passaged coxsackie B4 virus [104]. Glucose tolerance tests were performed before and after infection, and an elevation of the glucose tolerance curve and marked depression of the insulin secretion curve were seen only in the coxsackie B4 virus-infected patas monkeys. The rhesus, cynomolgus, and cebus monkeys did not show any changes in insulin or blood glucose levels after coxsackie B4 viral infection.

As coxsackie B4 virus produced abnormalities in glucose tolerance tests and impaired insulin secretion in only the patas monkey, genetic factors must therefore be critical for the development of diabetes in monkeys infected with coxsackie B4 virus. The genetic differences amongst the hosts may also explain the development of diabetes only in some strains of mice after encephalomyocarditis (EMC) viral infection; SJL/J, SWR/J, DBA/1J, and DBA/ 2J strains are susceptible to EMC-induced diabetes, whereas C57BL/6J, CBAI/J, and AKR/J mouse strains areresistant. Results from genetic and *in vitro* viral attachment studies showed that susceptibility to EMC virus- induced diabetes is determined by a single autosomal recessive gene that is inherited in a Mendelian mode.The gene may operate by modulating the expression of viral receptors on beta cells in genetically susceptible mice [68].

In most cases where it has been possible to demonstrate that enterovirus infection triggers the development of islet cell autoantibodies, an increased frequency of high-risk HLA DQB1 genotypes (0201/0302) among the seroconverters, or the presence of at least one HLA class II allele that confers susceptibility to type 1 diabetes, has been shown. This pointing to the possibility that enterovirus infection could be a risk factor in those individuals genetically susceptible to the development of type 1 diabetes. For example, In Finnish population genetic susceptibility for type 1 diabetes is common (the incidence of type 1 diabetes is the highest in the world) and in this kind of situation enterovirus infections might be more dangerous than elsewhere (in people having different genetic background).

However, the results obtained by Craig and co-workers [26] have demonstrated a more aggressive enterovirus-induced subgroup of autoimmune type 1 diabetes that is associated with reduced genetic predisposition to diabetes in nonwhite children. A lack association between HLA genotype and enterovirus infection in children with β-cell autoimmunity or diabetes was reported also in Finnish and white children [121]. Moderate or high risk HLA DR alleles were found in only 2 of 6 enterovirus RNA-positive adults with type 1 diabetes in a French study [5]. In addition, the development of type 1 diabetes in the case reported by us is therefore consistent with this body of previous work. Because enterovirus RNA has been detected in subjects with both high- and low-risk HLA alleles it has been postulated that enterovirus infections may initiate β-cell destruction in patients with low-risk HLA alleles and accelerate the process in patients with high-risk HLA alleles [77].

In this review, we have attempted to summarize the possible role of enterovirus in the pathogenesis of type 1 diabetes. From the results of the above research, it is speculated that enteroviruses, as one non-genetic factor, are implicated in the expression of the disease.

Acknowledgements

Special thanks to my friends and family and for their encouragement and interest in my work, and to my son Diego, you are my inspiration and your presence really completes my life.

References

[1] Adams SF. The seasonal variation in the onset of acute diabetes. *Arch Intern Med* 1926;37:861-4.

[2] Akerblom HK, Vaarala O, Hyoty H, Ilonen J, Knip M. Environmental factors in the etiology of type 1 diabetes. *Am J Med Genet* 2002;30:18-29.

[3] Al-Hello H, Davydova B, Smura T, Kaialainen S, Ylipaasto P, Saario E, et al. Phenotypic and genetic changes in coxsackievirus B5 following repeated passage in mouse pancreas in vivo. *J Med Virol* 2005;75:566-74.

[4] Amedei A, Bergman M, Appelmelk B, Azzurri A, Benagiano M, Tamburini C et al. Molecular mimicry between Helicobacter pylori antigens and H+, K+ --adenosine triphosphatase in human gastric autoimmunity. *J Exp Med* 2003;198:1147.

[5] Andreoletti L, Hober D, Hober-Vandenberghe C, Belaich S, Vantyghem MC, Lefebvre J, et al. Detection of coxsackie B virus RNA sequences in whole blood samples from adult patients at the onset of type I diabetes mellitus. *J Med Virol* 1997;52:121-7.

[6] Atkinson M, Bowman MA, Campbell L, Darrow BL, Kaufman DL, MaClaren NK. Cellular immunity to a determinant common to glutamate decarboxylase and coxsackie virus in insulin-dependent diabetes. *J Clin Invest* 1994;94:2125-9.

[7] Atkinson M, Maclaren N. The patogénesis of insulin dependent diabetes mellitus. *New Engl J Med* 1994;24:1428-36.

[8] Bae Y, Yoon J. Determination of diabetogenicity attributable to a single amino acid Ala-776, on the polyprotein of encephalomyocaerditis virus. *Diabetes* 1993;42:435-43.

[9] Banatvala JE, Bryant J, Schernthaner G, Borkenstein M, Schober E, Brown D, et al. Coxsackie B, mumps, rubella, and cytomegalovirus specific IgM responses in patients with juvenile-onset insulin-dependent diabetes mellitus in Britain, Austria, and Australia. *Lancet* 1985;1:1409-12.

[10] Banatvala JE. Insulin-dependent (juvenile-onset, type 1) diabetes mellitus Coxsackie B viruses revisited. *Prog Med Virol* 1987;34:33-54.

[11] Barrett-Connor E. Is insulin-dependent diabetes mellitus caused by coxsackievirus B infection? A review of the epidemiologic evidence. *Rev Infect Dis*1985;7:207-15.

[12] Berger MM, See DM, Aymard M, Lina B. Demonstration of persistent enterovirus in the pancreas of diabetic mice by in situ polymerase chain reaction. *Clin Diagn Virol* 1998;9:141-3.

[13] Bopegame S, Petrovicova A. In vitro infection of mouse pancreatic islet cells with Coxsackie viruses. *Acta Virol* 1994;38:251-5.

[14] Bowles N, Dubowitz V, Sewry C, Archard L- Dermatomyositis, polymyositis and Coxsackie-B-virus infection. *Lancet* 1987;i:1004-7.

[15] Bowles N, Richardson P, Olsen E, Archard L. Detection of Coxsackie-B-virus-specific RNA sequences in myocardial biopsy samples from patients with myocarditis and dilated cardiomyopathy. *Lancet* 1986;i:1120-2.

[16] Buesa-Gomez J, de la Torre JC, Dyrberg T, Landin-Olsson M, Mauseth RS, Lernmark A, et al. Failure to detect genomic viral sequences in pancreatic tissues from two children with acute-onset diabetes mellitus. *J Med Virol* 1994;42:193-7.

[17] Caggana M, Chan P, Ramsingh A. Identification of a single aminoacid residue in the capsid protein VP1 of coxsackievirus B4 that determines the virulent phenotype. *J Viral* 1993;67:4797-803.

[18] Cainelli F, Manzaroli D, Renzini C, Casali F, Concia E, Vento S. Coxsackie B virus-induced autoimmunity to GAD does not lead to type 1 diabetes. *Diabetes Care* 2000;23:1021-22.

[19] Chatterjee NK, Nejman C, Gerling I. Purification and characterization of a strain of coxsackievirus B4 of human origin that induces diabetes in mice. *J Med Virol* 1988;26:57-69.

[20] Chehadeh W, Kerr-Conte J, Pattou F, Alm G, Lefebvre J, Wattre P, et al. Persistent infection of human pancreatic islets by coxsackievirus B is associated with alpha interferon synthesis in beta cells. *J Virol* 2000;74:10153-64.

[21] Chehadeh W, Weill J, Vantyghem MC, Alm G, Lefebvre J, Wattre P, et al. Increased level of interferon-alpha in blood of patients with insulin-dependent diabetes mellitus: relationship with coxsackievirus B infection. *J Infect Dis* 2000;181:1929-39.

[22] Chueca M, Oyarzabal M, Reparaz F, Garagorri JM, Sola A. Incidence of type 1 diabetes mellitus in Navarre, Spain (1975–1991). *Acta Paediatr* 1997;86:632-7.

[23] Clements GB, Galbraith DN, Taylor KW. Coxsackie B virus infection and onset of childhood diabetes. *Lancet* 1995;346:221-3.

[24] Couper JJ. Environmental triggers of type 1 diabetes. *J Paediatr Child Health* 2001;37:218-20.

[25] Coutant R, Carel JC, Lebon P, Bougneres PF, Palmer P, Cantero-Aguilar L. Detection of enterovirus RNA sequences in serum samples from autoantibody-positive subjects at risk for diabetes. *Diabet Med* 2002;19:968-9.

[26] Craig ME, Howard NJ, Silink M, Rawlinson WD. Reduced frequency of HLA DRB1*03-DQB1*02 in children with type 1diabetes associated with enterovirus RNA. *J Infect Dis* 2003;15:1562-70.

[27] Craig ME, Silink M, Howard NJ, Rawlinson WD. Genotyping of enteroviruses in children at diagnosis of Type 1 diabetes (Abs). *26th Ann Meeting International Society for paediatric and adolescent diabetes,* ISAPD, Los Angeles (Abstract) 2000.
[28] Craighead J, Mc Lane M. Diabetes Mellitus: induction in mice by encephalomyocarditis virus. *Science* 1968;162:913-5.
[29] Craighead J, Steinke J. Diabetes mellitus-like syndrome in mice infected with encephalomyocarditis virus. *Am J Pathol* 1971;63:119-34.
[30] Craighead J, Steinke J. Temporary diabetes in mice caused by encephalomyocarditis virus. *Clin Res* 1969;17:380.
[31] D'Alessio DJ. A case-control study of group B coxsackie IgM antibody prevalence and HLA-DR antigens in newly diagnosed cases of insulin-dependent diabetes mellitus. *Am J Epidemiol* 1992;135:1331-8.
[32] Dahlquist G, Blom L, Holmgrem G, Hagglof B, Larsson Y, Sterky G, et al. The epidemiology of diabetes in Swedish children 0-14 years-a six-year prospective study *Diabetologia* 1985;28:802-8.
[33] Dahlquist G, Frisk G, Ivarsson SA, Svanberg L, Forsgren M, Diderholm H. Indications that maternal coxsackie B virus infection during pregnancy is a risk factor for childhood- onset IDDM. *Diabetologia* 1995;38:1371-3.
[34] Dahlquist G. Viruses and other perinatal exposure as initiating events for B-cell destruction. *Ann Med* 1997;29:413-7.
[35] Dahlquist GG, Bowman JE, Juto P. Enteroviral RNA and IGM antibodies in early pregnancy is a risk factor for childhood onset IDDM. *Diabetes Care* 1999;22:364-5.
[36] Dahlquist GG, Forsberg J, Hagenfeldt L, Boman J, Juto P. Increased prevalence of enteroviral RNA in blood spots from newborn children who later developed type 1 diabetes: a population-based case-control study. *Diabetes Care* 2004;27:285-6.
[37] Dahlquist GG, Ivarsson S, Lingberg B, Forsgren M. Maternal enteroviral infection in pregnancy is a risk factor for childhood IDDM-A population based case control study. *Diabetes* 1995;44:408-13.
[38] Dalhquist G, Kalen B. Time-space clustering of time at birth in childhood onset diabetes. *Diabetes Care* 1996;19:328-32.
[39] Davydova B, Harkonen T, Kaialainen S, Hovi T, Vaarala O, Roivainen M. Coxsackievirus immunization delays onset of diabetes in non-obese diabetic mice. *J Med Virol* 2003;69:510-20.
[40] Dippe S, Bennet P, Miller M, Maynard J, Berquist K. Lack of causal association between Coxsackie B4 virus infections and diabetes. Lancet 1975;14:1314-7.
[41] Editorial. Dilated cardiomyopathy and enteroviruses. *Lancet* 1990;336:971-2.
[42] Eggers HJ. Accomplishments and challenges in picornavirology as observed by a medical doctor. *Clin Diagnostic Virol* 1998;9:67-76.
[43] Fohlman J, Friman G. Is juvenile diabetes a viral disease? *Ann Med* 1993;25:569-74.
[44] Forrest JM, Menser MA, Harley JD. A twenty five year follow up of congenital rubella. *Lancet* 1967;ii:1347-50.
[45] Foulis AK, Farquharson MA, Cameron SO, McGill M, Schonke H, Kandolf R. A search for the presence of the enteroviral capsid protein VP1 in pancreases of patients

with type 1 (insulin-dependent) diabetes and pancreases and hearts of infants who died of coxsackieviral myocarditis. *Diabetologia* 1990;33:290-8.

[46] Foulis AK, Farquharson MA, Meager A. Immunoreactive alpha interferon in insulin secreting beta cells in Type 1 diabetes. *Lancet* 1987;ii:1423-27.

[47] Foulis AK, McGill M, Farquharson MA, Hilton DA. A search for evidence of viral infection in pancreases of newly diagnosed patients with IDDM. *Diabetologia* 1997;40:53-61.

[48] Foy CA, Quirke P, Lewis FA, Futers TS, Bodansky HJ. Detection of common viruses using the polymerase chain reaction to assess levels of viral presence in type 1 (insulin-dependent) diabetic patients. *Diabet Med* 1995;12:1002-8.

[49] Foy CA, Quirke P, Willians D, Lewis FA, Grant PJ, Eglin R et al. A search for candidate viruses in type 1 diabetic pancreas using the polymerase chain reaction. *Diabet Med* 1994;11:564-9.

[50] Friman G, Fohlman J, Frisk G, Diderholm H, Ewald U, Kobbah M, et al. An incidence peak of juvenile diabetes. Relation to Coxsackie B virus immune response. *Acta Paediatr Scand* 1985; Suppl 320:14-9

[51] Frisk G, Diderholm H. Antibody responses to different strains of coxsackie B4 virus in patients with newly diagnosed type 1 diabetes mellitus or aseptic meningitis. *J Infection* 1997;34:205-10.

[52] Frisk G, Fohlman J, Kobbah M, Ewald U, Tuvemo T, Diderholm H, et al. High frequency of Coxsackie B virus-specific IgM in children developing type 1 diabetes during a period of high diabetes morbidity. *J Med Virol* 1985;17:219-27.

[53] Frisk G, Friman G, Tuvemo T, Fohlman J, Diderholm H. Coxsackie B virus IgM in children at onset of type 1 (insulindependent) diabetes mellitus: Evidence for IgM induction by a recent or current infection. *Diabetologia* 1992;35:249-53.

[54] Frisk G, Nilsson E, Tuvemo T, Friman G, Diderholm H. The possible role of Coxsackie A and echo viruses in the pathogenesis of type 1 diabetes mellitus studied by IgM analysis. *J Infect* 1992;24:13-22.

[55] Gamble D, Taylor K. Seasonal incidence of diabetes mellitus. *Br Med J* 1969;3:631-3.

[56] Gamble DR, Kinsley MJ, Fitzgerald MG, Bolton R, Taylor KW. Viral antibodies in diabetes mellitus. *Br Med J* 1969;3:627-30.

[57] Gamble DR, Taylor KW, Cumming H. Coxsackie viruses and diabetes mellitus. *Br Med J* 1973;4:260-2.

[58] Gerling I, Nejman C, Chatterje N. Effect of coxsackievirus B4 infection in mice on expression of 64,000-Mr autoantigen and glucose sensitivity of islets before development of hyperglycemia. *Diabetes* 1988;37:1419-25.

[59] Glenson R, Kahn C, Funk I, Craighead J. Seasonal incidence of insulin dependent diabetes in Massachusetts, 1964-1973. *Int J Epidemiol* 1982;11:39-45.

[60] Grandien M, Forsgren M, Ehrnst A. Enteroviruses. In Lennette EH, Lennette DA, Lennette ET eds. *Diagnostic Procedures for Viral, Rickettsial, and Chlamydial Infections*. 7th ed. Washington, DC: American Public Health Association; 1995.p.279-97.

[61] Graves PM, Norris JM, Pallansch MA, Gerling IC, Rewers M. The role of enteroviral infections in the development of IDDM: limitations of current approaches. *Diabetes* 1997;46:161-8.

[62] Graves PM, Rotbart HA, Nix WA, Pallansch MA, Erlich HA, Norris JM, et al. Prospective study of enteroviral infections and development of beta-cell autoimmunity. Diabetes autoimmunity study in the young (DAISY). *Diabetes Res Clin Pract* 2003;59:51-61.

[63] Green A, Patterson CC. Trends in the incidence of childhoodonset diabetes in Europe 1989–1998. *Diabetologia* 2001;44:B3-B8.

[64] Green J, Casabonne D, Newton R. Coxsackie B virus serology and Type 1 diabetes mellitus: a systematic review of published case-control studies. *Diabet Med* 2004;21:507-14.

[65] Hadden DR, Connolly JH, Montgomery D, Weaver JA. Coxsackie B virus and diabetes. *Br Med J* 1972;4:729.

[66] Harkonen T, Lankinen H, Davydova B, Hovi T, Roivainen M. Enterovirus infection can induce immune responses that crossreact with beta-cell autoantigen tyrosine phosphatase IA-2/IAR.*J Med Virol* 2002;66:340-50.

[67] Harkonen T, Paananen A, Lankinen H, Hovi T, Vaarala O, Roivainen M. Enterovirus infection may induce humoral immune response reacting with islet cell autoantigens in humans. *J Med Virol* 2003;69:426-40.

[68] Harkonen T, Puolakkainen M, Sarvas M, Airaksinen U, Hovi T, Roivainen M. Picornavirus proteins share antigenic determinants with heat shock proteins 60/65. *J Med Virol* 2000;62:383-91.

[69] Hartig PC, Madge GE, Webb SR. Diversity within a human isolate of coxsackie B4: relationship to viral-induced diabetes. *J Med Virol* 1983;11:23-30.

[70] Haverkos HW, Battula N, Drotman DP, Rennert OM. Enteroviruses and type 1 diabetes mellitus. *Biomed Pharmacother* 2003;57:379-85.

[71] Hayashi K, Boucher D, Notkins A. Virus-induced diabetes mellitus. II. Relationship between β cell damage and hyperglycemia in mice infected with encephalomyocarditis virus. *Am J Pathol* 1974;75:91-102.

[72] Helfand RF, Gary HE, Freeman CY, Anderson LJ, Pallansch MA, Pittsburgh Diabetes Research Group. Serologic evidence of an association between enteroviruses and the onset of type 1 diabetes mellitus. *J Infect Dis* 1995;172:1206-11.

[73] Herrmann KL, Erdman DD. Diagnosis by serologic assays. In Lennette EH, Lennette DA, Lennette E, eds. *Diagnostic Procedures for Viral, Rickettsial, and Chlamydial Infections*. 7th ed. Washington, DC: American Public Health Association; 1995.p.121-38.

[74] Hierholzer J, Farris W. Follow up of children infected in a coxsackievirus B3 and B4 outbreak: no evidence of diabetes mellitus. *J Infect Dis* 1974;129:741-6.

[75] Hilton D, Fletcher A, Pringle J. Absence of Coxsackie viruses in idiopathic infalammatory muscle disease by in situ hybridization. *Neuropath Applied Neurobiol* 1994;20:234-42.

[76] Hiltunen M, Hyöty H, Karjalainen J, Leinikki P, Knip M, Lounamaa R, et al. Serological evaluation of the role of cytomegalovirus in the pathogenesis of IDDM: a prospective study. *Diabetologia* 1995;38:705-10.

[77] Hiltunen M, Hyoty H, Knip M, Ilonen J, Reijonen H, Vahasalo P, et al. Islet cell antibody seroconversion in children is temporally associated with enterovirus infections. Childhood Diabetes in Finland (DiMe) Study Group. *J Infect Dis* 1997;175:554-60.

[78] Hiltunen M, Lonnrot M, Hyoty H. Immunisation and type 1 diabetes mellitus: is there a link? *Drug Saf* 1999;20:207-12.

[79] Hober D, Chehadeh W, Weill J, Hober C, Vantyghem MC, Gronnier P, et al. Circulating and cell-bound antibodies increase coxsackievirus B4-induced production of IFN-alpha by peripheral blood mononuclear cells from patients with type 1 diabetes. *J Gen Virol* 2002;83:2169-76.

[80] Horwitz M, Fine C, Ilic A, Sarvetnick N. Requirements for viral-mediated autoimmune diabetes: beta-cell damage and immune infiltration. *J Autoimmun* 2001;16:211-7

[81] Horwitz M, Ilic A, Fine C, Rodriguez E, Sarvetnick N. Presented antigen from damaged pancreatic beta cells activates autoreactive T cells in virus-mediated autoimmune diabetes. *J Clin Invest* 2002;109:79-87.

[82] Horwitz MS, Bradley LM, Harbertson J, Krahl T, Lee J, Sarvetnick N. Diabetes induced by coxsackie virus: initiation by bystander damage and not molecular mimicry. *Nat Med* 1998;4:781-5.

[83] Hou H, Said C, Franchi D, Dockstader P, Chatterjee N. Antibodies to glutamic and decarboxylase and P2C peptides in sera from coxsackievirus B4-infected mice and IDDM patients. *Diabetes* 1994;43:1260-6.

[84] Hou J, Sheikh S, Martin DL, Chatterjee NK. Coxsackievirus B4 alters pancreatic glutamate decarboxylase expression in mice soon after infection. J Autoimmun 1993;6:529-42.

[85] Hovi T, Stenvik M, Rosenlew M. Relative abundance of enterovirus serotypes in sewage differs from that in patients. Clinical and epidemiological implications. *Epidemiol Infect* 1996;116:91-7.

[86] Hovi T. Molecular Epidemiology of enterovirus with special reference to their potential role in the etiology of insulin-dependent diabetes mellitus. A review. *Clin Diagn Virol* 1998;9:85-99.

[87] Huang X, Yuang J, Goddard A, Foulis J, James R, Lernmark A, et al. Interferon expression in the pancreases of patients with type I diabetes. *Diabetes* 1995; 44:658-64.

[88] Huff JC, Hierholzer JC, FarrisWA. An "outbreak" of juvenile diabetes mellitus: consideration of a viral etiology. *Am J Epidemiol* 1974;100:277-87.

[89] Hyoty H, Hiltunen M, Knip M, Laakkonen M, Vahasalo P, Karjalainen J, et al. A prospective study of the role of coxsackie B and other enterovirus infections in the pathogenesis of IDDM. Childhood Diabetes in Finland (DiMe) Study Group. *Diabetes* 1995;44:652-7.

[90] Hyoty H, Hiltunen M, Lonnrot M. Enterovirus infections and insulin dependent diabetes mellitus-evidence for causality. *Clin Diagn Virol* 1998;9:77-84.

[91] Hyöty H, Räsänen L, Hiltunen M, Lehtinen H, Huupponen T, Leinikki P. Decreased antibody reactivity to Epstein-Barr virus capsid in Type 1 (insulin dependent) diabetes mellitus. *APMIS* 1991;99:359-63.

[92] Hyoty H, Taylor KW. The role of viruses in human diabetes. *Diabetologia* 2002;45:1353-61.

[93] Hyöty H. Enterovirus infections and type 1 diabetes. *Ann Med* 2002;34:138-47.

[94] Ihm S, Lee K, McArthur R, Yoon J. Predisposing effect of anti-Beta-cell autoimmunity process in NOID mice on the induction of diabetes by environmental insults. *Diabetologia* 1990;33:709-12.

[95] Imagawa A, Hanafusa T, Makino H, Miyagawa JI, Juto P. High titres of IgA antibodies to enterovirus in fulminant type-1 diabetes. *Diabetologia* 2005;48:290-3.

[96] Imagawa A, Hanafusa T, Miyagawa J, Matsuzawa Y. A novel subtype of type 1 diabetes mellitus characterized by a rapid onset and an absence of diabetes-related antibodies. *New Engl J Med* 2000;342:301-7.

[97] Jefferson I, Smith M, Baum J. Insulin dependent diabetes in under 5 year olds. *Arch Dis Child* 1985;60:1144-8.

[98] Jenson A, Rosenberg H, Notkins A. Pancreatic islet-cell damage in children with fatal viral infections. *Lancet* 1980;2:354-8.

[99] Jones DB, Crosby I. Proliferative lymphocyte responses to virus antigens homologous to GAD65 in IDDM. *Diabetologia* 1996;39:1318-24.

[100] Juhela S, Hyoty H, Hinkkanen A, Elliott J, Roivainen M, Kulmala P, et al. T cell responses to enterovirus antigens and to beta-cell autoantigens in unaffected children positive for IDDM-associated autoantibodies. *J Autoimmun* 1999;12:269-78.

[101] Juhela S, Hyoty H, Roivainen M, Harkonen T, Putto-Laurila A, Simell O, et al. T-cell responses to enterovirus antigens in children with type 1 diabetes. *Diabetes* 2000;49:1308-13.

[102] Juhela S, Hyoty H, Uibo R, Meriste SH, Uibo O, Lonnrot M, et al. Comparison of enterovirus-specific cellular immunity in two populations of young children vaccinated with inactivated or live poliovirus vaccines. *Clin Exp Immunol* 1999;117:100-5.

[103] Jun H, Khil LY, Yoon JW. Role of glutamic acid decarboxylase in the pathogenesis of type 1 diabetes. *Cell Mol Life Sci* 2002;59:1892-901.

[104] Jun H, Yoon J. A new look at Virus in Type 1 Diabetes. *Diabetes Metabolism Research and Reviews* 2002;19:8-31

[105] Kang Y, Chatterjee NK, Nodwell NJ, Yoon JW. Complete nucleotide sequence of Coxsackie B4 virus of human origin that induces diabetes in mice and its comparison with the non-diabetogenic Coxsackie B4 JVB strain. *J Med Virol* 1994;44:353-61.

[106] Kaptur P, Thomas D, Giron D. Differing attachment of diabetogenic and nondiabetogenic variants of encephalomyocarditis virus to B-cells. *Diabetes* 1989;38:1103-8.

[107] Karjalainen J. Islet cell antibodies as predictive markers for IDDM in children with high background incidence of disease. *Diabetes* 1990;39:1144-50.

[108] Kaufman D, Erlander M, Clare-Salzler M, Atkinson N, Maclaren N, Tobin J. Autoimmunity to two forms of glutamate decarboxylase in insulin dependent diabetes mellitus. *J Clin Invest* 1992;89:283-92.

[109] Kawashima H, Ihara T, Ioi H, Oana S, Sato S, Kato N, et al. Enterovirus-related type 1 diabetes mellitus and antibodies to glutamic acid decarboxylase in Japan. *J Infect* 2004;49:147-51.

[110] King ML, Shaikh A, Bidwell D, Voller A, Banatvala JE. Coxsackie B virus-specific IgM responses in children with insulin-dependent (juvenile-onset/type 1) diabetes mellitus. *Lancet* 1983;1:1397-9.

[111] Klemetti P, Hyoty H, Roivainen M, Ilonen J, Savola K, Knip M, et al. Relation between T-cell responses to glutamate decarboxylase and coxsackievirus B4 in patients with insulin-dependent diabetes mellitus. *J Clin Virol* 1999;14:95-105.

[112] Knip M, Akerblom HK. Environmental factors in the pathogenesis of type 1 diabetes mellitus. *Exp Clin Endocrinol Diabetes* 1999;107:S93-100.

[113] Kondrashova A, Romanov A, Karvonen A, Reunanen A, Hyoty H. Incidence of type 1 diabetes in the Karelian Republic of Russia. *Diabetologia* 2000;43:A91.

[114] Kupila A, Muona P, Simell T, Arvilommi P, Savolainen H, Hamalainen A, et al. Feasibility of genetics and immunological prediction of Type I diabetes in a population based birth cohort. *Diabetologia* 2001;44:290-7.

[115] Landin-Olsson M, Karlsson A, Dahlquist G, Blom L, Lernmark A, Sundkvist G. Islet cell and other organ specific autoantibodies in all children developing type 1 (insulin-dependent) diabetes mellitus in Sweden during one year and in matched control children. *Diabetologia* 1989;32:387-95.

[116] Lauwers S, Bissay V, Rombaut B. Development of an enterovirus specific PCR method for the quantification of enterovirus genomes in blood of diabetes patients. *Clin Diagn Virol* 1998;9:135-9.

[117] Leff R, Love L, Miller F. Viruses in idiopathic infalammatory myopathies: absence of candidate viral genomes in muscle. *Lancet* 1992,339:1192-5.

[118] Lonnrot M, Hyoty H, Knip M, Roivainen M, Kulmala P, Leinikki P, et al. Antibody cross-reactivity induced by the homologous regions in glutamic acid decarboxylase (GAD 65) and 2C protein of coxsackievirus B4. *Clin Experimental Immunol* 1996;104:398-405.

[119] Lonnrot M, Knip M, Marciulionyte D, Rahko J, Urboinaite B, Moore W, et al. Enterovirus antibodies in relation to islet cell antibodies in two populations with high and low incidence of type 1 diabetes. *Diabetes Care* 1999;22:2086-8.

[120] Lonnrot M, Knip M, Roivainen M, Koskela P, Akerblom HK, Hyoty H. Onset of type 1 diabetes mellitus in infancy after enterovirus infections. *Diabet Med* 1998;15:431-4.

[121] Lonnrot M, Korpela K, Knip M, Ilonen J, Simell O, Korhonen S, et al. Enterovirus infection as a risk factor for beta-cell autoimmunity in a prospectively observed birth cohort: the Finnish Diabetes Prediction and Prevention Study. *Diabetes* 2000;49:1314-8.

[122] Lonnrot M, Salminen K, Knip M, Savola K, Kulmala P, Leinikki P, et al. Enterovirus RNA in serum is a risk factor for beta-cell autoimmunity and clinical type 1 diabetes: a prospective study. Childhood Diabetes in Finland (DiMe) Study Group. *J Med Virol* 2000;61:214-20.

[123] Maclaren NK, Alkinson MA. Insulin-dependent diabetes mellitus: the hypothesis of molecular mimicry between islet cell antigens and microorganisms. *Mol Med Today* 1997;3:76-83.

[124] Maclaren NK, Riley WJ, Winter WE, Silverstein JH. Is insulin-dependent diabetes mellitus a preventable disease? *Clin Invest Med* 1987;10:444-9.

[125] Marttila J, Hyoty H, Vilja P, Harkonen T, Alho A, Roivainen M, et al. T cell epitopes in coxsackievirus B4 structural proteins concentrate in regions conserved between enteroviruses. *Virology* 2002;293:217-24.

[126] Marttila J, Juhela S, Vaarala O, Hyoty H, Roivainen M, Hinkkanen A, et al. Responses of coxsackievirus B4-specific T-cell lines to 2C protein characterization of epitopes with special reference to the GAD65 homology region. *Virology* 2001;284:131-1.

[127] Menser M, Forrest J, Bransby R. Rubella infection and diabetes mellitus. *Lancet* 1978;i:57-60.

[128] Mertens TH, Gruneklee D, Eggers HJ. Neutralizing antibodies against Coxsackie viruses in patients with recent onset of type 1 diabetes. *Eur J Pediatr* 1983;140:293-4.

[129] Molbak A, Norgaard K, Christau B, et al. Incidence of type 1 (insulin-dependent) diabetes mellitus in Denmark, evidence of secular trend. (Abstract). *Diabetologia* 1987;30:559.

[130] Morens D, Pallansch M. Epidemiology. In: Rotbart H, ed. *Human Enterovirus Infections*. Washington, DC: American Society for Microbiology Press;1995.p.3-23.

[131] Morens DM, Pallansch MA, Moore M. Poliovirus and other enteroviruses. In: Belshe RB, ed. *Textbook of human virology*. St. Louis: Mosby Year Book; 1991.p.427-97.

[132] Moya-Suri V, Schlosser M, Zimmermann K, Rjasanowski I, Gurtler L, Mentel R. Enterovirus RNA sequences in sera of schoolchildren in the general population and their association with type 1-diabetes-associated autoantibodies. *J Med Microbiol.* 2005;54:879-83.

[133] Nelson PG, Arthur LJH, Gurling KJ, Gamble DR, Taylor KW. Familial juvenile onset. *BMJ* 1977;2:1126-7.

[134] Nelson PG, Pyke DA, Gamble DR. Viruses and the aetiology of diabetes: a study in identical twins. *Br Med J* 1975;4:249-51.

[135] Neu A, Kehrer M, Hub R, Ranke MB. Incidence of IDDM in German children aged 0–14 years. A 6-year population-based study (1987–1993). *Diabetes Care* 1997;20:530-3.

[136] Nigro G, Pacella M, Patane E, Midulla M. multi-system coxsackievirus B6 infection with findings suggestive of diabetes mellitus. *Eur J Pediatr* 1986;145:557-9.

[137] Niklasson B, Dobersen M, Peters C, Ennis W, Moller E. An outbreak of coxsackievirus B infection followed by one case of diabetes mellitus. *Scand J Infect Dis* 1985;17:15-8.

[138] Notkins A, Yoon J. Virus-induced diabetes in mice prevented by a live attenuated vaccine. *New Engl J Med* 1982;306:486.

[139] Oberste MS, Pallansch MA. Establishing evidence for enterovirus infection in chronic disease. *Ann N Y Acad Sci* 2003;1005:23-31.

[140] Oberste S, Maher K, Kennett M, Campbell J, Carpenter M, Schnurr D. Molecular epidemiology and genetic diversity of echovirus type 30 (E30): genotypes correlate with temporal dynamics of E30 isolation. *J Clin Microbiol* 1999;37:3928-33.

[141] Oldstone M, Nerenberg M, Southern P, Price J, Lewicki H. Virus infection triggers IDDM in a transgenic model: role of antiself (virus) immune response. *Cell* 1991;65:319-31.

[142] Onkamo P, Vananen S, Karvonen M, Tuomilehto J. Worldwide increase in incidence of Type I diabetes-The analysis of the data on published incidence trends. *Diabetologia* 1999;42:1395-1403.

[143] Orchard T, Becker D, Atchison R, La Porte R, Wagener D, Rabin B, et al. The development of type 1 (insulin dependent) diabetes mellitus: two contrasting presentations. *Diabetologia* 1983;25:89-92.

[144] Orchard TJ, Atchison RW, Becker D. Coxsackie infection and diabetes. *Lancet* 1983;2:631.

[145] Otonkoski T, Roivainen M, Vaarala O, Dinesen B, Leipala JA, Hovi T, et al. Neonatal Type I diabetes associated with maternal echovirus 6 infection: a case report. *Diabetologia* 2000;43:1235-8.

[146] Paananen A, Ylipaasto P, Rieder E, Hovi T, Galama J, Roivainen M. Molecular and biological analysis of echovirus 9 strain isolated from a diabetic child. *J Med Virol* 2003;69:529-37.

[147] Pallansch M. Epidemiology of coxsackie B viruses. In: Friedman H and Bendinelli M, ed. *Coxsackieviruses-a general update*. New York: Plenum Press;1988.p.399-417.

[148] Palmer JP, Cooney MK, Ward RH, Hansen J, Brodsky J, Ray C, et al. Reduced Coxsackie antibody titres in type 1 (insulin-dependent) diabetic patients presenting during an outbreak of Coxsackie B3 and B4 infection. *Diabetologia* 1982;22:426-9.

[149] Pennisi E. Teetering on the brink of danger. *Science* 1996;271:1665-7.

[150] Phillips WR, Pauli R. Simultaneous onset of insulin dependent diabetes in siblings. *Lancet* 1981:807.

[151] Podar T, Solntsev A, Karvonen M, Padaiga Z, Brigis G, Urbonaite B, et al. Increasing incidence of childhood-onset type I diabetes in 3 Baltic countries and Finland 1983–1998. *Diabetologia* 2001;44:B17-B20.

[152] Ramsingh AI, Chapman N, Tracy S. Coxsackieviruses and diabetes. *Bioessays* 1997;19:793-800.

[153] Ren R, Moss E, Rascaniello V. Identification of two determinants that attenuate vaccine related type 2 poliovirus. *J Virol* 1991;65:1377-82.

[154] Rewers M, LaPorte R, Walczak J, Dmochowski K, Bogaczynska E. Apparent epidemic of insulin-dependent diabetes mellitus in Midwestern Poland. *Diabetes* 1987;36:106-13.

[155] Rewers M, Stone R, LaPorte R, Drash A, Becker D, Walczak J , et al. Poison regression modeling of temporal variation in incidence of childhood insulin-dependent diabetes mellitus in Allegheny County, Pennsylvania, and Wielkopolska, Poland, 1970-1985. *Am J Epidemiol* 1989;129:569-81.

[156] Ritcher W, Mertens T, Schoel B, Muir P, Ritzkowsky A, Scherbaum W, et al. Sequence homology of the diabetes-associated autoantigen glutamate decarboxylase with Coxsackie B4-2C protein and heat shock protein 60 mediates no molecular mimicry of autoantibodies. *J Exp Med* 1994;180:721-6.

[157] Roep BO. Immunology of Diabetes Society T-cell Committee. Standardization of T-cell assays in Type I diabetes. *Diabetologia* 1999;42:636-7.

[158] Roivainen M, Knip M, Hyoty H, Kulmala P, Hiltunen M, Vahasalo P, et al. Several different enterovirus serotypes can be associated with prediabetic autoimmune episodes and onset of overt IDDM. *J Med Virol* 1998;56:74-8.

[159] Roivainen M, Rasilainen S, Ylipaasto P, Nissinen R, Ustinov J, Bouwens L, et al. Mechanisms of coxsackievirus-induced damage to human pancreatic beta-cells. *J Clin Endocrinol Metab* 2000;85:432-40.

[160] Roivainen M, Ylipaasto P, Savolainen C, Galama J, Hovi T, Otonkoski T. Functional impairment and killing of human beta cells by enteroviruses: the capacity is shared by a wide range of serotypes, but the extent is a characteristic of individual virus strains. *Diabetologia* 2002;45:693-702.

[161] Rossmann M, Palmenberg A. Conservation of the putative receptor attachment site in picornaviruses. *Virology* 1988;164:373-82.

[162] Rothwell P, Staines A, Smail P, Wadsworth E, McKinney P. Seasonality of birth of patients with childhood diabetes in Britain. *BMJ* 1996;312:1456-7.

[163] Sadeharju K, Lonnrot M, Kimpimaki T, Savola K, Erkkila S, Kalliokoski T, et al. Enterovirus antibody levels during the first two years of life in prediabetic autoantibody positive children. *Diabetologia* 2001;44:818-23.

[164] Sakurami T, Nabeya N, Nagaoka K, Matsumori A, Kuno S, Honda A. Antibodies to Coxsackie B viruses and HLA in Japanese with juvenile-onset type 1 (insulin-dependent) diabetes mellitus. *Diabetologia* 1982;22:375-7.

[165] Salminen K, Sadeharju K, Lonnrot M, Vahasalo P, Kupila A, Korhonen S, et al. Enterovirus infections are associated with the induction of beta-cell autoimmunity in a prospective birth cohort study. *J Med Virol* 2003;69:91-8.

[166] Salminen KK, Vuorinen T, Oikarinen S, Helminen M, Simell S, Knip M, et al. Isolation of enterovirus strains from children with preclinical Type 1 diabetes. *Diabet Med* 2004;21:156-64.

[167] Savolainen C, Hovi T, Mulders M. Molecular epidemiology of echovirus 30 in Europe: succession of dominant sublineages within a single major genotype. *Arch Virol* 2001;146:521-37.

[168] Schloot NC, Roep BO, Wegmann DR, Yu L, Wang TB, Eisenbarth GS. T-cell reactivity to GAD65 peptide sequences shared with coxsackie virus protein in recent-onset IDDM, post-onset IDDM patients and control subjects. *Diabetologia* 1997;40:332-8.

[169] Schloot NC, Willemen SJ, Duinkerken G, Drijfhout JW, de Vries RR, Roep BO. Molecular mimicry in type 1 diabetes mellitus revisited: T-cell clones to GAD65 peptides with sequence homology to Coxsackie or proinsulin peptides do not crossreact with homologous counterpart. *Hum Immunol* 2001;62:299-309.

[170] Schmidt WAK, Brade L, Munterfering H, Klein M. Course of Coxsackie B antibodies during juvenile juvenile onset diabetes. *Med Microbiol Immunol* 1978;164:291-8.

[171] See DM, Tilles JG. The pathogenesis of viral-induced diabetes. *Clin Diagn Virol* 1998;9:85-8.

[172] Siemiatycki J, Colle E, Aubert D, Campbell S, Belmonte M. The distribution of type 1 (insulin-dependent) diabetes mellitus by age, sex, secular trend, seasonality, time cluster, and space-time cluster: evidence from montreal, 1971-1983. *Am J Epidemiol* 1986;124:545-60.

[173] Smith CP, Clements GB, Riding MH, Bottazzo GF, Taylor KW. Simultaneous onset of type 1 diabetes mellitus in identical infant twins with enterovirus infection. *Diabet Med* 1998;15:515-7.

[174] Somoza N, Vargas F, Roura-Mir C, Vives Pi-M, Fernandez-Figueras M, Ariz A, et al. Pancreas in recent onset insulin-dependent diabetes mellitus. Changes in HLA, adhesion molecules and autoantigens, restricted T cell receptor V beta usage, and cytokine profile. *J Immunol* 1994;153:1360-77.

[175] Strikas R, Anderson L, Panker R. Temporal and geographic patterns of isolates of nonpolio enterovirus in the United States, 1970-1983. *J Infect Dis* 1986;153:346-51.

[176] Svensson J, Lindberg B, Jonsson B, Ericsson UB, Olofsson P, Hyoty H, et al. Intrauterine exposure to maternal enterovirus infection as a risk factor for development of autoimmune thyroiditis during childhood and adolescence. *Thyroid* 2004;14:367-70.

[177] Szopa T, Ward T, Dronfield D, Portwood N, Taylor K. Coxsackie B4 viruses with the potential to damage B cells of the islets are present in clinical isolates. *Diabetologia* 1990;33:325-8.

[178] Szopa TM, Titchener PA, Portwood ND, Taylor KW. Diabetes mellitus due to viruses-Some recent developments. *Diabetologia* 1993;36:687-95.

[179] Tauriainen S, Salminen K, Hyoty H. Can enteroviruses cause type 1 diabetes? *Ann N Y Acad Sci* 2003;1005:13-22.

[180] Tian J, Lehmann PV, Kaufman DL. T cell cross-reactivity between coxsackievirus and glutamate decarboxylase is associated with a murine diabetes susceptibility allele. *J Exp Med* 1994;1805:1979-84.

[181] Toth EL, Couch RM, Lee K-C, Martin LF. High incidence of IDDM over 6 years in Edmonton, Alberta, Canada. *Diabetes Care* 1997;20:311-3.

[182] Triantafilou K, Triantafilou M. Coxsackievirus B4-induced cytokine production in pancreatic cells is mediated through toll-like receptor 4. *J Virol* 2004;78:11313-20.

[183] Tull E, Roseman J, Christian C. Epidemiology of childhood insulin-dependent diabetes mellitus in the U.S. Virgin Island from 1979-1988: evidence of an epidemic in the early 1980´s and variation by degree of racial admixture. Diabetes Care 1991;14:558-64.

[184] Tuomilehto J, Karvonen M, Padaiga Z, Tuomilehto-Wolf E, Kohtamaki K. Epidemiology of insulin-dependent diabetes mellitus around the Baltic Sea. The DIABALT Study Group. *Horm Metab Res* 1996;28:340-3.

[185] Tuomilehto J, Karvonen M, Pitka¨niemi J, Virtala E, Kohtamaki K, Toivanen L, et al. Record-high incidence of Type I (insulin-dependent) diabetes mellitus in Finnish children. *Diabetologia* 1999;42:655-60.

[186] Tuomilehto J, Virtala E, Karvonen M, Lounamaa R, Pitkaniemi J, Reunanen A, et al. Increase in incidence of insulin-dependent diabetes mellitus among children in Finland. *Int J Epidemiol* 1995;24:984-92.

[187] Tuvemo T, Berg AK, Frisk G, Yin H. Enterovirus RNA is found in a majority of IDDM children at onset. *Ups J Med Sci* 2001;56:73.

[188] Tuvemo T, Dahlquist G, Frisk G, Blom L, Friman G, Landin-Olsson et al. The Swedish childhood diabetes study III: IgM against Coxsackie B viruses in newly diagnoses type 1 (insulin-dependent) diabetic children—no evidence of increased antibody frequency. *Diabetologia* 1989;32:745-7.

[189] Vaarala O, Hyoty H, Akerblom HK. Environmental factors in the aetiology of childhood diabetes. *Diabetes Nutr Metab* 1999;12:75-85.

[190] Varela-Calvino R, Ellis R, Sgarbi G, Dayan CM, Peakman M. Characterization of the T-cell response to coxsackievirus B4: evidence that effector memory cells predominate in patients with type 1 diabetes. *Diabetes* 2002;51:1745-53.

[191] Varela-Calvino R, Peakman M. Enterovirus and type 1 diabetes. *Diabet Metab Res Rev* 2003;19:431-1.

[192] Varela-Calvino R, Sgarbi G, Wedderburn LR, Dayan CM, Tremble J, Peakman M. T cell activation by coxsackievirus B4 antigens in type 1 diabetes mellitus: evidence for selective TCR beta usage without superantigenic activity. *J Immunol* 2001;167:3513-20.

[193] Varela-Calvino, R, Sgarbi, G., Arif S, Peakman, M. T Cell reactivity to the P2C nonstructural protein of a diabetogenic strain of coxsackievirus B4. *Virology* 2000;274:56-64.

[194] Viskari HR, Koskela P, Lo¨nnrot M, Luonuansuu S, Reunanen A, Baer M, et al. Can enterovirus infections explain the increasing incidence of type 1 diabetes? *Diabetes Care* 2000;23:414-6.

[195] Viskari H, Ludvigsson J, Uibo R, Salur L, Marciulionyte D, Hermann R, et al. Relationship between the incidence of type 1 diabetes and enterovirus infections in different European populations: results from the EPIVIR project. *J Med Virol* 2004;72:610-7.

[196] Viskari HR, Ludvigsson J, Uibo R, Salur L, Marciulionyte D, Hermann R, Soltesz G, et al. Relationship between the incidence of type 1 diabetes and maternal enterovirus antibodies: time trends and geographical variation. *Diabetologia* 2005;48:1280-7.

[197] Vreugdenhil GR, Batstra MR, Aanstoot HJ, Melchers WJ, Galama JM. Analysis of antibody responses against coxsackie virus B4 protein 2C and the diabetes autoantigen GAD 65. *J Med Virol* 1999;59:256-61.

[198] Vreugdenhil GR, Geluk A, Ottenhoff T, Melchers W, Roep B, Galama J. Molecular mimicry in diabetes mellitus: the homologous domain in Coxsackie B virus protein 2C and islet autoantigen GAD65 is highly conserved in the Coxsackie B-like enteroviruses and binds to the diabetes associated HLA-DR3 molecule. *Diabetologia* 1998;41:40-6.

[199] Vreugdenhil GR, Schloot NC, Hoorens A, Rongen C, Pipeleers DG, Melchers WJ, et al. Acute onset of type I diabetes mellitus after severe echovirus 9 infection: putative pathogenic pathways. *Clin Infect Dis* 2000;31:1025-31.

[200] Vreugdenhil GR, Wijnands PG, Netea MG, van der Meer JW, Melchers WJ, Galama JM. Enterovirus-induced production of pro-inflammatory and T-helper cytokines by human leukocytes. *Cytokine* 2000;12:1793-96.

[201] Wagenknecht L, Roseman J, Herman W. Increased incidence of insulin-dependent diabetes mellitus following an epidemic of coxsackievirus B5. *Am J Epidemiol* 1991;133:1024-31.

[202] Waldhoer T, Schober E, Tuomilehto J. Long-term patterns in seasonality of insulin-dependent diabetes mellitus diagnosis in Austrian children. *J Clin Epidemiol* 1997;50:159-65.

[203] Wen L, Wong F, Tang J, Chen N, Altieri M, David C, et al. In vivo evidence for the contribution of human histocompatibility leukocyte antigen (HLA)-DQ molecules to the development of diabetes. *J Exp Med* 2000,191:97.

[204] Wong F, Wen L. What can the HLA transgenic mouse tell us about autoimmune diabetes? *Diabetologia* 2004;47:1476.

[205] Wucherpfennig KW, Strominger JL. Molecular mimicry in T cell mediated autoimmunity: viral peptides activate human T cell clones specific for myelin basic protein. *Cell* 1995;80:695-705.

[206] Yin H, Berg AK, Tuvemo T, Frisk G. Enterovirus RNA is found in peripheral blood mononuclear cells in a majority of type 1 diabetic children at onset. *Diabetes* 2002;51:1964-71.

[207] Yin H, Berg AK, Westman J, Hellerstrom C, Frisk G. Complete nucleotide sequence of a Coxsackievirus B-4 strain capable of establishing persistent infection in human pancreatic islet cells: effects on insulin release, proinsulin synthesis, and cell morphology. *J Med Virol* 2002;68:544-57.

[208] Yin H, Frisk G. Genomic structure of a "diabetogenic" CB4 strain-VD2921. *Ups J Med Sci* 2001;106:83.

[209] Ylipaasto P, Klingel K, Lindberg A, Otonkoski T, Kandolf R, Hovi T, et al. Enterovirus infection in human pancreatic islet cells, islet tropism in vivo and receptor involvement in cultured islet beta cells. *Diabetologia* 2004;47:225-39.

[210] Yoon J, Austin M, Onodera T, Notkins A. Isolation of a virus from the pancreas of a child with diabetes ketoacidosis. *N Engl J Med* 1979;300:1173-9.

[211] Zanone MM, Favaro E, Conaldi PG, Greening J, Bottelli A, Perin P, et al. Persistent infection of human microvascular endothelial cells by coxsackie B viruses induces increased expression of adhesion molecules. *J Immunol* 2003;171:438-6.

[212] Zinkernagel R, Cooper S, Chambers J, Lazzarini R, Hengartner H, Arnheiter H. Virus-induced autoantibody to a transgenic viral antigen. *Nature* 1999;345:68-71.

[213] Zurbriggen A, Thomas C, Yamada M, Roos R, Fuginami R. Direct evidence of a role of aminoacid 101 of VP1 in central nervous system disease in Theiler's murine encephalomyelitis virus infection. *J Virol* 1991;65:1929-37.

Chapter IV

Our Contributions to the Association Between Enterovirus Infections and Type 1 Diabetes

***Eduardo Cabrera-Rode*[1,*] *and Luis Sarmiento-Pérez*[2]**

[1]Department of Immunology of Diabetes, National Institute of Endocrinology, Havana, Cuba;

[2]Department of Virology, PAHO/WHO Collaborating Center for Viral Diseases, "Pedro Kouri" Tropical Medicine Institute, Havana, Cuba.

Abstract

One of the major disease hallmarks in type 1 diabetes is the presence of islet cell autoantibodies, present in over 90% of cases and defined by indirect immunofluorescence or, more recently, by reactivity to at least three molecularly defined islet autoantigens, insulin autoantibodies, glutamic acid decarboxylase antibodies and insulinoma-associated-antigen-2 autoantibodies. The Cuban experience in the field of the viral aetiology of type 1 diabetes has provided a clear link between the epidemics of enterovirus and islet cell autoimmunity. Public health surveillance strategies in Cuba have identified 3 epidemics of echovirus (a member of the enterovirus genus) since 1986, during each of which a high proportion of patients have gone on to develop evidence of an autoimmune reaction to islet β cells. Moreover, the epidemic enterovirus strains showed subtle differences in the nature of islet cell autoimmunity they induced. We also report of a 12-year-old girl that developed pancreatic autoimmunity and type 1 diabetes after enteroviral infection. The data obtained from Cuba support the hypothesis

---

* Correspondence concerning this article should be addressed to:
Eduardo Cabrera-Rode. Department of Immunology of Diabetes, National Institute of Endocrinology, Zapata and D, Havana 10 400, Cuba; fax: 53-7-333417; email: *diabetes@infomed.sld.cu*.
Luis Sarmiento Pérez, Department of Virology, PAHO/WHO Collaborating Center for Viral Diseases, "Pedro Kouri" Tropical Medicine Institute, Autopista Novia del Mediodía, km 6, PO Box, 601, Marianao 13, Havana, Cuba; fax: 53-7-2046051; email: sarmiento@ipk.sld.cu or *lsarmientop@yahoo.com*.

that enterovirus infections may be involved in the pathogenesis of type 1 diabetes and are in agreement with the view that the autoimmune mechanisms in the type 1 diabetes are indeed different from the LADA subjects.

Keywords: enterovirus, echovirus, islet cell associated antibodies, type 1 diabetes, epidemic, latent autoimmune diabetes.

As has been shown in chapter III, the "enteroviral aetiology" of type 1 diabetes is a credible disease mechanism but is difficult to conduct and interpret. Taking into account that large-scale and explosive epidemics can be caused by enteroviruses, they represent an opportunity to study the relation between enteroviral infection, pancreatic autoimmunity and development type 1 diabetes. The opportunistic study of enterovirus epidemics in Cuba and their relationship to islet cell autoimmunity and type 1 diabetes mellitus has been analyzed in three previous reports in which various types of enterovirus were associated to a varying degree with the acute development of islet cell autoimmunity. In a fourth report we analyzed the possible influence of enteroviral infections in the emergence of latent autoimmune diabetes in adults.

I. Echovirus 4 and Type 1 Diabetes Mellitus (*ReportI*)

The first evidence of an association between the presence of islet cell antibodies (ICA) and a meningoencephalitis epidemic caused by echovirus was published in Cuba in 1990 [9,24,58,59,60]. In this study, 48 out of 133 (36.1 %) infected children during an epidemic of echovirus 4 occurred in Cuba in 1986 were ICA positive [58].

At that time, Uriarte and colleagues also found that a significant proportion of the infected children developed temporary glucose intolerance [9,56,60]. It has been shown that β cells from mice infected with echovirus 4 (isolated strains from children of the previously mentioned epidemic) produced less insulin and had reduced synthesis of total proteins [56]. Such changes were related to alterations in their blood glucose concentrations.

Subsequently, studies in Cuba demonstrated that type 1 diabetic patients showed a significantly higher frequency of neutralizing antibodies to echovirus 4 than non-diabetic control subjects [18]. In this study, serum samples were obtained from newly (less than 6 months) diagnosed patients with type 1 diabetes (n=33), healthy offspring of parents with type 1 diabetes mellitus without ICA (n=43) and ICA negative normal subjects without diabetes family history (n=57). The offspring of type 1 diabetic group was included to recruit the highest number of young subjects carrying HLA-associated type 1 diabetes susceptibility genes and lacking pancreatic β cells autoimmunity.

Mean duration of diabetes, mean/median age and range as well as sex distributions of the different groups are described in Table 1. Groups were matched for geographical location (all living in Havana city), time of sampling (blood samples were collected during the spring of 1999) and socio-economic status.

Table 1. Age, sex distribution and diabetes duration of the studied group

Group	N	Mean	Median	Minimum	Maximum	Sex distribution Male/female gender ratio	Duration of diabetes Days Mean
Control	57	8.3	8	1	16	1.28	-
ODM1	43	7.7	7	1	18	1.04	-
T1DM	33	10.7	11	3	19	0.91	25
Total	133	8.7	8	1	19	1.11	-

Reprinted from reference [18].

The neutralizing antibodies to coxsackieviruses A9, B1, B2, B3, B4, B5, B6 and echoviruses 4, 6, 9, 11 were measured in all sera. Whole blood samples were also obtained to perform class II HLA typing in offspring of type 1 diabetic patients.

This study showed that type 1 diabetic patients exhibit a higher frequency (21.2 %, p<0.01) of neutralizing antibodies to echovirus 4 in relation to controls (1.8 %), although there were no differences comparing with offspring of type 1 diabetic patients (20.9 %) (Table 2).

Table 2. Frequency (%) of positive neutralizing antibodies (dilution 1/10 of the serum) for the studied virus. P<0.01 vs control.

Groups	Age groups (years)	N	CVA9	CVB1	CVB2	CVB3	CVB4	CVB5	CVB6	E4	E6	E9	E11
Control	1-6	17	58.8	29.4	41.2	70.6	64.7	17.6	0.0	0.0	35.3	47.1	35.3
	7-12	32	84.4	65.6	71.9	78.1	87.5	21.9	3.1	0.0	68.8	56.3	59.4
	13-19	8	100.0	87.5	87.5	87.5	100.0	25.0	0.0	12.5	62.5	62.5	75.0
	Total	57	78.9	57.9	64.9	77.2	82.5	21.1	1.8	1.8	57.9	54.4	54.4
	1-6	18	83.3	66.7	61.1	38.9	55.6	44.4	16.7	11.1	72.2	55.6	55.6
ODM1[1]	7-12	18	88.9	50.0	83.3	66.7	77.8	44.4	5.6	22.2	55.6	55.6	66.7
	13-19	7	100.0	85.7	85.7	71.4	100.0	0.0	14.3	42.9	71.4	71.4	57.1
	Total	43	88.4	62.8	74.4	55.8	72.1	37.2	11.6	20.9*	65.1	58.1	60.5
	1-6	7	85.7	57.1	71.4	28.6	100.0	28.6	14.3	0.0	71.4	57.1	57.1
	7-12	12	100.0	58.3	66.7	66.7	91.7	41.7	8.3	16.7	50.0	66.7	50.0
	13-19	14	92.9	57.1	78.6	71.4	92.9	28.6	0.0	35.7	78.6	85.7	64.3
T1DM[2]	Total	33	93.9	57.6	72.7	60.6	93.9	33.3	6.1	21.2*	66.7	72.7	57.6
(p)[3]			<0.01	0.059	<0.01	<0.05	<0.01	>0.05	>0.05	<0.01	>0.05	0.056	>0.05

[1] Healthy offsprint of parents with type 1 diabetes. [2] Type 1 diabetes.

[3] Relation between the frequency of neutralizing antibodies and age: Chi-squared test for trend.

Reprinted from reference [18].

Healthy offspring carrying type 1 diabetes HLA DR susceptibility genes were also exposed to echovirus 4 (15.0 %) indicating that the interaction between these genetic and environmental factors does not totally lead to the autoimmune process. However, it is possible that the diabetogenicity of certain echovirus 4 strains may vary and these strains cannot be distinguished by the neutralization assay. Type 1 diabetic and offspring of type 1 diabetic groups could also share type 1 diabetes-related non-HLA-DR genes of susceptibility to echovirus 4 infections. These data support the multifactorial etiology hypothesis of this pathology.

On the other hand, no differences were found as we compared the overall frequency of neutralizing antibodies to all enteroviruses between the groups. Sex had no effect on the frequency of enterovirus infections among all groups studied. Age was associated with higher frequencies of neutralizing antibodies to most enteroviruses. High frequencies of neutralizing antibodies to most of the enterovirus were found in the control group. Thus, the Cuban population displays high frequencies of exposure to enterovirus, despite the low incidence of type 1 diabetes reported for Cuba (3.0 per 100.000 population) [13,17]. Accordingly, the Cuban data together with the finding reported in the chapter III about the correlation between the epidemiology of enterovirus infections and type 1 diabetes on population level [34,64,65] reinforce the proposed polio hypothesis according to which the complications of enterovirus infections become more common in an environment with a decreased rate of infections. To date, there are no reports on the frequency of type 1 diabetes susceptibility genes in Cuban population; however, several studies have shown that HLA-DR3 and HLA-DR4 haplotypes are associated with type 1 diabetes in Hispanic populations. Genetic typing for susceptibility markers for type 1 diabetes in Cuban population would give crucial information whether the population genetic susceptibility justifies the low observed incidence.

Similar, albeit less well documented studies on echovirus outbreaks in Glasgow [19] and Poland [48], give broad support to this "epidemic echovirus → islet autoimmunity → metabolic disturbance" pattern. In Glasgow, 17 patients from an echovirus 4 outbreak were studied. The group's mean insulin levels were transiently increased following infections, and one subject showed ICA positivity just after infections, with the ICA titer declining at follow up.

II. Type 1 Diabetes Islet Associated Antibodies in Subjects Infected by Echovirus 16 *(Report II)*

From April to September 2000, an epidemic of aseptic meningitis spread throughout Cuba, with 16.943 reported cases. Most of the patients were children under 15 years old. The highest incidence corresponded to infants of less than 1 year of age, followed by the 1- to-9-year-old group, and none of the infant cases were neonates. Vomiting (91.5 %), headache (88.1 %), and fever (72.8 %) were the predominant clinical manifestations; few patients had diarrhoea (11.8%) or skin rash (6.8 %) [51]. None of the infected children had altered blood fasting glucose concentrations.

To establish the outbreak-associated enterovirus, 54 cerebrospinal fluid, 76 fecal samples and, 31 paired sera from the acute and convalescent phases were obtained from 98 children with symptoms suggestive of aseptic meningitis. The children were admitted in different hospitals in 11 of Cuban's 14 provinces. We applied both, the conventional methods for diagnosis of enterovirus and our own-developed reverse transcriptase-nested polymerase chain reaction assay of cerebrospinal fluid specimens [51,52].

The sensitivity (0.01 tissue culture infective dose, $TCID_{50}$) and specificity of our enterovirus-RNA detection assay [51] allowed us to detect specific enterovirus RNA sequences in 46.3% (25 of 54) of the cerebrospinal fluid specimens.

For enterovirus isolation, 200 μl of cerebrospinal fluid and fecal specimens were inoculated in duplicate into tubes covered with monolayers of fibroblastic diploid embrionary human cells and monkey kidney cells. From the 76 fecal specimens inoculated, 45 (59.2 %) induced cytopathic effect. This cytophatic effect was only evident in the fibroblastic diploid embrionary human cell monolayers while monkey kidney cells remained invariable. Viral isolation was possible from all the tubes showing cytopathic effect.

All strains from the epidemic were identified as echovirus 16 by a neutralization test using the Lim-Benyesh-Melnick antisera pools. To corroborate the infecting serotype the presence of a fourfold or greater increase of the type-specific virus-neutralizing antibody titers between the sera specimens from the acute and the convalescent phase was determined. It was found that 54.8 % of the patiens' sera exhibited a significant rise of neutralizing antibody titer against the isolated strains. The geometric mean titer of the first and second sera was 1; 3.4, and 1; 22.4, respectively.

All Cuban aseptic meningitis epidemic cases from the year 2000 were associated with echovirus 16. None were caused by other agents. Before this epidemic, echovirus16 isolates from patients with viral meningitis had never been recognized in Cuba. This was the first evidence in the world of a large-scale epidemic by echovirus 16.

To determine whether the emergent infection by echovirus 16 that occurred in Cuba during the year 2000 was related to the presence of type 1 diabetes associated autoantibodies, 38 sera samples from children and adolescents were studied. We obtained the sera samples in the acute and convalescent stage (age ranged from 11 to 156 months, 86±49; mean ± SD) randomly selected from a large-scale echovirus 16 meningitis epidemic throughout the country [52]. The acute serum was taken five/five to six (median/ range) days after the beginning of the infection (at onset of the clinical symptoms), and the convalescent serum when the patients recovered completely 30/29 to 35 (median/range) days after the beginning of the infection.

We determined the presence of neutralizing antibodies against echoviruses serotypes 4, 6, 9, 11, 16 and 30 in these sera [67]. Sera samples from 80 healthy children and adolescents (age ranged from 11 to 153 months, 88±47; means ± SD), who were serologically verified as negative for neutralizing antibodies to echovirus 16, were also used. These sera were paired for sex, age, location of residence and time of sample collection in relation to children and adolescents who were infected by echovirus 16.

The presence of ICA, insulin autoantibodies (IAA), glutamic acid decarboxylase antibodies (GADA) and tyrosine phosphatase antibodies (IA2A) were determined in all sera using international workshop-validated assay [4,8,20,54,61,63]. Measurement of thyroid microsomal antibodies and parietal gastric cells antibodies were also carried out in subjects infected in order to show the specific pancreatotoxic activity of this infection [5].

The analysis of neutralizing antibodies to echoviruses 4, 6, 9, 11, 16 and 30 during the meningitis epidemic showed a high frequency of neutralizing antibodies to echovirus 16 at the convalescent stage compared to the acute stage of the infection (p=0.0006) (Table 3).

Notably, in the convalescent (but not the acute stage of the infection), ICA seroconversion was demonstrated, as well as the emergence of IAA and GADA to a minor degree, but not with IA2A concentrations. The islet cell autoimmunity is clearly epidemic and infection-associated, since no serum samples from 80 uninfected subjects serologically negative for neutralizing antibodies to echovirus 16 had ICA, and only one was GADA positive (similar to reported background population prevalence of GADA) (Table 4).

Table 3. Frequency of neutralizing antibodies against different echovirus serotypes in children and adolescents affected by viral meningitis infection.

Stage	E4 + (%)	E6 + (%)	E9 + (%)	E11 + (%)	E16 + (%)	E30 + (%)
1	3 (7.9)	14 (36.8)	23 (60.5)	21 (55.2)	6 (15.8)	9 (23.7)
2	4 (10.5)	18 (47.3)	26 (68.4)	22 (57.8)	21 (55.2)[a]	10 (26.3)

Stage 1: Acute infection of meningitis during the epidemic by echovirus 16.
Stage 2: Convalescence of meningitis infection by echovirus 16.
a p = 0.0006 vs stage 1. Reprinted from reference [8].

Table 4. Frequency of islet cell antibodies (ICA), glutamic acid decarboxylase antibodies (GADA) and tyrosine phosphatase antibodies (IA2A) in children and adolescents affected by echovirus 16 infection.

Autoantibodies	Stage 1 +/n (%)	Stage 2 +/n (%)	Control +/n (%)
ICA	5/38 (13.1)	35/38 (92.1)[a]	0/80 (0.0)
IAA	0/38 (0.0)	19/38 (50.0)[a]	0/80 (0.0)
GADA	0/38 (0.0)	11/38 (28.9)[bc]	1/80 (1.2)
AIA2	0/38 (0.0)	0/38 (0.0)	0/80 (0.0)

Stage 1: Acute infection of meningitis during the epidemic by echovirus 16.
Stage 2: Convalescence of meningitis infection by echovirus 16.
Control: Negative for neutralizing antibodies to echovirus 16.
n: Total of subjects. a p< 0,0001 vs stage 1 and control b p = 0,0004 vs stage 1 c p< 0,0001 vs control. Reprinted from reference [8].

Table 5. ICA titers in children and adolescents affected by echovirus 16 according the stage of infection.

Stage	ICA <40 UJDF + (%)	ICA ≥ 40 UJDF + (%)
1 (n=5)	5 (100.0)	0 (0.0)
2 (n=35)	26 (74.3)	9 (25.7)

Stage 1: Acute infection of meningitis during the epidemic by echovirus 16

Stage 2: Convalescence of meningitis infection by echovirus 16.
n: Total of ICA positive subjects. Reprinted from reference [8].

The titres of neutralizing antibodies to echovirus 16 were correlated with the ICA titres, both in the acute and convalescent stages (r=0.91; *p*<0.0001, r=0.55, *p*=0.0003 respectively) of echovirus 16 infection (Figure 1). An increase in the frequency of high ICA titres was shown in the convalescent stage although no statistical differences were found compared to those of the acute stage of infection (Table 5).

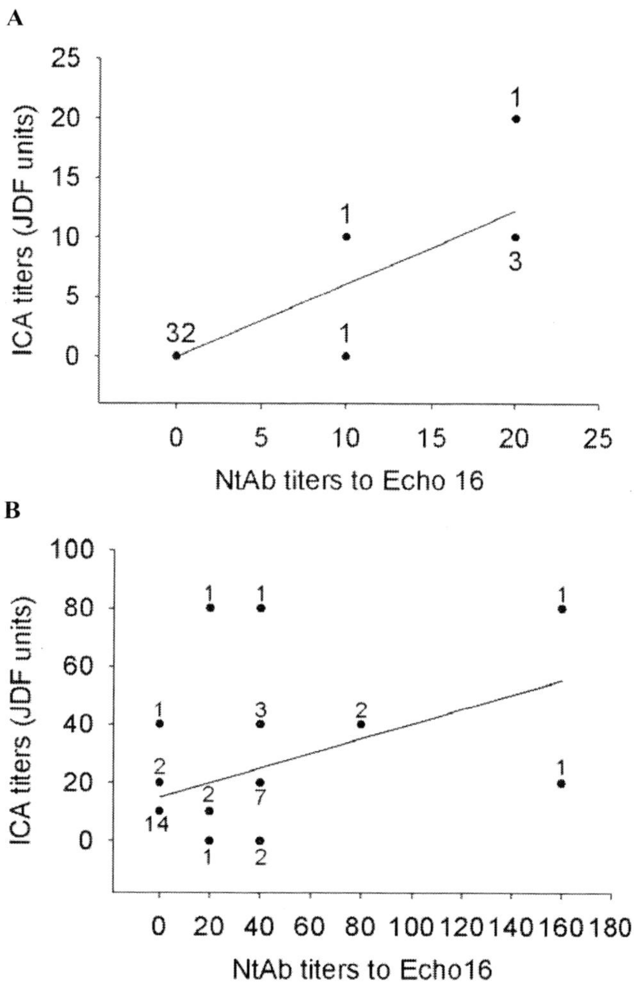

Figure 1 (A, B). A Correlation of ICA and neutralizing antibodies (NtAb) to echovirus16 levels during the acute stage of meningitis infection (r =0.91, p<0.0001) and B In the convalescence stage of meningitis infection by echovirus 16 (r = 0.55; p = 0.0003). Reprinted from reference [8].

The presence of high ICA titres in the subjects could indicate the existence of an important specific immune response against antigenic components of β-cells during infection by echovirus 16. We also found the highest frequencies of GADA in high titre ICA positive sera during the convalescent stage of echovirus 16 infection. GADA were positive in 19.2 %

(5/26) of subjects with ICA less than 40 JDFU and in 66.6 % (6/9) of subjects with ICA greater than or equal to 40 JDFU (*p*=0.0146). The presence of IAA was also higher in subjects with ICA greater than or equal to 40 JDFU (77.7 %, 7/9) in contrast to subjects with ICA less than 40 JDFU (30.7%, 8/26; *p*=0.0216). In addition, IAA frequency was higher in GADA positive subjects (81.8 %, 9/11) compared to GADA negative subjects (29.6 %, 8/27; *p*=0.0049). Accordingly, the high frequencies of IAA and GADA in subjects with high ICA titres in the convalescent stage of the infection might be a reflection of the severity of the β-cell damage. The increase in ICA titres does not seem to reflect a general response of autoantibodies since the presence of thyroid microsomal antibodies and parietal gastric cells antibodies were not detected during the infection.

According to our results, echovirus 16 could be involved in an autoimmune induction against β-cell antigens, due to the fact that the presence of neutralizing antibodies to echovirus 16 was associated with the appearance of or increases in islet-associated antibody concentrations. Our findings showed the first evidence of an association of echovirus 16 with the presence of antibodies related to type 1 diabetes (ICA, IAA and GADA). Echovirus 16 could be another serotype to be included in the list of enteroviruses related to type 1 diabetes and could be involved in initiating the destruction of β-cells in subjects with high genetic risk of developing type 1 diabetes.

Based on limited virologic surveillance data, the isolation of echovirus 16 is relatively uncommon worldwide. For example, U.S. enterovirus surveillance data for the period 1994-1998 indicated that the annual frequency of echovirus 16 isolation ranged from 5 to 3 isolation per year (Centers for Diseases Control and Prevention, unpub.data). The last Cuban outbreak of aseptic meningitis associated with echovirus 16 infections occurred in Tajimi City, Gifu prefecture, in 1984. Diverse etiologic agents (coxsackievirus B1, coxsackievirus B4, and coxsackievirus B5) were also reported during the outbreak [40].

Echovirus 16 isolates associated with sporadic cases of aseptic meningitis have not been frequently reported in previous years, probably because of the difficulties in tissue culture propagation [39]. Given the lack of adequate viral diagnostic laboratories and the difficulty in isolating echovirus 16 strains, it is tempting to speculate that there must be more echovirus 16 activities around which is not being noted. Genotypes of echovirus 16, which are potentially diabetogenic might be "silently" circulating in different world regions. Therefore, those populations with high frequency of type 1 diabetes might be endemically exposed to this virus.

It will be important that further epidemiological studies are carried out with special reference to the exposure to echovirus 16 in countries with high incidences of type 1 diabetes in addition to other studies elucidating how the echovirus 16 infection could contribute to the pathogenesis of type 1 diabetes.

III. Islet Cell Related Antibodies and Type 1 Diabetes Associated with Echovirus 30 Epidemic: A Case Report (*Report III*)

From June to November 2001, an epidemic of aseptic meningitis spread throughout Cuba, with 14.477 reported cases. Most of patients were children under 15 years old. The age-specific peak incidence corresponded to 1-to-4-years-old group, followed by infants of less than 1 year of age. Vomiting, headache and fever were the predominant clinical manifestations. No deaths related to aseptic meningitis were reported and all patients recovered completely.

To establish the etiological association of an enterovirus with this epidemic, 86 children (from 6 out of Cuba's 14 provinces) with symptoms suggestive of aseptic meningitis were studied. Children/specimen correspondence is described as follows: 35/cerebrospinal fluid, 43/feces, 7/feces and paired sera and 1/paired sera.

Serum samples were obtained from 5 males and 3 females, age ranged from 11 to 156 months, 55.4 ± 49.4; mean ± SD. The acute serum was taken five/five to six (median/range) days after the beginning of the infection (at onset of the clinical symptoms), and the convalescent serum when the patients recovered completely 30/29 to 35 (median/range) days after the beginning of the infection.

Virologic studies using the methods as described before identified echovirus 30 as the cause of the epidemic occurred in 2001. The analysis of neutralizing antibodies to 13 enterovirus serotypes most frequently isolated during the last 30 years in Cuba showed that all sera exhibited a rise of neutralizing antibody titres against the isolated strains (Table 6). The geometric mean titres of the first and second sera were 1: 14.1; and 1: 113.1, respectively (Table 6). No other viral agent was detected during the epidemic of the year 2001.

Table 6. Titres of neutralizing antibodies against different enterovirus serotypes in the eight case samples. Values are expressed as geometric means.

Stage	CVB1	CVB2	CVB3	CVB4	CVB5	CVB6	CVA9	E4	E6	E9	E11	E16	E30
1	4.7	16.3	21.8	5.1	6.1	3.9	67.2	2.2	12.6	33.7	18.3	6.9	14.1
2	4.7	23.7	28.2	5.6	8.2	4.2	80.0	2.9	14.9	47.5	23.8	8.1	113.1*

Stage 1: Acute infection of meningitis during the epidemic by echovirus 30.

Stage 2: Convalescence of meningitis infection by echovirus 30.

Eightfold increase of type-specific virus - neutralizing antibody titres between acute- and convalescent-phase. Reprinted from reference [6].

Previous studies in Cuba have estimated the circulation of enterovirus in patients with meningitis [3,38,51,52]. Echovirus 30 was reported as the cause of a large nationwide outbreak of aseptic meningitis occurred in 1994 [3]. Echovirus 30 has been the predominant enterovirus serotype associated with large outbreaks of aseptic meningitis during the last 40-year period in different parts of the world [42]. According to several reports from the National Enterovirus Surveillance System in the United States, echovirus 30 is one of the most frequently isolated enterovirus in the United States, comprising 6.8 % of all reported enterovirus isolations from 1970 to 1983 [55] and 9.5 % of enterovirus isolated from 1993 to 1996 [42]. Large outbreaks of echovirus 30-associated meningitis occurred in the United States in the years 1959/1960, 1968/1969, 1981/1982, 1993 and 2001 [11,12,27,32,33,42,44,55]. Echovirus 30 widespread dissemination was also reported in Europe during 2000/2001. Echovirus 30 was associated with outbreaks of aseptic meningitis in France, Islandia, Kosovo, The Netherlands, United Kingdom, Gales, Escocia and Germany in year 2000 [14]. There were also notifications of echovirus 30 isolations associated with meningitis outbreak in United Kingdom, Germany and Ireland in year 2001.

Despite Rovainen and co-workers have shown that some echovirus 30 strains can replicated in islets *in vitro* [49], widespread circulations of echovirus 30 elsewhere [12,42,52] have not been linked with increased incidence of human type 1 diabetes. To assess whether the occurrence of the epidemic is associated with the presence of antibodies associated with type 1 diabetes, the same 8 paired sera abovementioned were screened for diabetes-associated antibodies.

Sera from infected children were matched with at least two control sera (selected from 300 healthy children) for age, sex, date of collection and location. A total of 20 controls (13 males and 7 females, age ranged from 11 to 156 months, 55.1 ± 44.5; mean ± SD) were serologically verified as negative for neutralizing antibody to echovirus 30 and had no family history of diabetes. All subjects, or their parents, gave their informed consent to be studied, and the local Ethical Committee approved the protocol.

Determination of the presence of neutralizing antibodies to enteroviruses (echoviruses 4, 6, 9, 11, 16, 30, and coxsackieviruses A9, B1, B2, B3, B4, B5, B6), ICA, IAA, GADA and IA2A were performed in all sera. Measurement of thyroid microsomal antibodies and parietal gastric cells antibodies were only carried out in subjects infected in order to show the specific pancreatotoxic activity of this infection.

The appearance of neutralizing antibodies to echovirus 30 in the convalescent stage was associated with the occurrence of ICA (Table 7). ICA presence was higher during the convalescent stage of infection (7 out of 8; 87.5 %) than the acute stage (0 out of 8, $P < 0.01$) and the control group (0 out of 20, $P < 0.0001$). In contrast, we did not find positivity to IAA, GADA and IA2A in any of the stages (Table 7). High ICA titres (≥ 40 JDF units) were shown in 42.8 % (3 out of 7) of ICA positive subjects. None of the 8 matched sera obtained during the echovirus 30 epidemic were positive for thyroid microsomal antibodies or parietal gastric cells antibodies (Table 7).

We also reported of a 12-year-old girl without family history of diabetes that developed pancreatic autoimmunity and type 1 diabetes 8 months after the echovirus 30 epidemic [6].

In November 2001, a 12 years old girl of mixed origin (mulatto) commenced to show clinic symptoms of meningitis (intense headache of front-occipital origin, projectile-like vomiting, photophobia and fever). Physic examination, complementary analysis, evolution and epidemiological contest indicated the viral aetiology of meningitis of this subject.

Table 7. Frequency of neutralizing antibodies (NtAb), islet cell antibodies (ICA), insulin autoantibodies (IAA), glutamic acid decarboxylase antibodies (GADA), tyrosine phosphatase antibodies (IA2A), thyroid microsomal antibodies (TMA) and parietal gastric cells antibodies (PGA) in children and adolescents affected by echovirus 30 infection.

Antibodies	Stage 1 +/n (%)	Stage 2 +/n (%)	Control +/n (%)
NtAb	0/8 (0.0)	8/8 (100)[ab]	0/20 (0.0)
ICA	0/8 (0.0)	7/8 (87.5)[ab]	0/20 (0.0)
IAA	0/8 (0.0)	0/8 (0.0)	0/20 (0.0)
GADA	0/8 (0.0)	0/8 (0.0)	0/20 (0.0)
IA2A	0/8 (0.0)	0/8 (0.0)	0/20 (0.0)
TMA	0/8 (0.0)	0/8 (0.0)	0/20 (0.0)
PGA	0/8 (0.0)	0/8 (0.0)	0/20 (0.0)

Stage 1: Acute infection of meningitis during the epidemic by echovirus 30.
Stage 2: Convalescence of meningitis infection by echovirus 30. Control: Negative for neutralizing antibodies to echovirus 30. a $p < 0.01$ vs stage 1. b $p < 0.0001$ vs control. Reprinted from reference [6].

A random blood glucose concentration determined during the clinic symptoms of meningitis showed a value of 7.7 mmol/L. One fasting blood glucose determination during the convalescent phase was of 6.02 mmol/L. During this period the weight of the patient was 34 Kg.

High titres of neutralizing antibodies to echovirus 30 (1:80) were found in patient's serum suggesting this virus as the agent causing the aseptic meningitis. For the other epidemic enterovirus determined, only low titres of antibodies to coxsackievirus B2 and coxsackievirus A9 (1/10 and 1/20, respectively) were found. These results indicate that the adolescent was recently exposed neither to the former viruses nor to the rest of enteroviruses which frequently circulated in our country (Figure 2).

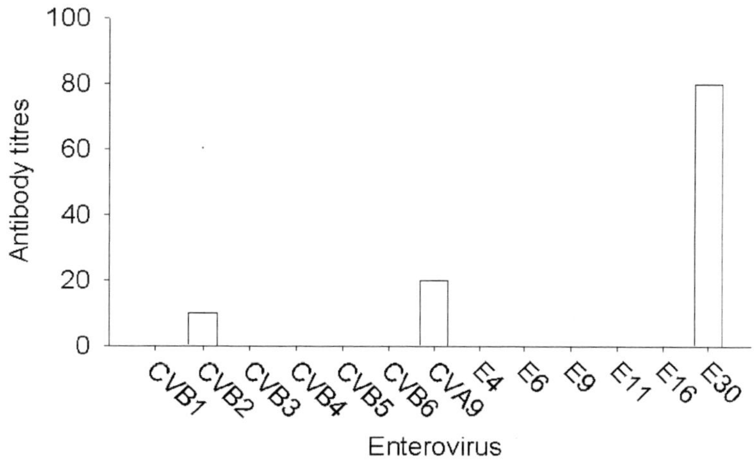

Figure 2. Titres of neutralizing antibodies against different enterovirus in the adolescent that developed type 1 diabetes after meningitis infection. Reprinted from reference [6].

After the meningitis episode the adolescent gained 5 Kg of weight in the subsequent 6 months. At month six after infection a fasting blood glucose determination was 4.02 mmol/L. Two months later, the subject started to show symptoms suggesting diabetes (polyuria, polydipsia, increased appetite and weight lost [3 Kg]). At this period, fasting and postprandial blood glucose concentrations were 12.1 and 18.9 mmol/L, respectively. Immediate hospitalization was decided to establish diabetes prognosis and treatment beginning.

Resulting glycaemic profile (in mmol/L) during hospitalization consisted in 6.02 at fasting, 8.2 before lunch and 4.55 before dinner. Since no ketosis was present the patient was treated with diet. Type 1 associated antibodies (ICA; IAA; GADA and IA2A) and C-peptide were measured aiming at determining the existence of pancreatic autoimmunity and to estimate insulin secretion. Results showed ICA titres of 160 JDFu and 13.9 U/mL of IA2A. IAA and GADA were negative. Thyroid microsomal antibodies and parietal gastric cells antibodies were also negative. Fasting C-peptide blood concentration was 1.1 ng/mL (normal values: 1.07-3.51 ng/mL). We also measured glycosylated haemoglobin and its value was 7.8 %. All these data demonstrated the type 1 diabetes diagnosis.

She was treated then with multiple doses of recombinant human insulin (Novo Nordisk). The insulin requirement was 0.2 $IU \cdot Kg^{-1} \cdot day^{-1}$ with dietetic treatment of 2200 kcal. After 3 months of insulin treatment, ICA and IA2A showed titres of 80 JDFu and 8 U/ml, respectively. IAA and GADA remained negative. Fasting glucose and C-peptide were 7.29 mmol/L and 0.8 ng/mL, respectively. The adolescent was found to carry the HLA DR 15(DR2)/DR7 and DQ 2/DQ6(DQ1) genotype which is not associated with an increased risk for type 1 diabetes.

The emergence of type 1 diabetes associated antibodies (ICA and AIA2) followed by clinical manifestations of the disease in the adolescent after meningitis infection by echovirus 30 and the presence of high frequencies of ICA during the convalescent phase in echovirus 30 meningitis epidemic of the year 2001, open the possibility that this virus could be an environmental factor that may trigger autoimmune diabetes. This fact appears to be relevant if we consider that genetic background (HLA-DR2/DR7 y DQ2/DQ6) of the adolescent has been described as a combination of strong and weak protection haplotypes for Caucasians [47]. However, the protective effect associated with these alleles is not absolute and may differ among ethnic groups [21,22,47]. Indeed, Craig and co-workers [15] reported a subgroup of non-white type 1 diabetic patients, who are at low genetic risk, in whom enteroviruses contribute to type 1 diabetes onset. Additional studies are required to examine the interaction between enteroviral infections and HLA and non HLA candidate genes, including those that may determine β-cell tropism of enteroviruses.

IA2A positivity has been widely accepted as the highest sensitive marker of disease progression [29,30]. Zanone and coworkers [68] have found that IA2A persistence can also be used as indicator of residual function of β-cells. Our findings support the former since IA2A titres of the newly onset type 1 diabetic adolescent decreased in parallel with C-peptide concentrations. Interestingly, echovirus 30 appeared to generate only ICA during the convalescent phase of the infection in most studied subjects; however, IA2A also emerged in the case developing type 1 diabetes. In either case, echovirus 30 β-cell tropism is demonstrated although appearance of IA2A is a reflection of the severity of β-cell damage.

Onset of type 1 diabetes mellitus after echovirus 30 infection and the paralleled ICA, and neutralizing antibodies seroconversion in the echovirus 30 infected subjects suggests a causal relationship between viral infection and type 1 diabetes in the case report presented here. However, we cannot exclude the possibility that echovirus 30 infection accompanying the developing of type 1 diabetes could be a temporal coincidence of two real but unlinked events.

The high ICA titres in 42.8% of our subjects could indicate the existence of a strong specific immune response against antigenic component of β-cells during infection by echovirus 30. The increased in ICA titres does not seem to reflect a general response of autoantibodies since the presence of TMA and PGA were not detected during infection.

Interestingly, no coincidence in type 1 diabetes associated antibody response pattern has been found among case reports (including ours) after enteroviral infections [43,66]. It has been demonstrated that echovirus 30 is capable to kill human β-cells or impair their function *in vitro*, however, these effects is not entirely defined by the serotype. These results reveal the existence echovirus 30 variants with differential diabetogenicity [49]. Thus, echovirus 30 strains circulating in Cuba during the year 2001 could be considered as one of the diabetogenic variant.

IV. Lack of Association of Latent Autoimmune Diabetes in adults (LADA) with Enterovirus Infection *(Report IV)*

Latent autoimmune diabetes in adults (LADA) is an autoimmune form of diabetes characterized by the presence of antibodies related to type 1 diabetes (ICA and/or GADA), HLA-DR, DQ associated genes, as well as, insulin deficiency [28,45]. At present, some have called this form of disease "slow-progressing type 1 diabetes" [28,45]. It is speculated that multiple etiological factors such as susceptibility genes and an abnormal immune response towards β-cells after exposure to some environmental factors not yet characterized [45] may initiate a common pathogenic pathway which results in immune mediated β-cell destruction. However, Pozzilli and Di Mario hypothesised that in the case of LADA, exposure to environmental factors damaging β-cells is less pronounced [45]. Certain viral infections, especially those caused by enteroviruses have been associated with the autoimmune process leading to clinical type 1 diabetes mellitus [8,18,25].

To assess whether LADA is also associated with enterovirus infections, sera of 1000 patients with an initial diagnosis of type 2 diabetes mellitus over 35 years of age were screened for ICA and GADA with antibody assays validated in international workshops [8]. A total of 34 antibody-positive patients (ICA/GADA) were identified [7]. These subjects were considered as LADA. Forty-four out of 966 autoantibody-negative subjects with classic type 2 diabetes mellitus, were also studied. Seventy-eight sera samples from healthy subjects, who were matched for age, geographical location and time of year in relation to LADA and type 2 diabetic subjects, were used as controls.

The frequency of enterovirus infections in each group was studied using a neutralization test [67] with 11 enterovirus serotypes most frequently isolated during the last 30 years in Cuba (echoviruses: 4, 6, 9, 11, and coxsackieviruses: A9, B1, B2, B3, B4, B5, B6). Statistical differences of frequencies among groups were analyzed using the Chi-square test.

High frequencies of neutralizing antibodies to most enteroviruses were found in all groups studied, suggesting a high exposure to these enterovirus types in the Cuban population (Table 8). No differences were found in the overall frequency of neutralizing antibodies to all enteroviruses between LADA, type 2 diabetic patients and healthy subjects (Table 8). However, a significantly higher frequency of neutralizing antibodies to coxsackievirus A9 (93.9 vs. 64.0%; $p = 0.003$) and coxsackievirus B4 (93.9 vs. 41.2%, $p = 0.006$) were found in newly diagnosed childhood-onset type 1 diabetes (n=33) [18] when compared with LADA subjects. These data indicate that enterovirus infection does not appear to be associated with LADA.

Table 8. Frequency of neutralizing antibodies against 11 enterovirus serotypes most frequently isolated during the last 30 years in Cuba.

Subjects	CVA 9	CVB1	CVB2	CVB3	CVB4	CVB5	CVB6	E4	E6	E9	E11
LADA (n=34)	64.0	50.0	55.8	58.8	41.2	20.0	20.6	26.3	64.7	79.4	58.9
T2DM* (n=34)	77.3	41.3	77.3	50.0	59.5	29.5	20.4	36.3	75.0	63.6	45.4
Healthy Subjects (n=78)	60.2	39.7	67.9	69.2	63.7	57.7	17.9	11.5	57.7	79.5	71.8

*T2DM: type 2 diabetic subjects. Reprinted from reference [50].

V. Summary of our Studies

Table 9 summarizes the epidemiology and islet autoimmunity in echovirus epidemics in Cuba. In summary, our studies provide further support for the association between enterovirus infections and type 1 diabetes. Echovirus has been isolated from patients with aseptic meningitis who, during the convalescent stage of their illness, seroconverted to islet cell antibody positivity. Moreover, there were subtle differences in the patterns of islet autoimmunity associated with each of the three different epidemics. The isolation of viruses with proven but varying potency in their ability to induce islet autoimmunity in man suggests that there is heterogeneity of the immune response against β-cell antigens after echovirus infection. We have hypothesized the generation of post-viral islet autoimmunity will depend upon a combination of two qualities; the ability of a virus to induce pro-inflammatory innate immune activation and the ability to cause β cell damage. These processes can initiate or accelerate autoimmune diabetes in those individuals genetically predisposed, through inheritance of genes that influence central and peripheral tolerance, as several diabetes-susceptibility genes are thought to [46,57,62].

Similar findings account for other infections by enteroviruses. A raise of ICA and IAA titres was described in a case report, in which maternal infection with echovirus 6 produced type 1 diabetes in the neonate [43]. The presence of enterovirus RNA has also been described in sera of pre-diabetic subjects and appeared to be associated with increases of ICA and GADA, but not in IAA or IA2 concentrations [35]. The presence of ICA, IAA and IA2A was observed after infection of enterovirus in a child participating in the Finish Diabetes Prediction and Prevention Trial [25]. Recently, a raise of GADA concentration was positively associated with an increase of neutralizing antibody titres to different CVB strains in newly onset type 1 diabetic subjects and their non-diabetic siblings [8]. Taken together, these studies suggest that the induction of islet cell associated antibodies seems to occur right after episodes of enterovirus infections. This can take place from weeks to years before diabetes is clinically evident [25].

The serological results obtained in Cuba indicate a strong temporal relationship between islet autoantibodies and exposure to echovirus, and prompt further important questions, such as the longevity of post-echovirus islet autoimmunity and the intriguing lack of IA-2 autoantibodies (often been associated with a progressive phase of prediabetes, heralding the clinical diagnosis of the disease). Specific questions will be whether there is antigen spreading to include additional islet autoantibody specificities over time (especially IA-2); or whether the autoimmune response is transient and wanes. Although, no follow-up of these children for diabetes has been reported, we predict that the post-echovirus islet autoimmunity detected in the original epidemics will not show persistence, and is unlikely to have shown spreading to include additional autoantibody specificities. This assertion is based on the fact that type 1 diabetes incidence in Cuba is low (3/100.000) [13,17]. Probably, the frequency of susceptibility genes could justifies the low incidence for type 1 diabetes although some apparently type 1 diabetes associated strains are highly prevalent in Cuba.

It is likely that β cell autoimmunity may remit and reappear in the course of viral infections. Evidence has accumulated that β-cell autoimmunity may remit without cause diabetes. Studies of schoolchildren with no familiar history of type 1 diabetes in the United States [37], Sweeden [31] and Finland [26] have reported ICA remission rates between 10 and 78 %. The prevalence of β cell autoimmunity in these children was as high as 0.7 to 4.1 %; however, only a minority of children with β-cell autoimmunity (one in three to eight) develops type 1 diabetes by the age of 15 years. A follow up study of children from a background population in with high ICA titres demonstrated that those person who remain persistently and strongly ICA positive have HLA genotype similar to those of diabetic patients. Thus, while β-cell autoimmunity may be triggered in anyone, the HLA genes may be crucial from progression from autoimmunity to type 1 diabetes [1,2,16,23,36,53].

The occurrence of echovirus epidemics associated with the appearance of islet autoimmunity in Cuba presents an exceptional opportunity to throw further light on the virus-host interaction. Our findings provide the first evidence of association of echovirus 4, echovirus 16 and echovirus 30 epidemic with diabetes-associated autoimmunity and development of type 1 diabetes [6,8,18]. Of note that, the occurrence of enterovirus infections and β-cells autoimmunity and/or diabetes in the same individuals do not automatically imply a causal relationship between the infections and the pathogenesis of type 1 diabetes. However, our findings are in line with other reports indicating a temporal association between enterovirus infections and the appearance of ICA. Temporal association is one of the key characteristics of a causal relationship, and hence our findings support the hyphothesis that enterovirus infections may induce β-cells autoimmunity.

Very little is known about the potential participation of virus in the aetiology of LADA. Our data suggest that enterovirus infection is not related to LADA, although our work does not discard the possible association between other viruses and this autoimmune disease. Thus, our results [50] are in agreement with the view that the autoimmune mechanisms in the type 1 diabetes are indeed different from the LADA subjects [28,45] and further investigations should be carried out to explain those differences.

Table 9. Summary of epidemiology and islet autoimmunity in echovirus epidemics in Cuba.

	YEAR OF EPIDEMIC		
	1986 [18]	2000 [8]	2001 [6]
Echovirus strain	4	16	30
Number of separate isolates obtained	14	47	43
Number of reported meningitis cases	~300.000	16.943	14.477
Percentage positive for ICA	36 %	92 %	87 %
Percentage positive for GAD65	ND[a]	28	0
Percentage positive for IA-2	ND	0	0
Percentage positive for IAA	ND	44	0

Reprinted from references [6, 8, 18].

VI. Perspectives

"The one thing sure about the future is that it is hard to predict". Precisely what happens will depend upon the strategy employed for the study of the association virus-diabetes. This review has revealed several aspects of the enteroviral etiology of type 1 diabetes about which additional knowledge could be of particular value in the pathogenesis of this autoimmune disease. To date, there are controversial results about the implications of enterovirus in human islet autoimmunity. It is not known in detail how enterovirus infections bring about the loss of insulin-producing β-cells, a phenomenon characteristic of the disease. Nevertheless, the evidence clearly warrants further investigation into this potential association.

The prospects for progress in this area are improving rapidly through several approaches. A great challenge for future research is a better understanding of the mechanisms and factors underlying type 1 generate promising research hypotheses. Exploration of the question how enteroviruses might interact with host factors may yield sufficient information to type 1 diabetes in a more complex manner than previously thought. The next works should clarify the link between the enterovirus and the development of islet autoimmunity, highlight the critical host-virus interactions and indicate the structural basis of this virulence, and then it will provide much needed impetus to the development of anti-enteroviral strategies that could be aimed at identifying, controlling and eradicating these harmful pathogens.

Future work could then extend the hypothesis that there are strain-related structural features through mutation studies, in which key structural areas of pathogenic strains are reverted to the less pathogenic form. This is facilitated by the recent description that infectious enterovirus virions can be generated from full-length viral cDNA in vitro [10,41].

By careful consideration of the unique feature of enteroviruses and their infections and how affect study design and data interpretation, as well as use of improved laboratory techniques, it should be possible in the near future to better understand correlation between enterovirus infection and type 1 diabetes.

In the future, immunization against enterovirus infections would be an applicable approach in the prevention of type 1 diabetes. If the association enterovirus-type 1 diabetes holds true then it would be possible to reduce the risk of developing type 1 diabetes by preventing enterovirus infections with a multivalent enterovirus vaccine that could be given to children soon after birth.

Acknowledgements

We wish to express our gratitude to Dr Oscar Diaz Horta who has been a valuable collaborator in our studies.

References

[1] Andreoletti L, Hober D, Hober-Vandenberghe C, Belaich S, Vantyghem MC, Lefebvre J et al. Detection of coxsackie B virus RNA sequences in whole blood samples from adult patients at the onset of type I diabetes mellitus. *J Med Virol* 1997;52:121-7.

[2] Andreoletti L, Hober D, Hober-vandenberghe C, Fajardy I, Belaich S, Lambert V, et al. Coxsackie B virus infection and Beta cell autoantibodies in newly diagnosed IDDM adult patients. *Clin Diagn Virol* 1998;9:125-33.

[3] Bello M, Mas P, Palomera R, Morier L, Avalos I, Sarmiento et al. Meningoencefalitis virales por enterovirus en el período 1990-1995. *Rev Arg Microbiol* 1997;29:176-83.

[4] Bonifacio E, Lampasona V, Genovese S, Ferrari M, Bosi E. Identification of protein tyrosine phosphatase-like IA2 (islet cell antigen 512) as the insulin-dependent diabetes-related 37/40k autoantigen and a target of islet-cell antibodies. *J Immunol* 1995;155:5419-26.

[5] Bottazzo GF, Florin-Christensen A, Doniach D. Islet-cell antibodies in diabetes mellitus with autoimmune polyendocrine deficiencies. *Lancet* 1974;2:1279-83.

[6] Cabrera E, Sarmiento L, Molina G, Pérez C, Arranz C, Galvan J. Islet Cell Related Antibodies and Type 1 Diabetes Associated with Echovirus 30 Epidemic: A Case Report. *J Med Virology* 2005;76:373-7.

[7] Cabrera-Rode E, Perich P, Díaz-Horta O, Tiberti C, Molina G, Arranz C, et al. Slowly progressing type 1 diabetes: persistence of islet cell autoantibodies is related to glibenclamide treatment. *Autoimmunity* 2002;35:469-74.

[8] Cabrera-Rode E, Sarmiento L, Tiberti C, Molina G, Barrios J, Hernández D, et al. Type 1 diabetes islet associated antibodies in subjects infected by echovirus 16. *Diabetologia* 2003;46:1348-53.

[9] Cabrera-Rode E. Prevalence of islet cell antibodies (ICA) in diabetes mellitus and other diseases in Cubans. *Autoimmunity* 1997;26:7-9.

[10]Cello J, Paul AV, Wimmer E. Chemical synthesis of poliovirus cDNA: generation of infectious virus in the absence of natural template. *Science* 2002;297:1016.

[11]Centers for Disease Control and Prevention. Non polio enterovirus surveillance-United States, 1993-1996. *Morbid Mortal Weekly Rep* 1997,46:748-50.

[12]Centers for Disease Control and Prevention. Outbreaks of aseptic meningitis associated with echoviruses 9 and 30 and preliminary surveillance reports on enterovirus activity - United States, 2003. *Morbid Mortal Weekly Rep* 2003;52:761-4.

[13]Collazo F, Diaz O, Hernandez I. Epidemiologic behaviour of insulin dependent diabetes mellitus in children younger than 15 years of old. Cuba, 1990-1993. *Rev Cub Endocrinol* 1993;8:119-25.

[14]Communicable Disease Surveillance Centre. Viral meningitis associated with increase in echovirus type 13. *Commun Dis Rep CDC Weekly* 2000;10:277-80.

[15]Craig ME, Howard NJ, Silink M, Rawlinson WD. Reduced frequency of HLA DRB1*03-DQB1*02 in children with type 1 diabetes associated with enterovirus RNA. *J Infect Dis* 2003;187:1562-70.

[16]D'Alessio DJ. A case-control study of group B coxsackievirus immunoglobulin M antibody prevalence and HLA-DR antigens in newly diagnosed cases of insulin-dependent diabetes mellitus. *Am J Epidemiol* 1992;135:1331-8.

[17]Diaz O, Carvajal F, Fernández L, Rodríguez J. Epidemiology of type 1 diabetes mellitus in children younger than 15 years old. Evidence of season variation. *Invest Biochem* 1983;2:316-25.

[18]Diaz-Horta O, Bello M, Cabrera-Rode E, Suaréz J, Mas P, García I, et al. Echovirus 4 and Type 1 Diabetes Mellitus. *Autoimmunity* 2001;34:275-81.

[19]Dronfield D, Taylor K. Changes in serum insulin and islet cell antibodies following an outbreak of Echovirus 4 in Glasgow. *Diabet Med* 1993,10:S41.

[20]Grubin CE, Daniels T, Toivola B, Landin-Olsson M, Hagopian W, Li L, et al. A novel radioligand binding assay to determine diagnostic accuracy of isoform-specific glutamic acid decarboxylase antibodies in childhood IDDM. *Diabetologia* 1994;37:344-50.

[21]Hermann R, Knip M, Veijola R, Simell O, Laine AP, Akerbloom HK, et al. Temporal changes in the frequencies of HLA genotypes in patients with type 1 diabetes – indication of an increased environmental pressure? *Diabetologia* 2003;46:420-5.

[22]Heward JM, Mijovic CH, Kelly Ma, Morrison E, Barnett AH. HLA-DQ and DRB1 polymorphism and susceptibility to type 1 diabetes in Jamaica. *Eur J Immunogenet* 2002;29:47-52.

[23]Hiltunen M, Hyoty H, Knip M, Ilonen J, Reijonen H, Vahasalo P, et al. Islet cell antibody seroconversión in children is temporally associated with enterovirus infections. Childhood Diabetes in Finland (DiMe) Study Group. *J Infect Dis* 1997;175:554-60.

[24]Hyoty H, Hiltunen M, Lonnrot M. Enterovirus infections and insulin dependent diabetes mellitus--evidence for causality. *Clin Diagn Virol* 1998;9:77-84.

[25]Hyoty H, Taylor KW. The role of viruses in human diabetes. *Diabetologia* 2002;45:1353-61.

[26]Karjalainen J. Islet cell antibodies as predictive markers for IDDM in children with high background incidence of disease. *Diabetes* 1990;39:1144-50.

[27]Kleinman H, Cooney M, Nelson C, Owen R, Boyd L, Swanda G. Aseptic meningitis and paralytic disease due to a newly recognized enterovirus. *JAMA* 1964;187:90-5.

[28]Kobayashi T, Maruyama T, Shimada A, Kasuga A, Takei I, Tanaka S, et al. Insulin intervention to preserve β cells in slowly progressive insulin dependent (Type 1) diabetes mellitus. *Annals NY Acad Sci* 2002; 958;117-30.

[29]Krischer JP, Cuthbertson DD, Yu L, Orban T, Maclaren N, Jackson R, et al. Screening strategies for the identification of multiple antibody-positive relatives of individuals with type 1 diabetes. *J Clin Endocrinol Metab* 2003;88:103-8.

[30]Kulmala P, Savola K, Reijonen H, Veijola R, Vähäsalo P, Karjalainen J, et al. Genetic markers, humoral autoimmunity, and prediction of type 1 diabetes in siblings of affected children. Childhood Diabetes in Finland Study Group. *Diabetes* 2000;49:48-58.

[31]Landin-Olsson M, Karlsson A, Dahlquist G, Blom L, Lernmark A, Sundkvist G. Islet cell and other organ specific autoantibodies in all children developing type 1 (insulin-dependent) diabetes mellitus in Sweden during one year and in matched control children. *Diabetologia* 1989;32:387-95.

[32]Lennette H, Schmidt N, Magoffin R, Dennis J, Wiener A. The price virus. An unidentified enterovirus isolated from patients with central nervous system disease. *Proc Soc Exp Biol Med* 1962;110:769-75.

[33]Likoski W, Emmons R, Davis E, Thompson R. Epidemiology of echovirus 30 aseptic meningitis. *Health Serv Rep* 1972;87:638-42.

[34]Lonnrot M, Knip M, Marciulionyte D, Rahko J, Urboinaite B, Moore W, et al. Enterovirus antibodies in relation to islet cell antibodies in two populations with high and low incidence of type 1 diabetes. *Diabetes Care* 1999;22:2086-8.

[35]Lonnrot M, Korpela K, Knip M, Ilonen J, Simell O, Korhonen S, et al. Enterovirus infection as a risk factor for beta-cell autoimmunity in a prospectively observed birth cohort: the Finnish Diabetes Prediction and Prevention Study. *Diabetes* 2000;49:1314-8.

[36]Luppi P, Alexander A, Bertera S, Noonan K, Trucco M. The same HLADQ alleles determine either susceptibility or resistance to different coxsackievirus-mediated autoimmune diseases. *J Biol Regul Homeost Agents* 1999;13:14-26.

[37]Maclaren N, Horne G, Spillar R, Brown L, Silverstein J, Shah S, et al. The feasibility of using ICA to predict IDDM in U.S. school children. *Diabetes* 1990;39:122A.

[38]Mas P, Comellas M, Marrero, Jacobo M, Palomera R. Meningoencefalitis por enterovirus en Cuba. Estudio de 14 años. *Rev Cubana Pediatr*1992;64:16-21.

[39]Melnick J, Wenner H, Phillips C. Enterovirus. In: Lenette E and Schmidt N, ed. *Diagnostic procedures for viral, rickettsial and chlamydial infections*. 5th ed. Washington, DC: American Public Health Association Inc; 1979.p.471-534.

[40]Miwa C, Watanabe Y. Diversity of etiological agent associated with aseptic meningitis-a survey on an epidemic in Tajimi City, Gifu Prefecture in 1984. *Kansenshogaku Zasshi* 1990;64:794-801.

[41]Molla A, Paul AV, Wimmer E. Cell-free, de novo synthesis of poliovirus. *Science* 1991;254:1647.

[42]Oberste S, Maher K, Kennett M, Campbell J, Carpenter M, Schnurr D. Molecular epidemiology and genetic diversity of echovirus type 30 (E30): genotypes correlate with temporal dynamics of E30 isolation. *J Clin Microbiol* 1999;37:3928-33.

[43]Otonkoski T, Rovainen M, Vaarala O, Dinesen B, Leipälä JA, Hovi T, et al. Neonatal type 1 diabetes associated with maternal echovirus 6 infection: a case report. *Diabetologia* 2000;43:1235-8.

[44]Plager H, Decher W. A newly – recognized enterovirus isolated from cases of aseptic meningitis. *Am J Hyp* 1963;77:26-8.

[45]Pozzilli P, Di Mario U. Autoimmune diabetes not requiring insulin at diagnosis (Latent autoimmune diabetes of adult). *Diabetes Care* 2001;24:1460-7.

[46]Pugliese A, Zeller M, Fernandez A, Zalcberg L, Bartlett RJ, Ricordi C, et al. The insulin gene is transcribed in the human thymus and transcription levels correlated with allelic variation at the INS VNTR-IDDM2 susceptibility locus for type 1 diabetes. *Nat Genet* 1997;15:293.

[47]Redondo MJ, Fain PR, Eisenbarth GS. Genetic of type 1A diabetes. *Recent Prog Horm Res* 2001;56:69-89.

[48]Rewers M, LaPorte R, Walczak M, Dmochowski K, Bogaczynska E Apparent epidemic of insulin-dependent diabetes mellitus in Midwestern Poland. *Diabetes* 1987;36:106.

[49]Rovainen M, Ylipaasto P, Savolainen C, Galama J, Hovi T, Otonkoski T. Functional impairment and killing of human beta cells by enterovirus: the capacity is shared by a wide range of serotypes, but the extend is characteristic of individual virus strains. *Diabetologia* 2002;45:693-702.

[50]Sarmiento L, Cabrera-Rode E, Diaz-Horta O. Lack of Association of Latent Autoimmune Diabetes in Adults (LADA) with Enterovirus Infection. *Autoimmunity* 2004;37:245-6.

[51]Sarmiento L, Mas P, Goyenechea A, Palomera R, Morier L, Capo V, et al. First epidemic of echovirus 16 meningitis in Cuba. *Emerg Infect Dis* 2001;7:887-9.

[52]Sarmiento L. Enteroviral meningitis and emergence of rare enterovirus types: Cuban experience. In: Strong P, ed. *Focus on meningitis research*. New York: Nova Science Publishers;2004.p.1-14.

[53]Schernthaner G, Banatvala JE, ScherbaumW, Bryant J, Borkenstein M, Schober E, et al. Coxsackie B virus– specific IgM responses, complement-fixing islet-cell antibodies, HLA DR antigens, and C-peptide secretion in insulin-dependent diabetes mellitus. *Lancet* 1985;2:630-2.

[54]Schmidli RS, Colman PG, Bonifacio E. Disease sensitivity and specificity of 52 assays for glutamic acid decarboxylase antibodies. The second international GADAb workshop. *Diabetes* 1995;44:636-40.

[55]Strikas R, Anderson L, Parker R. Temporal and geographic patterns of isolates of nonpolio enterovirus in the United States, 1970-1983. *J Infect Dis* 1986;153:346-51.

[56]Szopa TM, Titchener PA, Portwood ND, Taylor KW. Diabetes mellitus due to viruses - some recent developments. *Diabetologia* 1993;36:687-95.

[57]Ueda H, Howson J, Esposito L, Heward J, Snook H, Chamberlain G, et al. Association of the T-cell regulatory gene CTLA4 with susceptibility to autoimmune disease. *Nature* 2003;423:506.

[58]Uriarte A, Cabrera-Rode E, Ventura R, Vargas J. Islet cell antibodies and Echo 4 virus infection. *Diabetologia*1987;30:590.

[59]Uriarte A, Cabrera-Rode E, Ventura R, Vargas J. Alteraciones pancreatoespecíficas de la inmunidad en niños infectados con virus ECHO-4. *Rev Cub Pediatr* 1990;62:359-63.

[60]Uriarte A, Molina G, Cabrera-Rode E, Ventura R, Vargas J, Vera M. Estudio prospectivo en niños con alto riesgo de diabetes tipo 1 como secuela de infección por virus ECHO-4. 1986-1989. *Rev Cub Endocrinol* 1991;2:34-43.

[61]Vardi P, Dib SA, Tuttleman M, Connelly JE, Grinbergs M, Radizabeth A, et al. Competitive insulin autoantibody assay. Prospective evaluation of subjects at high risk for development of type 1 diabetes mellitus. *Diabetes* 1987;36:1286-91.

[62]Verdaguer J, Amrani A, Anderson, Schmidt D, Santamaria P. Two mechanisms for the non-MHC-linked resistance to spontaneous autoimmunity. *J Immunol* 1999;162:4614.

[63]Verge CF, Stenger D, Bonifacio E, Colman P, Pilcher C, Bingley P, et al. Combined use of autoantibodies (IA-2 autoantibody, GAD autoantibody, insulin autoantibody, cytoplasmic islet cell antibodies) in type 1 diabetes: Combinatorial Islet Autoantibody Workshop. *Diabetes* 1998;47:1857-66.

[64]Viskari H, Ludvigsson J, Uibo R, Salur L, Marciulionyte D, Hermann R, et al. Relationship between the incidence of type 1 diabetes and enterovirus infections in different European populations: results from the EPIVIR project. *J Med Virol* 2004;72:610-7.

[65]Viskari HR, Koskela P, Lo¨nnrot M, Luonuansuu S, Reunanen A, Baer M, et al. Can enterovirus infections explain the increasing incidence of type 1 diabetes? *Diabetes Care* 2000;23:414-6.

[66]Vreugdenhil GR, Schloot NC, Hoorens A, Rongen C, Pipeleers DG, Melchers WJ, et al. Acute onset of type I diabetes mellitus after severe echovirus 9 infection: putative pathogenic pathways. *Clin Infect Dis* 2000;31:1025-31.

[67]WHO/EPI/01. Manual for the virological investigation of polio, Geneva, Switzerland *WHO/EPI/GEN/97.01* 1997:44-51.

[68]Zanone MM, Catalfamo E, Pietropaolo SL, Rabbone I, Sacchetti C, Cerutti F, et al. Glutamic acid decarboxylase and ICA512/IA2 autoantibodies as disease markers and relationship to residual beta-cell function and glycemic control in young type 1 diabetic patients. *Metabolism* 2003;52:25-9.

INDEX

A

B

C

D

E

F

G

H

J

K

L

M

N

O

P

T

U

V